Job Stressors and Mental Health

A Proactive Clinical Perspective

Job Stressors and Mental Health

A Proactive Clinical Perspective

Karen Belkić, M.D., PhD
Adjunct Professor of Preventive Medicine
Physician Specialist in Internal Medicine

Čedo Savić, M.D., PhD
Primarius Attending Physician
Physician Specialist in Neurology and Psychiatry

World Scientific

NEW JERSEY • LONDON • SINGAPORE • BEIJING • SHANGHAI • HONG KONG • TAIPEI • CHENNAI

Published by

World Scientific Publishing Co. Pte. Ltd.

5 Toh Tuck Link, Singapore 596224

USA office: 27 Warren Street, Suite 401-402, Hackensack, NJ 07601

UK office: 57 Shelton Street, Covent Garden, London WC2H 9HE

Library of Congress Cataloging-in-Publication Data

Belkic, Karen, 1952– author.

Job stressors and mental health : a proactive clinical perspective / by Karen Belkic, Cedo Savic.

p. ; cm.

Includes bibliographical references and index.

ISBN 978-9814525558 (hardcover : alk. paper)

I. Savic, Cedo, author. II. Title.

[DNLM: 1. Stress, Psychological--Case Reports. 2. Burnout, Professional--psychology--Case Reports. 3. Job Satisfaction--Case Reports. 4. Mental Disorders--etiology--Case Reports. 5. Occupational Diseases--prevention & control--Case Reports. 6. Work--psychology--Case Reports. WM 172.4]

RC454

616.89--dc23

2013021399

British Library Cataloguing-in-Publication Data

A catalogue record for this book is available from the British Library.

Printed in Singapore by World Scientific Printers.

Dedication

This book is dedicated to our patients and to our colleagues, physicians, towards a healthier working life.

Contents

Preface

This book is the result of our long-term clinical and scientific experience and collaboration. These have developed in a number of settings in several countries. We have increasingly come to appreciate the importance of the work environment for our patients' well-being. We also see that within our own profession, the work environment impacts profoundly upon physicians' health. Taken together, these observations have lead us over the years to develop a proactive approach, whereby we as clinicians could more effectively examine, understand and improve our own and our patients' work conditions. The body of epidemiological evidence linking job stressors to adverse mental health outcomes, as reviewed in Chapter 2 of this book, is large and continually growing. The scope of the problem, in human terms, as well as economic is enormous. The biological underpinnings through cognitive ergonomics and brain research, as reviewed in Chapter 3, are very strong, further justifying a focus upon job stressors in relation to mental health. Having reviewed the current standard of care within the area of work fitness and occupational rehabilitation in Chapter 4, we come, however, to a striking incongruity. Namely, that despite the epidemiological evidence and sophisticated knowledge concerning the mechanisms by which stressors impact upon the central nervous system, current practice is still far from protecting the mental health of working populations. Particularly lacking has been the means to effectively ameliorate those work stressors that trigger or exacerbate mental health disorders. In Chapter 5, we present the Occupational Stressor Index, the OSI, our own methodology by which patients, including our colleagues can be helped to return to healthier working conditions. In the subsequent portion of the book through a series of clinical case studies, reflective of our own experience within the realm of neuropsychiatry, we illustrate this approach in practice. Integrating this experience with our clinical and research perspectives in occupational and preventive medicine, we then suggest certain promising avenues for the future.

Acknowledgements

We would like to express deep appreciation to our families, our teachers and our colleagues for their support, inspiration and dialogue. We greatly appreciate the willingness of our patients as well as participants in our research studies, to share their concerns and experiences with us. Many librarians have also cooperated and helped us over the years; most recently, thanks are due to the librarians at the Karolinska Institute Library (KIBIC). We have also communicated with many clinicians and researchers throughout the world about the OSI, and we appreciate their queries and interest.

The scientific research of Dr. Karen Belkić has been supported over the years by a number of research foundations. These include the Swedish Working Life Fund, the Center for Social Epidemiology, the Swedish Medical Research Council (Vetenskapsrådet), Stockholm's County Council through FoUU (Forskning, Utveckling och Utbildning) at the Karolinska Hospital, the Signe and Olof Wallenius Foundation, the Center for Gender Medicine, the Sweden Cancer Foundation (Cancerfonden), the Karolinska Institute Fund and Gustav the Fifth Jubileum Fund. We are very grateful for this support.

We thank the staff at World Scientific Publishers for their cooperation, and in particular, to Ms. Joy Quek for helpful feedback in layout preparation.

Thank you, Dr. Saša Savić, for your help.

Our very special thanks are due to Primarius Dr. Ljiljana Savić and to Professor Dževad Belkić who have understood the scientific, clinical and humanitarian goals of this endeavor, and have provided indispensable support and insight during the many years required to realize this work.

Karen (Edinger) Belkić, MD, PhD
Adjunct Professor of Preventive Medicine
Physician Specialist in Internal Medicine

Čedo Savić, MD, PhD
Primarius Attending Physician
Physician Specialist in Neuropsychiatry

List of Panels and Table

List of Figures

Chapter 1

Work as a Potential Source of Meaning versus of Stress: Implications for Mental Health

According to Professor Dr. Viktor Frankl, psychiatrist and neurologist, the human being's foremost quest is for meaning, without which life becomes empty, a void. Frankl considers lack of meaning to be the primary cause of psychological distress in the modern era [Frankl 1963]. Professor Frankl founded the school of "Logotherapy," based upon the premise that finding and creating meaning in their lives will help patients recover from various manifestations of mental ill-health.

One of the most important potential sources of meaning in life is through work. Work can help fill a human being's life with a sense of achievement, with dignity and with a structure. Work is one of the ways by which human beings can feel that they have made a difference, that it has mattered that they have been alive. To paraphrase Professor Bertil Gardell [1987], a pioneer in the efforts to humanize the work environment: work is one of the most important potential sources of social and psychological well-being, which can provide much of the meaning and structure in adult life.

On a much more obvious level, the majority of adults depend upon their work in order to survive, to meet their own needs, as well as those of their families, to earn their "daily bread." In that sense, having a stable job is the basis of a secure life, which besides being essential for bare biological existence, can contribute to psychological well-being.

Unfortunately, however, a large number of jobs fall short of this potential. Rather, the contemporary work environment has all too often become the locus in which employed people spend many of their waking hours performing activities that are demanding, constraining, and otherwise stressful. Some work activities may even seem pointless.

Reflecting pressures of global competition, trends in working life are towards increasing job demands, longer working hours and job instability. Growing dependence on computer technology, which could improve working life, has *actually* led to heavier workload and increased pressure. The toll of unhealthy work upon mental well-being is a primary concern.

Professor Dr. Lennart Levi, one of the founders of stress medicine, considers that work-related mental health problems are among the major causes of morbidity and premature death in much of the developed world [Levi 2006].

What can a clinician do to help solve these problems?
That is the theme of this book.

1.1 The Need for an Integrative Clinical Approach

Besides conventional biomedical therapy directed towards the cure or at least palliation of disease, a more integrative clinical approach is increasingly aimed at promoting a healthier balance between the patient and his or her surroundings. Particularly with regard to mental health disorders, it is coming to be appreciated that ill-health has not only biological but also psychosocial determinants.

The roots of such an integrative clinical approach have existed since antiquity. Now, with the expansion of our scientific sophistication, the possibilities are fully at our reach to much more deeply explore the enormous complexity and innumerable interconnections among the environment, the human nervous system and the target organs affected by disease.

Notwithstanding these insights, we still very frequently miss the mark. Namely, we too often fail to realize that the fundamental source of the patient's psychological distress is beyond the strictly biomedical domain. Neither prevention nor even adequate treatment is possible within that isolated framework.

Not surprisingly, the common tendency to over-medicalize problems that are actually of a psychosocial nature is, therefore, all too often unsuccessful [Savić 1993]. Problems such as, for example, prolonged sickness absence, job-related exhaustion, low motivation for work tasks, or, on the other hand, excessive involvement in work with attendant anxiety and tension, often cannot be solved by the clinician and patient alone.

Yet, as will be amply illustrated in this book, the clinician, particularly the neuropsychiatrist, is in a key position to provide an interface between the patient and work environment.

1.1.1 *Preventing and overcoming demoralization: a critical task*

Numerous experts in the field, have placed the prevention of demoralization as one of the critical tasks of modern psychiatry [Connor & Walton, 2011] [Cherny, 2010] [Gabel, 2012] [Kissane, *et al.*, 2010] [Perakis, 2010] [Sansone & Sansone, 2010]. This concern about demoralization as well as the stigma surrounding mental health is shared by Professor Norman Sartorius, former director of the World Health Organization Division of Mental Health, and former president of the World Psychiatric Association [Kissane *et al.*, 2010]. Demoralization is characterized by a psychological state of fear, dysphoria, loss of self-confidence and self-respect, along with feelings of hopelessness, isolation, and the inability to face new situations. Demoralization can occur as a consequence of somatic disease or fear of disease, but it can also arise without any relation to real or imagined pathology. Countering and preventing demoralization is an essential component of the physician-patient relationship and the therapeutic process. In other words, helping the patient to regain self-confidence and self-respect, as well as to evoke feelings of hope and optimism, even under very difficult circumstances, are as vital, and sometimes even more so than the actual biomedical treatment.

Within the context of mental ill-health which has developed in relation to a stressful work environment, the starting point for recovery is to bring about some change in work conditions, sometimes even relatively small, that can help initiate a positive feedback loop. Thereby, the patient begins, typically with the aid of psychotherapy and sometimes also medication, to regain a sense of control over his or her working life, returning to productive and active engagement in job tasks. Returning to work, under healthier conditions, can thereby be viewed as an integral part of overcoming demoralization.

1.2 Insights from Cognitive Neuroscience

Defining these "healthier conditions" of work is within the domain of cognitive neuroscience, or more specifically, cognitive ergonomics, informed by brain research. Tremendous strides have made in our understanding of the human nervous system. This knowledge can be used to help create working conditions that are in harmony with human needs.

As stated in the Tokyo Declaration on Work-Related Stress and Health [Tokyo Declaration, 1998]:

> "The growth of neuroscience and stress science has allowed elucidation of the links between social structures and processes (at work and outside it), the way in which these are perceived and appraised and the resulting interaction between the central nervous system and other organ systems to promote or counteract workers' health, based on a bio-psycho-social approach to all relevant aspects of the [human] – environment ecosystem and its dynamics" (p. 2).

1.2.1 *Work stressors vs. the stress response: a key distinction*

One of the major stumbling blocks in this area has been the lack of distinction between the *stressors*, namely the objective characteristics of a given set of working conditions, and *stress* or how the individual perceives and responds to these stressors. We paraphrase the formulation of Professor Walter Rohmert [1971] as a helpful starting point for clarification. He clearly distinguishes the evaluation of work from the assessment of the individual worker, whom he terms the "human operator." The independent factors of work are the stressors. These stressors can potentially elicit a stress response in a given individual. The physiological, psychological and social reactions of a given individual upon exposure to these stressors are the dependent variable. The nature of this stress response is related not only to stressors, but also to the characteristics of the given person. The various phases and physiological components of the stress response have been described in the seminal works of Cannon [1914] and of Selye [1976], as well as of Folkow [1988] Frankenhauser and Johansson [1986], Henry [1992], Kagan and Levi [1974] [Levi, 1972], Wolf [1995], *inter alia.*

The distinction between stressors and the stress response is of utmost importance, especially for occupations in which many of the most taxing stressors are not readily apparent. It is here, as we will demonstrate, that insights from cognitive neuroscience prove to be invaluable.

1.3 The Aims and Organization of this Book

We have chosen the title of this book to reflect our fundamental aim: to explore the relation between exposure to job stressors and mental health. This is done with the primary intention of developing a new clinical approach, one which takes a proactive stance, emphasizing the need for creating work conditions that are more in harmony with the needs of the human being. Pivotal to this endeavor is to provide an integrative and comprehensive methodology for assessing work stressors and ameliorating them whenever possible. This methodology, the Occupational Stressor Index, the OSI, is our own [Belkić 1989] [Belkić 2003] [Belkić & Savić, 2008]. We have successfully applied the OSI over the years in the context of prevention-oriented clinical practice within neurology and psychiatry, as well as within cardiology, oncology and other medical disciplines.

We the authors, as clinicians ourselves, have a special interest in and affinity with our colleagues, our fellow physicians [Savić 2002] [Belkić & Nedić, 2007]. This is motivated by a number of considerations that we will discuss in detail later on. At this juncture, suffice it to say that the working conditions and mental health of physicians will be strongly emphasized throughout the book.

We would also like to emphasize that gender considerations are woven into the entire book. Gender medicine is coming to be appreciated not only as a specialty in itself, but also an approach that is needed for all aspects of medicine. Gender is a key effect modifier that warrants consistent attention in research on the work environment and health [Belkić, Landsbergis *et al.*, 2004] [Messing 2000] [Nedić, Belkić, *et al.*, 2008a].

Part I of this book sets the stage. In ***Chapter 2***, we first present the leading sociological models used to assess the work environment and then review the epidemiologic evidence concerning job stressors and psychosomatic health and ill-health, emphasizing mental health outcomes, as well as salient somatic co-morbidities. Included are considerations of various aspects of "work deprivation": unemployment, prolonged sick leave, job insecurity as well as retirement.

The evidence presented in Chapter 2 justifies proceeding further to examine the "econeurologic" mechanisms by which work stressors impact upon the central nervous system, the theme of ***Chapter 3***. In order to do so, we needed to present some basic information about how the brain receives and handles information: the aversions and affinities of the human nervous system in relation to the environment. Illustrations are provided to facilitate this aim, and, hopefully, to spark interest and curiosity to delve further. This also represents a unified vantage point from which various types of stressors: mental, physical and ergonomic, can be considered in concert, with respect to their effect upon the central nervous system. Our methodological focus is electroencephalography in its various applications, in particular, event-related potentials. In the latter part of Chapter 3 neurophysiological processes are examined in direct relation to psychiatric and neurologic disorders. We segue to a review of the current standard of care concerning work fitness and occupational rehabilitation in ***Chapter 4***. Again, the focus is upon mental health, but there is also much to be learned from return to work considerations for patients with cancer, cardiovascular disease and rheumatologic/musculoskeletal disorders, *inter alia*. Since pulmonary medicine offers perhaps the most advanced approach to assessing work fitness, work-related respiratory disorders and occupational hygiene, albeit for physical-chemical rather than psychosocial/ergonomic exposures, we devote a portion (4.3.5) to that topic. Special considerations concerning work fitness and public safety are also discussed in Chapter 4.

Chapter 5 is devoted to a full presentation of the Occupational Stressor Index: its theoretical and physiological basis derived from cognitive ergonomics and brain research and also incorporating salient aspects the sociological models, the organization of the OSI as a two-dimensional matrix, the generic versus specific OSI instruments for physicians and certain other occupations. Its reliability and validity including empirical results among physicians and certain other occupations are also reviewed. The clinical validity of the OSI is discussed in the concluding section of Chapter 5 (5.4.4), thus leading us into Part II.

Part II of this book contains eight clinical case studies. The major diagnosis for nearly all of these patients is psychiatric or neurologic. The first and concluding case studies are of physicians, and the fourth clinical case is an oncology nurse who has been afflicted with breast cancer and suffers from sleep disturbances. The OSI is applied to each of the case studies, both for baseline assessment of the work environment and for formulating and implementing modifications. ***Chapter 6*** provides a more detailed introduction to the clinical case studies.

In **Part III** a novel clinical approach to mental health is introduced, in which the work environment is the focus. On the basis of Parts I and II, we suggest that there is a need for new subspecialty: Occupational Neuropsychiatry. In Part III, we envision how this expertise could contribute to healthier, more humane work environmentsfor patients with mental health disorders, as well as more broadly for working populations.

Part I –Background

Evidence, Mechanisms, Current Standard of Care and Methodology

Chapter 2

The Work Environment's Impact on Mental Health: Epidemiologic Evidence

In his seminal series of papers, Professor Sven Hernberg [1980] [1981] [1984], Editor Emeritus of the Scandinavian Journal of Work Environment & Health [Rantanen 2000], explained why it is that epidemiologic evidence linking work exposures to disease outcomes is generally biased towards the null. This is especially true for longitudinal studies, the most difficult to carry out, and, when positive, providing the strongest confirmatory evidence. Our more recent systematic review [Belkić, Landsbergis, *et al.*, 2004] confirms Hernberg's conclusions. The "healthy worker effect" [McMichael 1976] must be particularly taken into account, whereby selection factors strongly attenuate existing associations whenever the referent group is comprised of the general population (working as well as not working, where the latter are generally less healthy).

The published data reviewed in this chapter have been systematically sought, with null findings presented, when found. Publication bias, i.e. the greater likelihood of null findings remaining unpublished, could conceivably be operative [Boissel & Haugh 1993]. However, a substantial number of null findings have been published concerning the relation between work stressors and various health outcomes, and we are also aware of some strongly positive studies that actually remained unpublished [Belkić, Landsbergis, *et al.*, 2004].

2.1 Sociological Models to Assess the Association between the Psychosocial Work Environment and Health Outcomes

Etiologic research has demonstrated a strong relationship between workplace stressors and a number of adverse health outcomes. In this empirical research, the deleterious psychosocial job exposures have been most frequently assessed through generic instruments from the Job Strain [Karasek 1979] and Effort-Reward Imbalance [Siegrist 1996] Models, based heavily upon sociological theory.

Stressors associated with modern working life have long been suspected of leading to ill-health [Cooper & Marshall 1976] and [Kagan & Levi 1974].

In reviewing how this area developed, Karasek and Theorell [1990] emphasized that the question of whether the social organization of work caused serious illness would require strong empirical evidence of such associations. Furthermore, they noted that evidence which relied merely upon subjective perceptions, for example, reported dissatisfaction with one's job, would be insufficient to motivate the policy decisions needed to redress hazards related to psychosocial exposures. It was clear that this evidence would be much more difficult to accumulate compared to that for physical or chemical work exposures, where the cause of injury was often clearly work-related. The key obstacle was, in fact, the theoretical conceptualization, modeling and measurement of workplace stressors.

2.1.1 *Job strain*

In 1979 a pioneering breakthrough came when the Job Strain (Demand-Control) Model [Karasek 1979] was introduced. This model was developed for work environments in which the stressors are:

> "chronic, not initially life-threatening and the product of sophisticated human organizational decision making. In decision-making the controllability of the stressor is critical, and it becomes more important as increasingly complex and integrated social organizations develop, with ever more complex limitations on individual behavior" [Karasek & Theorell 2000] (p.78).

The Job Strain Model contains two dimensions: psychological demands, and decision-making latitude, which is a combined measure of control over task performance and skill utilization, Panel 2.1.

Job strain occurs when one is overloaded from psychological work demands and at the same time deprived of control over one's work environment. This untoward combination is predicted to give rise to increased risk of stress-related illness.

A second hypothesis generated from The Job Strain Model is that high demands together with high levels of decision-making latitude lead to the "active learning" of new, adaptive behaviors such as better coping. These positive behaviors would then purportedly lead to improved health [Karasek 1990]. Jobs with low demands and low decision-making latitude were classified as "passive," whereas "relaxed jobs" are defined as having low demands and high decision-making latitude [Karasek & Theorell 1990].

A third dimension, social support, was later added to the Job Strain Model by Johnson and Hall [1988], yielding the expanded Demand-Control-

Support Model. When workers are faced with job strain, or other types of adverse working conditions, by a dynamic process they would seek to improve these conditions via "collective control" which comes from joint, supportive efforts. This, and other types of social support at work, can help protect against ill health. On the other hand, when faced with high psychological demands and low decision-latitude, workers who are also socially isolated at work are in the worst situation and this would be particularly dangerous for their health.

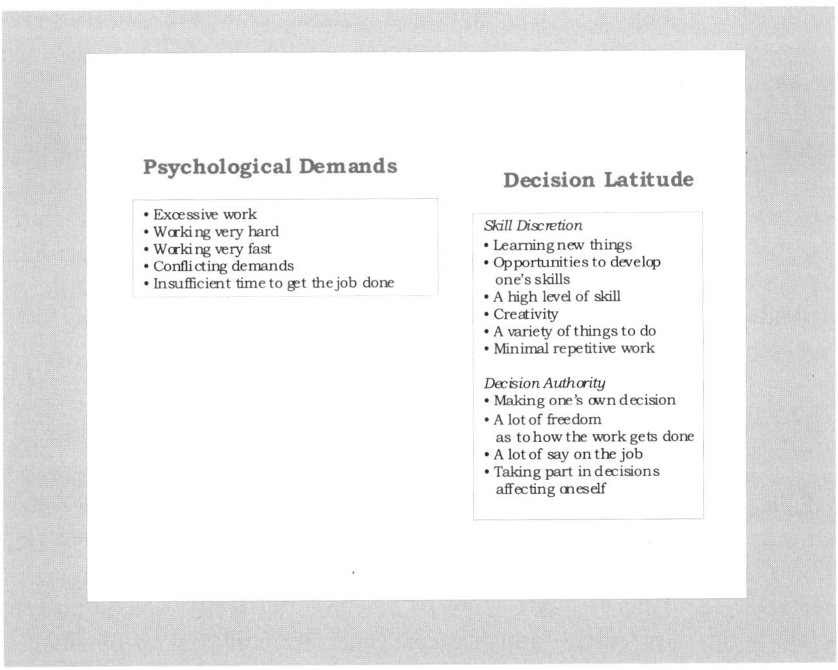

Panel 2.1 Components of Karasek's Job Strain Model, where high psychological demands plus low decision-making latitude lead to job strain, based on Ref. [Karasek *et al.*, 1982].

The Demand-Control-Support model is not only theoretically plausible, but it also has good face validity. The model is readily embraced by working people, who confirm that these concepts coincide well with their real life experience. As stated by Karasek and Theorell [2000]:

> "The ... model is useful educationally when a worksite is being explored. The model has great face value, and the employees immediately grasp the

importance of it in the practical exploration of the psychosocial work environment" (p. 78).

Questionnaires can be used to assess self-reported exposure to job strain. The dimensions are operationalized by short, generic instruments, such as the Job Content Questionnaire (JCQ) or the Psychosocial Job Strain Questionnaire (PSJSQ) [Johnson & Hall 1988][Karasek, *et al.*, 1998] [Landsbergis *et al.*, 2000] [Theorell *et al.*, 1988]. The psychometric properties of the scales as assessed via these instruments are good and the questionnaires have been validated in a number of languages and cultural settings [Karasek *et al.*, 1998] [Landsbergis *et al.*, 2000]. The questionnaires are easily administered and thereby particularly amenable for epidemiological investigations.

Exposure to Job Strain or Iso-Strain can also be inferred from occupational title alone. This method is termed "imputation" and utilizes data linkage systems that have been developed in the U.S. and in Sweden [Johnson & Stewart 1993] [Schwartz 2000]. External assessment of job characteristics via, for example an expert observer is yet another method for obtaining exposure data about job strain. (For an in-depth discussion of methodological issues concerning the Job Strain Model, see Ref. [Landsbergis *et al.*, 2000]).

2.1.2 *Effort reward imbalance*

The Effort-Reward Imbalance Model is another, complementary sociological approach for considering psychosocial work stressors [Siegrist *et al.*, 1991] [Siegrist 1996]. The Effort-Reward Imbalance (ERI) model is based upon the concept of reciprocity between the effort made and rewards received. The latter include material rewards, as well as appreciation, opportunities for career advancement and possibilities to obtain job security. According to the ERI model, efforts can be extrinsic (job demands and obligations) as well as intrinsic (over-commitment to work by the individual). The extrinsic components of the ERI model are displayed in Panel 2.2.

Compared with the Job Strain Model, which focuses more upon control over the immediate work process (i.e., decision-making latitude), the Effort-Reward Imbalance model emphasizes macro-level, longer-term control as reflected in rewards such as income, recognition and chances for job advancement. As we have pointed out, [Belkić, Schnall, *et al.*, 2000]:

"Key dimensions are shared by the Job Strain and ERI Models: both control as well as challenge (demands) are an integral part of each. However, control varies—from micro (task) level in the former, to macro level in the latter. The nature of the challenge varies from model to model, but there is a challenge of some kind in each" (p. 310).

Extrinsic Effort

- Constant time pressure due to heavy workload
- Many interruptions and disturbances on the job
- Pressured to work overtime
- Physically demanding work
- Job has become increasingly demanding

Rewards

Esteem
- Respect from supervisors
- Respect from colleagues
- Respect and prestige based on efforts and achievements
- Adequate support in difficult situations
- Not treated unfairly

Monetary Gratification/Security and Career Opportunities
- Adequate salary/income given efforts and achievements
- No undesirable change at work
- Promotion prospects
- Job security
- Job reflects education and training
- Adequate work prospects given efforts and achievements

Panel 2.2 Extrinsic components of the Siegrist and Peter's Effort Reward Imbalance (ERI) Model where high effort plus low rewards lead to ERI, based on Ref. [Siegrist & Peter 1999].

The ERI Model also has good face validity, its scales have good internal consistency, and questionnaires have been validated in a number of countries [Landsbergis *et al.*, 2000] [Li *et al.*, 2005].

2.2 The Work Environment and Mental Health Outcomes

There has been a long-standing interest in the relationship between the work environment and mental health. Even before the Job Strain Model was introduced, Cooper and Marshall [1976] postulated that a number of work stressors interacting with individual characteristics, would lead to behaviors such as smoking, absenteeism, escapist use of alcohol and to job dissatisfaction which, in turn, would eventuate in mental ill health. A large body of epidemiological investigation has examined exposure to Job

Strain, Effort Reward Imbalance and other work stressors in relation to mental health, risk behaviors well as other health outcomes.

In 2006 Stansfeld and Candy [2006] performed a meta-analytical review of eleven longitudinal investigations from several European countries and Canada, that overall included nearly 75 000 employees of various profiles. They concluded that the association between exposure to job strain and/or effort reward imbalance and common mental disorders was robust and consistent. These authors also found that low decision latitude, low social support, high psychological demands as well as job insecurity were predictive of common mental disorders.

More recently, a construct termed "relational or organizational justice" was introduced, to reflect whether management provides fair treatment, support, recognition and sufficient information to the employees whom they supervise [Ferrie *et al.*, 2006]. Low organizational justice was found to be a significant, independent predictor of future minor psychiatric morbidity (caseness (4/5) from the General Health Questionnaire (GHQ)) among over 10 000 white collar civil servants of both genders in the U.K. [Ferrie 2006]. Moreover, diminution in organizational justice was associated with an elevated risk of GHQ caseness at 1 to 4 year follow-up. On the other hand, the risk of psychiatric morbidity fell in association with increased organizational justice [Ferrie *et al.*, 2006]. Insufficient organizational fairness has also been linked to burnout in a one-year longitudinal study of 466 administrative staff a large North American university [Maslach & Leiter 2008].

2.2.1 *Depression, burnout and related mental health disorders*

Among the common mental health disorders, depression and burnout have been most often singled out in association with untoward working conditions. The International Labor Organization has pointed to the changes in the labor market associated with economic globalization as a link to the high prevalence of depression and burnout seen in many countries [Gabriel & Liimatainen 2000]. These disorders are recognized to be highly prevalent in the workplace [Bender & Farvolden 2008].

Conceptually, the entity of burnout[1] is actually linked to work conditions. As a construct, burnout is complex, placing the individual

[1] The most central dimension of burnout is exhaustion, with possible other features including cynicism or disengagement, as well as lack of efficacy at work/a diminished sense of personal accomplishment (See Appendix A section 3).

within the larger framework of his or her relation to the work environment [Maslach *et al.*, 2001] [Shirom 2011]. It has been emphasized that global market pressures, job insecurity, excessive demands to work long hours, as well as the need to keep pace with the rapidly developing informational technologies, *inter alia*, are such that burnout is likely to be a major social problem in the years to come [Shirom 2011].

Several large-scale longitudinal studies have demonstrated a significant association between exposure to job strain and depression. At 1-year follow-up of over 10 000 male and female electrical company employees in France, depressive symptoms were significantly predicted by baseline exposure to job strain, after adjustment for relevant confounders [Niedhammer *et al.*, 1998]. Among male and female civil servants in the U.K. having low decision latitude was associated with depression (assessed with the GHQ) assessed four to eight years later [Griffin *et al.*, 2002]. A two-year follow-up study of public employees from Denmark who were not depressed at baseline also suggests a possible association between new incidence of depression and low decision latitude, with a "dose-response" pattern, although the confidence intervals were very wide, compatible as well with the null hypothesis [Grynderup *et al.*, 2012].

Among male but not female employees in Alberta Canada working 35 to 40 hours/week and without current or lifetime major depressive disorders, at one year follow-up, exposure to job strain showed a significant multivariate relation to major depressive episodes[2] assessed by the World Health Organization Composite International Diagnostic Interview (CIDI) [Wang, Patten *et al.*, 2012]. For both male and female participants, job insecurity was also a significant predictor of incident depression. Among the female participants, high effort reward imbalance was a significant multivariate predictor of incident major depressive episodes in that study [Wang, Patten *et al.*, 2012].

Other longitudinal data also implicate exposure to effort reward imbalance with risk of depression. In a 1-year follow-up of over 1000 Belgian employees [Godin *et al.*, 2005], a significant association between ERI and depression (using Symptom Checklist-90, SCL-90) was found in both

---

[2] Depressive episodes are characterized by apathy, loss of energy and depressed mood lasting for at least two weeks, as well as a number of possible additional symptoms including low self-esteem, suicidal thoughts, sleep disturbances, *inter alia* (See Appendix A section 1).

men and women. Interestingly, for men the odds ratio (OR) was highest with new exposure (non-exposure at baseline and exposure at follow-up), whereas among women the OR was highest with cumulative exposure (exposure both at baseline and at follow-up). Over-commitment, the intrinsic component of ERI also appears to be a significant contributor to depression, according to detailed analyses of longitudinal data from Norway [Innstrand *et al.*, 2012].

Cross-sectional findings from the Canada, Czech Republic, Russia, and Poland reveal that exposure to job strain and to effort-reward imbalance, are associated with depressive symptoms [Pikhart *et al.*, 2002] [Wang, Smailes *et al.*, 2012]. A case-control study using the Danish Psychiatric Central Research Register to compare 14 166 psychiatric patients with 58 060 controls revealed that in women an elevated risk of depression was related to high emotional demands (Incidence rate ratio (IRR) 1.39, 95% CI 1.22–1.58) and to working with people (IRR 1.15, 95% CI 1.01–1.30) [Wieclaw *et al.*, 2008].

Exposure to job strain has also been associated with burnout or vital exhaustion in cross-sectional studies among nurses in the U.S. and Canada [Bourbonnais *et al.*, 1998] and teachers in the U.K. [Cropley *et al.*, 1999]. Nurses in Germany exposed to effort-reward imbalance had high levels on two of the three core dimensions of burnout [Bakker *et al.*, 2000]. In the above-cited 1-year follow-up study of over 1000 Belgian employees [Godin *et al.*, 2005], a significant association between ERI and chronic fatigue was also reported with a similar pattern to that of depression: for men the odds ratio was significant only for new exposure (non-exposure at baseline and exposure at follow-up), whereas among women the OR was significant only with cumulative exposure (exposure both at baseline and at follow-up).

Long work hours have also been examined in relation to exhaustion and depression. In a review through 2003, the evidence was considered positive for various measures of fatigue and long work hours, but inconsistent for depression in the limited data available [van der Hulst 2003]. In a Canadian study [Shields 1999] which was not included in the review of Ref. [van der Hulst 2003], long work hours were found to be significantly associated with depressive episodes at five year follow-up in female, but not male employees [Shields 1999]. An earlier review of the health consequences of long work hours [Spurgeon *et al.*, 1997] noted a dearth of evidence concerning overtime work *per se* in relation to burnout and depression, and mental health outcomes in general. A few more recent large-scale cross-sectional studies from Norway [Kleppa *et al.*, 2008] and Japan

[Nakata 2011] among employees in various sectors indicate that long work hours or overtime work are significantly associated with depression, assessed respectively using the Hospital Anxiety and Depression Scale and the Center for Epidemiologic Studies Depression Scale (CES-D). This relation appears to be dose-dependent [Kleppa *et al.*, 2008] and due to sleep deprivation [Nakata 2011]. Although not seen in the detailed analyses of Shields [1999], in some studies there may be confounding between overtime work and exposures to psychosocial job stressors that require further examination [Kawada 2011].

A study from Krakow, Poland of 126 intensive care nurses reveals that those who worked longer working shifts (12 hours) had significantly higher mean emotional exhaustion scores (using the Maslach Burnout Inventory) compared to those working 8-hour shifts [Iskra-Golec *et al.*, 1996]. The authors note that this increased exhaustion was seen despite the fact that the nurses who worked the longer shifts had more days off than their colleagues who worked shorter shifts.

Longitudinal data from a nationally-representative U.K. study reveal that men and women who undertook night work, particularly after 4 years duration, were significantly more likely to show symptoms of depression (according to GHQ) compared to those who had not worked nights for extended periods [Bara & Arber 2009]. Based upon a dichotomous query ("Did you feel down every day over the last two weeks?") as an indicator of depression, results from the Maastricht cohort study [Driesen *et al.*, 2011] (1998-2008) reveal a small but significant relation (OR = 1.37 95% CI 1.01 – 1.86) between depression and shift work among men aged 45 or above. After adjustment for demographic and other work-related factors, these results became statistically insignificant. However, selection factors as well as non-differential misclassification based upon the manner in which depression was assessed are major biases to the null. Among surgeons, night shift work as well as long work hours show an independent association with burnout [Shanafelt *et al.*, 2009].

Shift work is increasingly becoming recognized as a risk factor not only for mental health outcomes, but also for a number of somatic diseases, as will be briefly reviewed later in this Chapter. Shift work disorder, although not yet in the International Classification of Disease, is now included in the International Classification of Sleep Disorders [Rosenberg 2011] (see Appendix A, Section 3). The estimated prevalence among those who work night or rotating shift appears to be at least 20% [Roth 2012].

The importance of occupational stressors in the etiology of depression among working populations is further corroborated by a comprehensive intervention study carried out among Japanese blue-collar workers [Kawakami *et al.*, 1997]. The 1-year intervention program was comprised of 4 components: 1) improving machine speed and performance to diminish the need for overtime work, 2) diminishing the number of checkpoints requiring starting and stopping the machines in order to lower psychological demands, 3) providing on-the-job training when possible to improve skill acquisition and 4) bolstering the supervisors' training and availability for the employees' needs. Zung self-rated depression scores fell significantly among the intervention group, whereas these scores remained unchanged among the referents.

2.2.2 *Suicide risk*

Suicide risk is a major concern among persons suffering from depression and/or burnout. As noted, suicidal thoughts are a frequent concomitant of depression. Such thoughts must be taken with utmost seriousness, as a sensitive and specific indicator of actual risk of suicide [Galfavy *et al.*, 2008] [Mann *et al.*, 2008]. However, querying about suicide in the framework of epidemiological studies is very delicate. In contrast to other aspects of mental ill-health such as depression and burnout, it has been pointed out that "suicide remains nearly as stigmatized as ever" [Sudak *et al.*, 2008]. It is therefore likely that the actual prevalence of suicidal thoughts or history of suicide attempts is underestimated. Studies examining suicidal thoughts or actual attempts in relation to the work environment are quite sparse, and longitudinal data from working populations are lacking.

A major work-related stressor which has been examined in relation to suicide risk is harassment. Harassment, mobbing or other degrading experiences at work have been linked to suicidal thoughts in the general working population [Leymann 1996], as well as among university hospital physicians in Italy and Sweden [Fridner *et al.*, 2009] [Fridner *et al.*, 2011]. Harassment at work has also been associated with actual suicide attempts among female physicians in the U.S [Frank & Dingle 1999] (see Subsection 2.2.4.1). Some data, though less consistent, implicate long work hours [Gyorffy *et al.*, 2005], role conflict [Fridner *et al.*, 2011] and low control over working conditions [Fridner *et al.*, 2011] with suicidal thoughts among physicians. On the other hand, social support, in the form of meetings, other help with difficulties at work or confidential discussions appears to be protective against suicidal thoughts among university hospital physicians, based upon our cross-sectional data [Fridner *et al.*, 2009] [Fridner *et al.*, 2011].

Certain occupational groups have been identified as being at risk for suicide. The most consistent data are for health professionals [Aasland *et al.*, 2001][Center *et al.*, 2003] [Gunnarsdottír & Rafnsson 1995] [Herner 1993] [Hawton *et al.*, 2011] [Petersen & Burnett 2008][Schernhammer & Colditz 2004][Stack 2004][Torre *et al.*, 2005][Wolfersdorf 2007], particularly nurses and female physicians [Center *et al.*, 2003][Gunnarsdottír & Rafnsson 1995][Petersen & Burnett 2008][Schernhammer & Colditz 2004] Wolfersdorf 2007]. Recent data from the U.S. indicate that job-related problems were significantly more frequently found among physicians compared to other occupations [Gold *et al.*, 2012]. Dentists are also cited as an at-risk group among health professionals [Sancho & Ruiz 2010]. Among industrial occupations in the U.S., miners, transportation workers, and construction workers were found to be at highest risk for completed suicide based upon death certificates [Liu & Waterbor 1994]. Similar findings are reported from Australia [Andersen *et al.*, 2010]. Farmers in the U.K., the U.S. and Australia (males) have also been reported to be at increased risk of suicide [Boxer *et al.*, 1995] [Liu & Waterbor 1994] [Andersen 2010]. However, data from Sweden indicate that rates of attempted suicide among male farmers were lower than among other economically active men in the same geographic area [Thelin 1991]. There are substantial data supporting an increased risk of suicide among persons working in semi-skilled and unskilled jobs, as well as in those without an occupation [Andersen *et al.*, 2010] [Mäki & Martikainen 2009] [Mustard *et al.*, 2010].

2.2.3 *Anxiety disorders*

Anxiety is among the most common of the mental health disorders, with an overall estimated point prevalence of approximately 2 to 5% in population studies from the U.S., U.K. and Sweden [Gorman 2000] [Horwath & Weissman 2000]. Women up until the age of about 40 appear to be particularly at risk for anxiety disorders compared to men and to women above age 40 [Horwath & Weissman 2000]. The generic symptom of anxiety has been well recognized for centuries, and until fairly recently was viewed as a single entity. Later, subdivisions of anxiety were made. Using the ICD-10 classification, these include phobic anxiety, panic disorder and generalized anxiety disorder [WHO 1993] (See Appendix A, Section 1). Anxiety disorders are strongly associated with occupational disability [Horwath &

Weissman 2000]. Therefore, the healthy worker effect is likely to be particularly pronounced. Notwithstanding the strong bias to the null, there are longitudinal as well as cross-sectional data indicating significant associations between work stressors and anxiety.

Exposure to effort reward imbalance was also significantly associated with anxiety (evaluated with the SCL-90) in the above-cited 1-year follow-up study of male and female Belgian employees [Godin *et al.*, 2005]. Over-commitment is likely to contribute to anxiety, according to the detailed longitudinal analysis from Norway [Innstrand *et al.*, 2012]. In the earlier cited study, male and female civil servants in the U.K. with low decision latitude at work were also at risk for anxiety (assessed with the GHQ) four to eight years later [Griffin *et al.*, 2002].

A cross-sectional survey of over 22 000 employed Canadians revealed that the highest quadrant of the JCQ (isostrain plus physical exertion and job insecurity) was associated with an adjusted OR of 1.84 (95% CI = 1.3, 2.59) for current anxiety disorders assessed via the standardized interview (World Mental Health-Composite International Diagnostic Interview, WMH-CIDI) [Wang 2006]. In the earlier cited case-control study from the Danish Psychiatric Central Research Register comparing 14 166 psychiatric patients to 58 060 controls, low job control was found to be associated with an increased risk of anxiety disorders in men (IRR 1.40, 95% CI 1.24–1.58) [Wieclaw *et al.*, 2008].

Primary and secondary school teachers considered to be in the high job strain category were at significant risk for clinical anxiety (assessed by the Revised Clinical Interview Schedule, CIS-R) compared to their colleagues in the low-strain category in a cross-sectional study from the U.K. [Cropley *et al.*, 1999]. High job strain and low social support showed a significant, multivariate association with anxiety in a cross sectional study of nurses and accountants of both genders from the U.K. [Evans & Steptoe 2002].

Besides job strain and ERI, other work stressors potentially leading to anxiety. These include night shift work, which is noted to severely disrupt not only biological rhythm but also family life and other aspects of social life [Costa 2003]. Having one or more nights on-call per week was significantly associated with self-reported "excessive anxiety" in a cross-sectional study of over 700 general practitioners in the U.K. [Chambers & Belcher 1994]. The earlier-cited longitudinal investigation of night shift work in the U.K. [Bara & Arber 2009] also revealed a significant association to anxiety. In the earlier cited study from Norway [Kleppa *et al.*, 2008], overtime work showed a significant cross-sectional relation to anxiety.

2.2.4 *Occupations at risk for adverse mental health outcomes*

We will now review occupations identified to be at risk for adverse mental health outcomes, with a focus upon potentially contributory work stressors. These data should be viewed in light of a particularly strong healthy worker effect with respect to mental health disorders, which biases results towards the null [Belkić, Landsbergis, *et al.*, 2004]. In other words, in training, hiring and retention into most of these highly stressful professions, there is a marked selection of mentally very healthy persons, since such persons are more likely to be productive and adaptable to difficult work situations [van Dijk 1995].

2.2.4.1 *Health professionals*

Notwithstanding the above-noted strong selection factors, physicians and nurses, especially early in their careers, are reported to have a high prevalence of mental ill-health, most notably depression and burnout [Arigoni *et al.*, 2010] [Baldwin & Rudge 1995] [Campbell *et al.*, 2010] [Grassi & Magnani 2000] [Kushnir *et al.*, 2004] [Olkinuora *et al.*, 1992] [Schweitzer 1994] [Tyssen 2007]. Moreover, the prevalence of physician burnout seems to be increasing [Kushnir *et al.*, 2004] [Arigoni *et al.*, 2010]. A recent study from the U.S. indicates that burnout appears to be significantly more common among physicians, than among other working adults. In that study, physicians in the "frontline of care access": family medicine, general internal medicine and emergency medicine were particularly at risk for burnout [Shanafelt *et al.*, 2012].

Other studies have indicated that surgeons and anesthesiologists are prone to burnout [Balch & Shanafelt 2010] [Lesić *et al.*, 2009] [Nyssen *et al.*, 2003] [Shanafelt *et al.*, 2009], with e.g. prevalence rates reportedly of approximately 40% among U.S. surgeons [Shanafelt *et al.*, 2009]. As mentioned, frequent night call and overtime work were independently associated with burnout in that cross-sectional study of U.S. surgeons [Shanafelt *et al.*, 2009].

Burnout is also recognized as a major problem for psychiatrists. Violence from patients and patient suicide are noted to be among the specific precipitating job stressors [Kumar *et al.*, 2005].

Non-specialists may also be vulnerable to burnout, according to a Finnish study of a representative sample of 671 physicians [Olkinuora *et al.*, 1992]. In that study, physicians who often cared for patients with chronic, incurable or end-stage disease were prone to burnout, as well. Corroborative of that finding is that burnout is recognized to occur in a sizable proportion of oncology staff [Sherman *et al.*, 2006]. Role conflict has also been identified as a contributor to burnout among physicians and other health professionals [Piko 2006] [Tunc & Kutanis 2009]. Being single-handed, having paperwork for several evenings per week, having no hobbies and, as mentioned earlier, having one or more night calls per week were among the factors associated with adverse mental health outcomes among a sample of over 700 general practitioners in the U.K. [Chambers & Belcher 1994].

According to the Job Strain Model, physicians are among those whose occupations fall into the "active" quadrant [Karasek & Theorell 1990], which, as discussed, is hypothesized to promote healthy modes of coping and mental well being [Karasek & Theorell 1990] [Karasek & Theorell 2000]. A more in-depth evaluation from a longitudinal study of U.S. physicians reveals that there is, in fact, substantial variance in decision-making latitude and, furthermore, that low control among physicians is significantly associated with psychiatric distress [Johnson *et al.*, 1995]. Broadly concordant findings are seen among Italian male university hospital physicians, whose demand levels were exceedingly high as a result of performing their work for long hours with minimal vacation. On the other hand, they also had increased control, because they could more often decide about scheduling work hours and amount of work. This increased control could reduce exposure to job strain and was associated with a decreased chance of harboring suicidal thoughts [Fridner *et al.*, 2011].

As discussed, health professionals are at increased risk for suicide [Aasland *et al.*, 2001][Center *et al.*, 2003] [Gunnarsdottír & Rafnsson 1995] [Hawton *et al.*, 2011] [Herner 1993][Petersen & Burnett 2008][Schernhammer & Colditz 2004][Stack 2004][Torre *et al.*, 2005][Wolfersdorf 2007]. In one of the cited Finnish studies [Olkinuora *et al.*, 1992] altogether 22% of the male and 26% of the female physicians had contemplated or attempted suicide. In our study, approximately 12% of male and 14% of female university hospital physicians admitted to suicidal thoughts within the last year, with about 5% of the Swedish physicians declining to answer the query [Fridner *et al.*, 2009][Fridner *et al.*, 2011]. Given the particular stigma surrounding mental illness among health professionals [Jamison 2006], these figures are likely underestimates of the actual prevalence of recent suicidal ideation.

Among studies that have addressed physician suicide and the work environment, most have reported significant associations with occupational factors [Frank 1999][Fridner *et al.*, 2009][Fridner *et al.*, 2011][Gyorffy *et al.*,

2005] [Herner 1993] [Lindfors *et al.*, 2009] [Shanafelt *et al.*, 2011]. As described earlier, the most consistent findings are reported for harassment and other forms of belittlement or degradation [Frank & Dingle 1999][Fridner *et al.*, 2009][Fridner *et al.*, 2011]. While prospective studies concerning suicide among physicians are lacking, longitudinal data from a large, nationally representative sample of US medical students indicate that experiencing belittlement was a correlate of suicidal thoughts [Frank *et al.*, 2006]. When medical schools did not adequately handle the stressors faced by these medical students, the likelihood of suicidal thoughts was significantly increased [Compton *et al.*, 2008]. These results indicate that harassment or having degrading experiences impacts upon suicide risk very early in medical training, and that measures are needed to protect these future physicians.

Our findings also indicate that physicians who had recent suicidal ideation had very often also thought about a method by which to do so [Fridner *et al.*, 2009]. In other words, physicians who have had recent suicidal thoughts are indeed at risk for carrying this out. Health professionals are generally more aware of these methods than the general population [Hem *et al.*, 2000]. Therefore, suicidal thoughts should be taken extremely seriously in this population.

2.2.4.2 *Teachers*

Mental health disorders, particularly burnout, depression and anxiety have been receiving increasing attention among teachers, with a number of work-related factors implicated [Messing *et al.*, 1997] [van der Berghe & Huberman 1999]. These disorders are of particular concern given that a very large percentage (in the U.S. an estimated 50%) of all teachers leave the profession within the first five years [Pas *et al.*, 2012].

Teachers and counselors at the pre-college levels in the U.S. were found to be among the four occupations with a significant adjusted odds ratio (2.85, 95% CI = 1.2 – 6.8) for major depression using DSM III criteria measured by the National Institute of Mental Health Diagnostic Interview Schedule [Eaton *et al.*, 1990].

In a longitudinal study [Schonfeld 1992] of 255 first-year female teachers in New York City, CES-D-assessed depression was significantly higher among those with the most difficult conditions (threat of personal injury, vandalism, overcrowding, unmotivated pupils, lack of disciplinary enforcement against unruly pupils). Among 352 nursery school teachers and guidance workers in homes for mentally retarded children in Japan, labor-related problems and the feeling of being overburdened were significant multivariate predictors of depression, using the Zung scale [Takeda 1994]. As noted earlier, job strain among teachers has been reported to be a significant multivariate correlate of anxiety [Cropley *et al.*, 1999]. Inverse associations have been reported between social support from coworkers with both anxiety and depression [Mahan *et al.*, 2010] and it has been suggested that strong staff relationships and support among colleagues would be protective against burnout [Pas *et al.*, 2012].

The concomitants and manifestations of anxiety and burnout appear to be quite gender-specific among teachers [Forcella *et al.*, 2009] [González-Morales 2010] [Vercambre *et al.*, 2009]. However, difficulties with pupils were identified in cross-sectional analyses as significant correlates of all three burnout dimensions (emotional exhaustion, reduced personal accomplishment and depersonalization) in both male and female teachers in a nationwide French study [Vercambre *et al.*, 2009].

Voice disorders are also highly prevalent among teachers and a major cause of sick leave. Psychological disturbances (anxiety, major depression and phobia) are reportedly significant correlates of these voice disorders, and therefore are likely to contribute to disability [Nerrière *et al.*, 2009].

2.2.4.3 *Professional drivers*

Professional drivers have been noted to be at risk for psychological distress [Orris *et al.*, 1997] [Duffy & Mc Goldrick 1990]. Exposure to accidents and violence render them a potential at-risk group for post-traumatic stress disorder, PTSD (see Appendix A, Section 1) [van Dijk 1995]. Among a representative sample of 228 male and 54 female city bus drivers in Montreal, 68% had been exposed to at least one traumatic event at work, and of these, 70% had multiple exposures [Brunet *et al.*, 1998]. A more recent study of Canadian urban mass transit operators indicates that approximately 15% of those exposed to traumatic events at work subsequently developed PTSD [Vedantham *et al.*, 2001].

Several studies have examined the mental health consequences of specific traumatic events, such as person-under train accidents among subway or other rail drivers and involvement in rescue during disasters. Particularly because of poor preparation for these traumatic events, among the outcomes noted can be depression, drug use, long term sick leave as well as PTSD [Johnson *et al.*, 2005] [Theorell *et al.*, 1992] [Theorell *et al.*, 1994]. On the other hand, the incidence of PTSD and other psychiatric disorders after "person under train" events was observed to be low in among French train drivers. In France, these events are treated as occupational accidents and the drivers are given temporary sick leave (usually short) and receive needed medical follow-up [Cothereau *et al.*, 2004]. Driving the train away alone in the aftermath of a person under train event was observed to be a work-related risk factor for PTSD [Cothereau *et al.*, 2004]. In another French study, city bus drivers who received early cognitive behavioral intervention after having been victims of aggression showed a statistically significant decrease in anxiety levels and intrusion of the traumatic memory compared to those who received usual medical-social care provided by the company [Andre *et al.*, 1997].

2.2.4.4 *Certain creative professions*

In their comprehensive review, which includes both historical/anecdotal as well as substantial epidemiological data, the overall conclusion of Goodwin and Jamison [2007] is that there appears to be an overrepresentation of persons in the arts and sciences with a tendency towards manic-depressive disorders[3]. These authors note

> "the tendency for highly accomplished individuals to be, almost by definition, inordinately productive and energetic creates a problem of another sort—bias towards under-diagnosis of the manic side of bipolar illness" (p. 382).

In a series of early studies of eminent scientists and artists, the most prominent traits were reportedly "the willingness and ability to work hard and to work long hours" (p. 399) [Goodwin & Jamison 2007].

Scientific activity among academic physicians has also been found to be a likely deterrent of seeking needed professional help for psychological distress. In our study [Fridner *et al.*, 2012] of 516 university hospital physicians with current signs of psychological distress, including 166 physicians with recent suicidal thoughts, being currently involved in scientific research showed the most powerful multivariate association with not having sought needed psychological help. We interpreted this finding as follows:

[3] Manic-depressive disorders or bipolar affective disorders are characterized by a switch to the opposite polarity, with mania or hypomania being manifested by an expansive, elevated mood with e.g. decreased need for sleep and feeling that one's thoughts are racing (see Appendix A, Section 1).

Scientific activity as critical for career advancement in academic medicine requires constant striving and competition to reach "the top": to publish, to attract funding and to maintain networks. On order to seek help for psychological distress one would need a very different mindset, recognizing one's own vulnerability. This could be perceived as a threat to one's competitive edge. In addition, the energy and time demands of scientific research may hamper seeking needed help for mental distress.

Among performing artists, anxiety may also be prevalent. Trait anxiety (STAI-T) was reported to be significantly higher among a small group of operatic chorus artists Australia compared to the general population [Kenny *et al.*, 2004]. It was suggested that being under constant social evaluation may heighten the baseline levels of anxiety among these performers. It is noteworthy that these artists were required to re-audition for their place in the chorus every year.

2.2.4.5 *Other occupational groups in whom mental distress is reported*

Air traffic controllers have been cited as a high-risk group for burnout [Potter 1987]. Among this occupational group, burnout is reportedly associated with several work-related factors, including having experienced a "near miss" in the past 3 years, working at the highest level of air traffic ("Level 5"), poor work organization, and lack of support from supervisors and co-workers [Landsbergis 1998].

A small cross-sectional study of firefighters in the U.S. reveals a significantly higher than expected prevalence of psychological distress [Boxer *et al.*, 1993]. Poor relationships with coworkers and supervisors were identified as a highly significant multi-variate correlate of depression assessed with the CES-D. Due to exposure to life threatening situations, firefighters and police officers are noted to be at risk for post-traumatic stress disorders [Heinrichs *et al.*, 2005] [Saijo *et al.*, 2012] [van Dijk 1995][Wagner *et al.*, 1998]. Studies among firefighters in Japan reveal a high prevalence of depressive symptoms (22.3%; based upon a CES-D $\geq$ 16). Among the potential contributory factors in cross-sectional multi-variate analysis were high variability in workload, intergroup conflict and role conflict [Saijo *et al.*, 2007]. Firefighters who worked 24-hours shifts were at higher risk for depression if they had shorter nap-time, although this association became non-significant in a fully adjusted model [Saijo *et al.*, 2008]. A study of 101 volunteer French firefighters indicates an association between dimensions of job strain and burnout, namely emotional exhaustion was predicted by high demands and lack of control, and depersonalization with high demands [Lourel *et al.*, 2008].

2.3 Neurological Disorders, Cognitive Function, Cerebrovascular Disease and Work-Related Exposures

2.3.1 *Headache*

Headaches are an extremely common disorder among the working population. In the U.K. alone, an estimated 90 000 persons are absent each day from work or school due to headache [Willcox & Hardy 2007]. The vast majority of headaches (an estimated 80%) are of the tension type, and about 10 to 15% being migraine. It is the latter which are particularly severe and incapacitating, accompanied by autonomic dysfunction and in some cases aura [Klimek 2011] (See Appendix A, Section 2).

While it is generally appreciated that psychosocial and physical stressors can trigger migraines, relatively little objective data are available in this regard. Overall, a large percentage of workers apparently attribute their headaches to work-related factors [Klimek 2011].

A cross-sectional study from Taiwan of 9 746 employed males and 5 599 employed females indicated a significant association between self-reported psychosocial job stressors and headache, as well as other subjective complaints, after adjusting for age and education [Cheng *et al.*, 2001].

Approximately 42% of 1 000 critical care nurses reported headaches during the past six months in a publication from Serbia [Milutinović *et al.*, 2012]. A significant cross-sectional association was found between the presence of headaches and the intensity of several stressors specific to their work as assessed by the Expanded Nursing Stress Scale [French *et al.*, 2000]. The latter included: exposure to death and dying, conflict with physicians, problems with peers, problems with supervisors, workload, uncertainty concerning treatment and relating to patients and their families. The highest level of significance was for problems with supervisors [Milutinović *et al.*, 2012].

2.3.2 *Epilepsy*

Epilepsy is a relatively common disorder which affects a large number of working people [Brown & Prevett 2007]. In the U.S. alone, it has been estimated that over two million people have been either diagnosed with epilepsy[4] or have experienced an unprovoked seizure [Strine *et al.*, 2005]. In the U.K. throughout working life, i.e. from the ages of 16 to 65, an estimated 40 cases of new seizures occur per 100 000 persons per year. The lifetime risk of having a seizure is reported to be approximately 2 to 5% [Brown & Prevett 2007]. Tonic-clonic seizures (generalized or secondarily generalized) are reportedly the most common type of epilepsy. Seizure frequency varies greatly among individuals; approximately 30% of persons have less than one seizure per year whereas an estimated 20% have more than one seizure per week [Brown & Prevett 2007]. A meta-analysis indicates that after a first tonic-clonic seizure the risk of recurrence over the subsequent two-years may be up to 40% [Berg & Shinnar 1991].

It has been generally reported that epilepsy impacts negatively upon employment, with high unemployment rates [Fisher, Vickrey *et al.*, 2000] [Klimek 2011] [Strine *et al.*, 2005] [Wada *et al.*, 2001]. Contrarily, in a study among a small group of adults with newly diagnosed unprovoked epileptic seizures, no adverse consequences upon employment *per se* were noted compared to healthy referents after 10 years [Lindsten *et al.*, 2002]. Nevertheless, the persons with epilepsy had a lower income compared to referents [Lindsten *et al.*, 2002].

Idiopathic generalized seizures occur most often in close proximity to the sleep-wake transition. It might therefore be postulated that shift work could provoke seizure activity. However, this postulation has not been confirmed by empirical evidence [Brown & Prevett 2007]. Selection factors may be important, since persons with epilepsy may choose to avoid shift work [Dasgupta *et al.*, 1982]. On the other hand, the sleep deprivation associated with night shift work is an established trigger of seizures in many persons [Brown & Prevett 2007].

The risk of triggering seizures by video display equipment is reportedly very low, even among persons with photosensitive epilepsy [Brown & Prevett 2007] [Savić & Rajšić 1996]. This may be due, in part, to the fact that photosensitive epilepsy is relatively uncommon among adults, being seen most often among children and adolescents [Savić & Rajšić 1996]. The association between psychosocial work stressors and epilepsy is anecdotal, although it is recognized that changes in arousal can affect neuronal discharges. In this regard, inactivity or underload may be a

---

[4] Epilepsy is defined as a tendency to recurrent unprovoked epileptic seizures. It can be classified by seizure type with the two main categories being partial and generalized [Brown & Prevett 2007] (see Appendix A, Section 2).

trigger although well-controlled data are lacking [Brown & Prevett 2007]. Although selection factors must be taken into account, the available evidence does not indicate that persons with epilepsy have an increased risk of accidents [Dasgupta *et al.*, 1982][US Department Labor 1948] [Brown & Prevett 2007].

2.3.3 *Cognitive function and work hours*

There has been limited examination of the effects of work hours upon cognitive function. A cross-sectional study [Proctor *et al.*, 1996] of male and female automotive workers in the U.S. revealed a significant multivariate relation between overtime work and impaired performance on neuropsychological tests of attention and task performance. Overtime work was defined as having worked longer than 8 hours per day or over 5 days per week in the 7 days immediately preceding the testing. Shift work and exposure to petroleum naphtha as well as sociodemographic and other covariates were included in the multivariate analysis. These well-controlled data corroborate a large body of observational studies indicating that long work hours are associated with poorer performance on the job, and that reducing work hours does not lead to lowered productivity [Spurgeon *et al.*, 1997]. In both men and women in the U.S., long work hours were significantly associated with recent accident risk. However, with adjustment for relevant covariates, this relation remained significant only for women [Wirtz *et al.*, 2012].

Night shift work has generally been associated high accident rates [Pokorny *et al.*, 1987]. For example, the effects of working nights *per se* have been investigated among physicians (pediatric residents). A significant association was found between errors of omissions and fatigue among the physicians working the floating night shift, but not among those working days [Cavallo *et al.*, 2003]. Time on task as well as shift work have been associated with accident risk among bus drivers [Pokorny 1987]. Clearly, the association between night shift work and accident risk is related, as least in part, to disturbed sleep, which is a well-established consequence of night shift work, due to disturbance of circadian rhythms [Åkerstedt 1990] [Åkerstedt *et al.*, 2007] [Tasto *et al.*, 1978] [Wehr 2000].

2.3.4 *Neuropsychiatric consequences of physical/chemical exposures*

Among the diagnoses recognized to be associated with work-place exposures are toxic encephalitis with exposure to lead, inorganic or organic mercury; Parkinson's disease secondary to manganese or carbon monoxide among welders, battery makers and the internal combustion engine industries; cerebellar ataxia from toluene or organic mercury; toxic neuropathy from exposure to arsenic, hexane, lead, mercury, acrylamide or ethylene oxide, as well as the noise effects on the inner ear from excessive noise exposure [Mullan & Murthy 1991]. Most toxic neuropathies have both sensory and motor components, with the exception of lead, which is associated with a purely motor neuropathy [Willcox & Hardy 2007]. There is some, albeit conflicting evidence that low-level exposure to organic solvents may be associated with a number of serious neurobehavioral outcomes, including psychosis and dementia [Gamble 2000] [Willcox & Hardy 2007]. Subtle neuropsychological abnormalities may be the long-term sequelae of acute exposure to organophosphates, although the evidence appears to be conflicting in this case, as well [Willcox & Hardy 2007].

2.3.5 *Occupational groups at risk for cerebrovascular disease*

Direct epidemiological data are lacking concerning risk of cerebrovascular disease and exposure to job strain, ERI or other stressors. Cerebrovascular disease (ICD I60-I69) was included in a few of longitudinal studies of job strain (or isostrain) and death from cardiovascular disease [Johnson *et al.*, 1989] [Karasek *et al.*, 1981] [Kivimäki *et al.*, 2002] (see section 2.5.1). While each of these studies reported significant positive associations, no separate risk estimates for cerebrovascular disease were given.

There are, however, epidemiological studies from Denmark reporting that professional drivers are at high risk for stroke [Tüchsen 1997] [Tüchsen *et al.*, 2006]. Compared to gainfully employed Danes of both genders, the standardized hospitalization rate for stroke among the combined category of professional drivers was significantly elevated. The excess risk was highest for cerebrovascular infarction and lowest for intracranial hemorrhage. Drivers in metropolitan areas were at significantly greater risk than those driving in rural areas; those carrying passengers had a higher risk compared to drivers carrying goods [Tüchsen *et al.*, 2006].

2.4 Unhealthy Behaviors Associated with Work Stressors

2.4.1 *Smoking*

Smoking has been identified as an unhealthy behavior associated with attempts to counteract negative emotions and the need to regulate arousal states [Landsbergis, Schnall, *et al.*, 1998]. Although the data are not entirely consistent, there is substantial evidence of a significant positive relation between exposure to job strain and smoking intensity [Belkić, Landsbergis, *et al.*, 2000]. Among men employed in a Japanese electrical factory, the number of cigarettes smoked per day was significantly associated with low control over the pace of work, and low social support at the worksite [Kawakami, *et al.*, 1998]. A 3-year longitudinal study reveals that increased decision-latitude was positively associated with smoking cessation among men [Landsbergis, Schnall *et al.*, 1998]. On the other hand, an association between exposure to job strain and smoking has not been observed among women [Brisson 2000], although job demands were found to be significantly related to smoking intensity among female employees in Minnesota [Hellerstedt & Jeffery 1997]. A large cross-sectional Dutch study revealed no association between smoking status and exposure to Job-Strain or isostrain relation in men or women [van Loon *et al.*, 2000].

In a cross-sectional study of Finnish public sector employees [Kouvonen *et al.*, 2005], persons exposed to ERI or to low rewards were significantly more likely to be smokers. Among smokers in that study, a significantly elevated risk of being a heavy smoker was found for exposure to Job Strain, as well as for ERI, and also for some components (low control, low rewards) of these work stressor models. Among German middle managers (all male) in a large industrial company, marked imbalance between efforts and rewards was associated with an age adjusted OR of 4.34 (95% CI = 1.5 – 12.54) for smoking ≥ 20 cigarettes per day [Peter *et al.*, 1991].

Studies among male workers in Sweden and female staff nurses in Japan indicate that night-shift work is associated with being a current smoker and/or with smoking more heavily [Kageyama *et al.*, 2005] [Karlsson *et al.*, 2003]. Long working hours (over 8 hours per day) have been associated directly with smoking intensity and inversely with smoking cessation among men working on Israeli kibbutzim [Westman *et al.*, 1985].

Our cross-sectional study [Belkić & Nedić 2007] of 112 female physicians indicates that heavy smoking had a significant multivariate association with problems hampering patient-care and the total burden from threat avoidant vigilance (see Chapter 5). Among policemen, exposure to disastrous events has been associated with tobacco use [Smith *et al.*, 2005]. The association between smoking and exposure to disastrous events is corroborated by studies in the general population events [Vlahov *et al.*, 2004]. In our cross-sectional study of male professional drivers we found a significant relation between smoking intensity and the overall burden of occupational stressors as assessed using the Occupational Stressor Index (OSI) (see Chapter 5) [Belkić *et al.*, 1996] [Emdad *et al.*, 1998a] [Greiner *et al.*, 1997].

2.4.2 *Obesity*

Obesity is another behaviorally mediated risk factor that may be associated with occupational stressors. In the U.S. Hispanic Health and Nutrition Examination Survey (HHANES) obesity, as assessed by detailed anthropometric measurements, was found to be significantly associated with exposure to job strain, decision authority and psychological demands (imputation method), after adjusting for age, education and smoking status [Georges *et al.*, 1992]. Among employed Danish men and women self-reported as well as imputed exposure to job strain were found to be associated with a significantly elevated body mass index (BMI) [Netterstrøm *et al.*, 1991]. In contrast, a number of other studies showed no relation between job strain or its major dimensions and BMI among men [Hellerstedt & Jeffery 1997] [Ishizaki *et al.*, 1996] [Landsbergis, Schnall *et al.*, 1998] [Reed *et al.*, 1989]. In our cross-sectional study of 69 male professional drivers, paradoxically, a significant inverse relation was found between self-reported job strain and self-reported BMI [Belkić *et al.*, 1996][Emdad *et al.*, 1998a]. However, long work hours showed a significant multivariate association with BMI among those drivers.

Diet and sedentary lifestyle, as the behaviors that contribute to obesity have also been directly examined in relation to job strain. Among nearly 2 000 male employees in Minnesota, a significant multivariate association was found between high fat diet and exposure to self-reported high psychological demands, as well as to job strain, although, as indicated above, no such associations were found for BMI [Hellerstedt & Jeffery 1997].

The findings among women concerning job strain in relation obesity, physical activity and diet have been mixed [Brisson 2000]. A significant multivariate association was found between BMI and exposure to job strain among nearly 2 000 female employees in the above-cited study from Minnesota [Hellerstedt & Jeffery 1997]. In the above-cited cross sectional study from Holland, no relation whatsoever was found between physical activity and exposure to Job-Strain or isostrain in women or in men [van Loon *et al.*, 2000]. However, psychological demands assessed by two questions about hectic and psychologically strenuous work yielded a significant risk for sedentary behavior among Swedish working women [Johansson *et al.*, 1991].

Our above-cited study [Belkić & Nedić 2007] of female physicians identified a number of work stressors that had a significant multivariate association with obesity and sedentary lifestyle. These include long work hours, restricted problem-solving strategy, insufficient help with clinical difficulties and supervisory responsibility. It has been emphasized that recreational physical activity requires time, planning and commitment; and that this is hampered by job demands that lead to fatigue and require long recovery times after work [Johansson *et al.*, 1991].

2.4.3 *Alcohol and drugs*

The data concerning work exposures and alcohol consumption and use of drugs are quite limited. A U.S. survey of over 8 500 male and female participants from the Epidemiologic Catchment Area Program of the National Institute of Mental Health using the Diagnostic Interview Schedule identified sales, production and laborer, transportation as occupational sectors with a significantly elevated risk for alcohol abuse or dependence. Occupational profiles associated with a significant risk for drug abuse or dependence included farming, production, operators and transportation [Roberts & Lee 1993].

A cross-section study of over 20 000 Belgian men and women employed in 25 companies indicates that exposure to isostrain is associated with a significant adjusted risk of benzodiazepine use [Pelfrene *et al.*, 2004]. In the above-cited Dutch study, no relation whatsoever was found between alcohol intake and exposure to job strain [van Loon *et al.*, 2000]. Neither job strain nor its components were found to be associated with alcohol consumption among nearly 2000, mainly male urban mass transit operators in San Francisco [Ragland *et al.*, 1995]. However, the frequency of problems on the job as well as depression did show a significant relation to the average number of drinks per week. Among 150 male Swedish engine drivers, alcohol consumption was significantly higher among those with musculoskeletal complaints (see section 2.5.4) [Gerdle & Hedberg 1988]. No significant associations were found among the few female physicians (5%) who reported consuming alcohol daily in our study [Belkić & Nedić 2007].

2.4.4 *Combined lifestyle related risk profile*

In addition to examining each behavioral risk factor separately, in our studies of physicians [Belkić & Nedić 2007][Belkić & Nedić 2012] we also created a favorable combined life-style related profile: not a current smoker, BMI < 28, regular recreational physical activity and no daily alcohol consumption. Among the 56 surgeons/anesthesiologists, lower night-shift work scores were associated with low lifestyle-related cancer/cardiovascular risk. A lower overall work stressor burden was associated with low risk among the other 135 physicians (see Chapter 5).

2.4.5 *Absenteeism and presenteeism*

Some significant associations have been found between work stressors and sick leave. In a cross-sectional study of over 3 500 Swedish postal workers [Voss *et al.*, 2004], bullying at the workplace, heavy lifting, unphysiological body position were work-related factors that showed a significant multivariate association with sick leave among the female employees. Among the males, anxiety about reorganization, heavy lifting, monotonous work and not being in a supervisory role were significantly associated with sick leave. A Finnish cross-sectional investigation of 856 municipal employees [Vahtera & Pentti 1996] revealed that among men, active jobs were associated with low sick leave and passive jobs with high sick leave, thus supporting the active learning hypothesis. Among the women with small households, the job strain hypothesis was supported: high strain jobs were associated with sick leave.

Women with large households had more sick leave episodes in association with job demands, irrespective of the levels of decision-making latitude. Women in active jobs took less sick leave insofar as they had support from their spouses or had a strong sense of coherence. The authors suggest that women in active jobs may be protected against role conflicts insofar as they receive adequate support from their husbands and that their sense of coherence is high. In the previously cited study of nurses and accountants in the U.K. [Evans & Steptoe 2002], a significant independent association was found between taking more than three sick days over the past 12 months and exposure to job strain. Lowered job strain in the intervention study of Japanese blue-collar workers [Kawakami *et al.*, 1997] was associated with a significant decrease in sick leave.

Among 15 256 Japanese men working in the manufacturing sector, low job control and high role ambiguity were found to be significant predictors of long-term sick leave due to depressive disorders after over five years of follow-up [Inoue *et al.*, 2010]. Peter and Siegrist [1997] found that low rewards together with lack of high effort were associated with sickness absence among middle managers in Germany. These authors interpret this finding as reflective of passive coping.

The problem of "sickness presence" or "presenteeism" has been observed frequently among physicians, namely going to work despite illness. Over 87% of the 200 U.K. physicians queried stated that they had gone to work when feeling "too unwell to carry out their duties to the best of their ability" [Waldron 1996]. In our study of 516 university hospital physicians who showed signs of psychological distress, 45% often went to work sick [Fridner *et al.*, 2012].

2.5 Other Health Outcomes Related to the Work Environment

We will now briefly review the epidemiological data concerning the relation between the work environment and certain other adverse health outcomes outside the explicit realm of neuropsychiatry. These are nevertheless relevant comorbidities and furthermore, illustrate in a broader framework how the work environment impacts upon psychosomatic health.

2.5.1 *Coronary heart disease, hypertension, other cardiovascular disease*

2.5.1.1 *Work stressors and cardiovascular disease (CVD)*

- Job strain has been the most widely evaluated *vis-à-vis* the impact of the psychosocial work environment upon CVD. Many studies reported positive findings, but some non-confirmatory longitudinal results, e.g. [Reed *et al.*, 1989] [Eaker *et al.*, 2004] spurred questions concerning the strength and consistency of the evidence. We systematically examined the empirical studies on job strain and CVD, using pre-defined criteria to assess methodological issues affecting internal validity, and identifying the likely direction in which the results were affected. We concluded that among men, there was strong and consistent evidence of an association between exposure to job strain and CVD, across study designs and across geographic lines. The data among women were sparser, not as consistent, but, as was found among men, the majority of studies, particularly longitudinal, are likely to have underestimated existing effects [Belkić, Landsbergis *et al.*, 2004]. Other elements of causal inference, particularly biological plausibility, are also supportive. Subsequently, Aboa-Éboulé and colleagues [2007] reported that chronic exposure to job strain was associated with a significant risk of acute recurrent cardiac events among 972 patients who returned to work after a first myocardial infarction (MI). At ≥ 2.2 years of follow-up the hazards ratio of recurrent coronary heart disease with chronic job strain exposure was 2.38 (95% CI = 1.37 – 4.13), after adjusting for 26 potential confounders. These results corroborate an earlier study of seventy-nine men who had suffered an acute MI that return to work at a high strain job is an independent predictor of subsequent lethal coronary events. The predictive strength of return to high-strain work was of comparable magnitude to degree of angiographically assessed coronary atheromatosis, and more powerful than left ventricular ejection fraction [Theorell *et al.*, 1991].

There is also strong empirical evidence linking job strain to hypertension [Belkić, Schnall *et al.*, 2001] [Brisson 2000] [Landsbergis, Schnall *et al.*, 1994] [Landsbergis, Schnall, *et al.*, 2008]. Cross-sectional and longitudinal data have accumulated, indicating that exposure to job strain is associated with significant elevations in ambulatory blood pressure (AmBP) of clinically important magnitude, greatest at work, but also at home and during sleep among heterogeneous working populations [LaFlamme *et al.*, 1998] [Melamed *et al.*, 1998] [Schnall, Schwartz *et al.*, 1992] [Schnall, Schwartz *et al.*, 1998]. The data on AmBP have been recently reviewed in a meta-analysis, concluding that exposure to job strain is a risk factor for elevated blood pressure [Landsbergis, Dobson *et al.*, 2013].

- Effort-reward imbalance is also implicated in a substantial body of longitudinal and cross-sectional studies, mainly among men, concerning acute MI, as well as CVD-related mortality. The effect sizes were similar or even larger than for job strain [Belkić, Landsbergis *et al.*, 2000][Brisson 2000][Kuper *et al.*, 2002] [Kivimäki *et al.*, 2006]. Cross sectional data indicate a significant relation between exposure to ERI and elevated blood pressure [Peter *et al.*, 1998]. An increased risk for the co-manifestation of elevated blood pressure and high LDL-cholesterol was found at 6.5-year follow-up of blue-collar workers exposed to ERI, after adjusting for age, body mass index, smoking and exercise [Siegrist 1991] [Siegrist *et al.*, 1996].
- The combined effects of exposure to job strain and effort-reward imbalance upon risk of acute MI have also been demonstrated in a large case-control study from Stockholm. Among men, exposure to job strain plus high extrinsic effort and low rewards, yielded a considerably higher adjusted effect estimate, OR = 2.02 (95% CI = 1.34 – 3.07), compared to being exposed only to job strain or only to ERI (1.42 and 1.30, respectively). Among women, only intrinsic effort (over-commitment) plus job strain yielded a combined effect [Peter *et al.*, 2002].
- Organizational injustice is implicated, as well. In a meta-analysis of the studies examining and incident coronary heart disease (CHD) reports relative risk of 1.47 (95% CI = 1.12 – 1.95), after adjusting for age, gender and several other covariates [Kivimäki *et al.*, 2006]. Overall, in that meta-analysis there was an estimated 50% excess risk of incident CHD among employees who faced work stress, defined as exposure to job strain, ERI and/or organizational injustice.

- Night shift work can be considered as a cardiovascular risk factor. Shift workers are estimated to have about a 40% increased CVD risk compared to day workers [Bøggild & Knutsson 1999] [Knutsson 2003]. In the Stockholm case-control study of myocardial infarction, night shift work versus day work, yielded an adjusted OR = 1.6 (95% CI 1.1 – 2.4) among men and 3.0 (95% CI 1.4 – 6.5) among women [Knutsson *et al.*, 1999].
- Long work hours have been associated increased prevalence of self-reported hypertension in a population-based study from California [Yang *et al.*, 2006]. Increased worksite blood pressure has been reported among physicians who worked long hours [Fialho *et al.*, 2006]. In our recent study, overweight female physicians who worked long hours (frequently > 42 hours/week or occasionally > 48 hours/week) were significantly more likely to have a clinical diagnosis of hypertension compared to their colleagues who were overweight, but did not work more than 40 hours/week [Nedić *et al.*, 2010]. In our study of city mass transit drivers, the *de facto* long work day when working the split shift, was associated with marked blood pressure spikes [Uglješić, Belkić, Bošković *et al.*, 1992]. A Japanese case-control study indicates ~three-fold increased risk of acute MI among men working 11 or more hours/day, compared to age-matched men of the same occupation [Sokejima & Kagamimori 1998]. Cardiovascular or cerebrovascular death due to long hours of demanding work, "*karoshi,*" is an established diagnosis in Japan [Shimomitsu & Odagiri 2000]. The relation between long work hours and CHD has been appreciated clinically elsewhere for many decades, as well [Michie &Cockcroft 1996] [Russek & Zohman 1958].
- The total burden of occupational stressors as assessed by the Occupational Stressor Index (OSI, see Chapter 5) was reported to be associated with risk of prevalent arterial hypertension in middle-aged men and women (age-adjusted OR = 1.58 (95% 1.49 – 1.68), 1.15 (1.10 – 1.21)) respectively, in a cross-sectional study of nearly 1 000 employees from Serbia [Djindjić *et al.*, 2012].

2.5.1.2 *Occupational groups at high risk of CHD and/or hypertension*

- Professional drivers are at very high risk for hypertension as well as CHD. The data have accumulated over four decades in various countries and despite strong selection against these diseases at hiring and subsequent re-licensing. A systematic compilation of the previous extensive reviews [Winkleby *et al.*, 1988] [Belkić, Savić, Theorell *et al.*, 1994][van Amelsvoort 1995] revealed that thirty-four of forty empirical studies on this topic showed a significant positive association between CHD or hypertension and professional driving [Belkić *et al.*, 1998]. Such a consistent and large body of evidence concerning hypertension and ischemic heart disease was not found for any other occupational group [Belkić *et al.*, 1998]. Acute cardiac events often occur prematurely, such that professional drivers are strikingly over-represented among series of young patients with MI [Belkić, Peruničić *et al.*, 1992] [Riecansky *et al.*, 1988] [Villarem *et al.*, 1982]. City mass transit drivers are especially at risk for CHD and hypertension [Alfredsson *et al.*, 1993] [Backman 1983] [Bigert *et al.*, 2002] [Bigert *et al.*, 2003] [Gustavsson *et al.*, 1996] [Michaels & Zoloth 1991] [Morris *et al.*, 1966] [Netterstrøm & Juel 1988] [Ragland *et al.*, 1987] [Ragland *et al.*, 1997] [Rosengren *et al.*, 1991]. Standard cardiac risk factors such as smoking, obesity and hyperlipidemia are frequently present among professional drivers. However, risk factor status does not consistently distinguish professional drivers from other groups at lower risk [Belkić, Savić, Theorell *et al.*, 1994]. Accounting for the major standard cardiac risk factors (age, serum cholesterol, blood pressure, smoking, body mass index, diabetes, positive parental history of CHD and physical activity) as well as socio-demographic factors, an OR of 3.0 (95% CI=1.8-5.2) was found for incident CHD after a mean of 11.8 years among male, middle-aged Gothenburg city bus and tram drivers compared to employed referents [Rosengren *et al.*, 1991].

- Emergency responders, including firefighters, police officers and emergency medical personnel also appear to be at increased risk for hypertension. An estimated 75% of emergency responders are reported to have prehypertension or hypertension [Kales *et al.*, 2009].

  Heart disease is the reported cause of 45% of deaths that occur on-duty among firefighters in the US. Fire suppression was associated with the highest risk of cardiac death while on duty [Kales *et al.*, 2007]. This appears to occur nearly exclusively among firefighters with underlying CVD [Kales *et al.*, 2003] [Soteriades *et al.*, 2011].

- In at least one empirical study other stressful occupational groups, including air traffic controllers, sea pilots, waiters/waitresses, and lower-ranking police officers are reported to be at increased risk for acute MI or CHD-related death, though the evidence is more sparse and somewhat conflicting [Belkić, Savić *et al.*, 1995] [Cobb & Rose 1973] [Hammar *et al.*, 1992] [Harrington 1972] [Nyström *et al.*, 1990] [Saarni *et al.*, 1996] [Sega *et al.*, 1998] [Tüchsen 2000] [Zorn *et al.*, 1977].
- Health professionals do not appear to be at increased risk of CHD or hypertension compared to other occupational groups [Carpenter *et al.*, 1997].. However, once hypertension develops, they may be at risk for complications, based upon a 7-year follow-up study of 160 physicians and nurses in the Vojvodina region of the former Yugoslavia [Nedić *et al.*, 2001].

  When compared to 122 hospital employees without clinical duties, the health professionals had a relative risk = 3.7 (95% CI = 1.6 - 8.6) for developing cardiovascular or cerebrovascular complications.

  These findings corroborate the special etiological importance of occupational stressors in the progression from hypertension to ischemic heart disease [Schwartz *et al.*, 1996] [Uchiyama *et al.*, 2005].

2.5.2 *Peptic ulcer disease and diabetes mellitus*

- Shift work appears to be linked to risk of peptic ulcer disease (PUD), and possibly also to diabetes mellitus (DM) [Knutsson 2003]. Recent data from a 9-year retrospective cohort study of 6 413 male employees, 805 of whom were shift workers indicate a strong independent relation between impaired glucose tolerance and night shift work [Oyama *et al.*, 2012]. Control of blood glucose was found to be significantly better among 120 day workers in Bangkok compared to 120 shift workers matched for age, duration of DM and use of hypoglycemic agents. The two groups did not differ significantly in BMI; however, there were significantly more shift workers with abnormal GHQ scores [Chalernvanichakorn *et al.*, 2008]. Working overtime was found to be a significant multivariate predictor of non-insulin dependent DM at follow-up in an 8-year longitudinal study from among male industrial workers in Japan [Kawakami *et al.*, 1999].
- Professional drivers may be at increased risk for peptic ulcer disease and diabetes mellitus, according to some investigations. Empirical studies have also revealed a significantly greater self-reported prevalence of symptoms characteristic of PUD (12%) among male urban bus drivers compared to other employed men (6%) [Netterstrøm & Juel 1990]. However, the risk of PUD over 6 years was not significantly increased among the drivers. A ten-year prospective study of male employees in Japan revealed a relative risk of 3.95 (95% CI = 1.1.5 – 13.6) among transport workers for developing non-insulin dependent DM, after adjusting for age and baseline differences in BMI, HbA1c and fasting blood glucose [Morikawa *et al.*, 1997].
- Air traffic controllers are possibly at high risk for these disorders. In the above-cited U.S. study comparing 4 325 ATC and 8 435 second class airmen [Cobb & Rose 1973], the ATC also had significantly higher point prevalence of diagnosed PUD and DM. The prevalence of PUD was significantly greater at the high-density towers, particularly among the younger age group.
- In the earlier-cited study from Serbia of Djindjić and colleagues [2012] the total OSI was found to be associated with prevalent Type 2 diabetes mellitus in middle-aged men and women (age-adjusted OR = 1.21 (95% CI: 1.15 – 1.45), 2.40 (95% CI: 1.67 – 3.45)), respectively.

2.5.3 *Vulnerability to malignancy*

- Toxic workplace exposures have the most data directly linked to risk of malignancy. In the U.S. toxic occupational exposures have been associated with approximately 4% of the attributable-risk for cancer [Cole & Rodu 2001]. Among the work-related exposures that are recognized to be causative agents for specific cancers are asbestos for mesothelioma, as well as cancers of the trachea, bronchus and lung; ionizing radiation for numerous malignancies including thyroid cancer, lymphoid and myeloid leukemia; benzidine for bladder cancer, chromium and cancers of the nasal cavity, trachea, bronchus and lung; to name a few [Adami *et al.*, 2002] [Mullan & Murthy 1991]. Some of the occupations for which specific cancers are recognized to be related to toxic work exposures include radiologists, agronomists, welders, foundry workers, chimney sweeps, and workers in the rubber industry, among many others [Mullan & Murthy 1991].

- Professional drivers are not included in the list of occupations with recognized work-related cancers [Mullan & Murthy 1991]. However, there are data from Denmark for truck drivers, indicating an increased risk of dying from multiple myeloma (standardized mortality ratio (SMR) = 439, 95% CI = 142 – 1024) and from lung cancer (SMR = 160, 95% CI = 126 – 200) [Hansen 1993]. It has been suggested that this may be related to exposure to diesel exhaust. A subsequent Swedish study showed an elevated relative risk for lung cancer among male short distance truck drivers, after adjusting for attributed smoking prevalence [Jakobsson *et al.*, 1997]. An elevated SMR for lung cancer has also been reported among Icelandic truck drivers [Rafnsson & Gunnarsdottír 1991].
- Until fairly recently, shift work and cancer had not been extensively investigated [Knutsson 2003]. However, an early British study reported a significantly elevated overall SMR for cancers compared to the general population [Taylor & Pocock 1972]. More recently, there have been some studies indicating an increased risk of breast cancer among women who work night shifts. A Danish case-control study reported an OR = 1.5 (95% CI = 1.3 – 1.7) for women aged 30 to 54 who worked mainly at night, adjusting for age, age of first and of last childbirth and number of children [Hansen 2001]. A 10-year follow-up of 78 562 female nurses showed that having worked least 3 night shifts/month for ≥ 30 years was associated with a relative risk of 1.36 (95% CI = 1.04 – 1.78) for breast cancer, after adjusting for numerous covariates, including age, age at menarche, parity, age at first birth, BMI at age 18, family history of breast cancer, benign breast disease, oral contraception, alcohol, age at menopause and post-menopausal hormone use [Schernhammer *et al.*, 2001]. The results from a more recent longitudinal Swedish study (mean follow-up 12.4 years) also indicate an increased risk of breast cancer among women with shift work including night work compared who worked only during the day (OR=2.02, 95% CI 1.03 – 3.95) [Knutsson *et al.*, 2012]. On the basis of the current evidence, including the experimental evidence that tumor growth is accelerated by suppression of melatonin secretion, it is recommended that women with previous or current breast cancer should be advised against working night shifts [Bonde *et al.*, 2012].

- Breast cancer risk has been reported to be elevated among certain occupations that entail night-shift work, such as flight attendants, radio and telegraph operators as well as nurses. However, it has been pointed out that carcinogenic exposures could also be contributory, e.g. ionizing radiation for airline cabin crew [Knutsson 2003]. A subsequent publication from the Nurse Health Study indicates an increased incidence of colorectal cancer associated with night shift work [Schernhammer *et al.*, 2003]. Rotating shift work has also been associated with a significantly increased risk of prostate cancer in a prospective study from Japan [Kubo *et al.*, 2006].
- The bio-behavioral model of malignant disease outlines multi-factorial pathways by which psychosocial factors and health behaviors interact with biological processes that, in turn, influence tumor physiology and resistance [Lutgendorf *et al.*, 2002]. However, in contrast to the strong evidence linking work-related toxic exposures to risk of several cancers and the emerging support for an association between night shift work and risk of breast and colon cancer, observational studies have yet to provide a coherent picture concerning the etiological relationship between occupational psychosocial exposures and cancer risk, *per se*.

2.5.4 *Musculoskeletal disorders*

The relationship between adverse psychosocial work conditions and musculoskeletal disorders is quite well established. Low social support at work, high psychological demands and high job strain have been significantly associated with soft tissue tenderness on physical examination in the central body regions in analyses stratified by gender, age and physical load at work [Toomingas *et al.*, 1997]. These results appear to confirm earlier studies regarding symptoms from the neck and back regions. Lean production and changes in the shop floor layout have been shown to increase risk of repetitive strain injury [Leslie & Butz 1998]. Exposure to job strain or its major dimensions has been associated with musculoskeletal symptoms among nurses and nurses' aides [Ahlberg-Hulten *et al.*, 1995] [Josephson *et al.*, 1997], municipal workers [Myers *et al.*, 1999], sales persons [Skov *et al.*, 1996], and among urban mass transit operators [Krause *et al.*, 1997a] [Krause *et al.*, 1998]. These associations remained significant after adjusting for physical factors in most of the studies. Working four or more hours per day at a video-display unit is estimated to carry an OR of approximately 2 for disorders of the hand and wrist. This is mediated through repetitive finger motion and sustained muscle loading. High work demand and poor workstation design further exacerbate the risk of upper extremity disorders [Punnett & Bergqvist 1997]. Thus, both physical ergonomic and psychosocial work factors need to be examined to properly address work-related musculoskeletal disorders [Carayon *et al.*, 1999].

Meat processing workers are listed as a group for whom in the U.S. carpal tunnel syndrome and mononeuritis multiplex are recognized to be occupationally-related due to cumulative trauma [Mullan & Murthy 1991]. In an intervention study, short rest breaks were demonstrated to ameliorate musculoskeletal discomfort ratings among meat-processing workers, while having no negative effect upon productivity [Dababneh *et al.*, 2001]. Empirical studies have also revealed an increased risk among professional drivers for musculoskeletal disorders [Backman 1983] [Hedberg 1988] [Krause 1997b].

> Up until here in this Chapter, we have focused upon the relation between working conditions *per se* with regard to mental health and other health outcomes. There are also mental health consequences of lacking employment or being in a precarious job situation. These will be briefly reviewed in the concluding section of this Chapter.

2.6 Mental Health Consequences of Job Insecurity, Precarious Employment, Unemployment and Retirement

The landmark studies of Jahoda and her colleagues [Jahoda *et al.*, 1933] during the Great Depression of the 1930's demonstrated the devastating psychological effects of mass unemployment. Subsequent research essentially corroborated and expanded these findings [Jahoda 1982] [Bohle *et al.*, 2001]. Risk behaviors such as smoking, physical inactivity and consequent obesity have been found to be significantly associated with being unemployed for over one year, in a cross-sectional study from Northern Sweden [Janlert *et al.*, 1991]. There are also substantial data linking unemployment with increased use of alcohol, illicit drugs as well as tobacco [Bohle *et al.*, 2001]. Recent longitudinal data from the U.S. among 13 451 persons aged 51 to 75 followed for 18 years indicate that the risk of acute myocardial infarction is particularly elevated within the 1st year of unemployment, after adjusting for numerous clinical, socioeconomic and behavioral risk factors [Dupre *et al.*, 2012].

With regard to studies of unemployment, there are many difficult methodological issues that arise, such that some questions about directionality of effects have been raised, especially with regard to cross sectional studies [Salm 2009]. Nevertheless, observations by many colleagues as well as our own clinical experience indicate that unemployment very often has a harmful impact upon mental as well as physical health. The mechanisms involved are noted to include: relative poverty, loss of self-esteem, untoward health-related behaviors and the impact of unemployment upon subsequent employment patterns [Bartley 1994]. Among persons who are unemployed, psychological distress is particularly pronounced with emotionally-focused coping patterns, namely self-blame and wishful thinking, as opposed to those who activate problem-solving coping strategies [Grossi 1999].

Major changes in the organization of work with the aim of increasing productivity have lead to what has been alternatively termed "lean production," "total quality management," "high-performance work organization," *inter alia* [Landsbergis *et al.*, 1999] [Belkić, Schnall *et al.*, 2000]. This has generally meant the collapse of the 4-quadrant Job Strain Model into two categories, active and high strain jobs, with the elimination of work with low demands, i.e. passive and relaxed jobs [Belkić, Schnall *et al.*, 2000]. In other words, the employees who stay on the job are frequently working harder in the face of downsizing with the elimination of many jobs.

Job insecurity is a direct consequence of these organizational changes, even among those who retain their jobs [Bohle *et al.*, 2001]. Besides the fact that such downsizing and restructuring frequently fail to improve the enterprise's financial standing and productivity, there is a well-documented "survivor effect" of demoralization and other deleterious effects upon mental health [Bohle *et al.*, 2001]. The earlier cited meta-analysis of studies through 2006 further corroborates the association between job insecurity and adverse mental health outcomes [Stansfeld & Candy 2006]. A recent study from the U.S. indicates a 50% increase in depressive symptoms among persons who had recently held temporary jobs [Quesnel-Vallé *et al.*, 2010]. Temporary employment was identified as a significant correlate of state anxiety among male teachers [Forcella *et al.*, 2009]. Similarly, a 1-year follow up study from South Korea, indicated that new onset of depression was significantly associated with change from permanent to precarious employment among women, although not among men. On the other hand, women, but not men, also showed a significant increase in new-onset depression with change from precarious to permanent employment [Kim *et al.*, 2012].

The risk of fatal accidents is also increased with downsizing [Landsbergis 2003]. Among the many reasons is that more senior workers often face mandatory early retirement. It is these "more experienced workers, who often play a critical role in maintaining informal safety rules, and to subtle but significant work practices" (p. 41) [Bohle *et al.*, 2001]. Cutting corners and longer work hours are also contributory factors.

Increasing numbers of people are employed in unstable jobs. These jobs often entail very high demands and low decision-making latitude [Quinlan *et al.*, 2001]. Thus, in addition to the direct deleterious consequences of insecure employment upon mental health as briefly summarized in this section, exposure to job strain and other untoward working conditions further impact negatively upon mental health.

We will now brief address retirement, which is recognized by clinicians to be complex, potentially affecting mental and somatic health. These issues are of particular concern for those with over-engagement in work, including those who are sickness present [Knežević 2011].

The path by which retirement occurs, especially whether this is through disability retirement, obviously needs to be taken into account [Robroek *et al.*, 2012]. On the one hand, compared with those who continued their employment, early voluntary retirement or statutory retirement at age 60 among civil servants from the Whitehall II cohort study was significantly associated with indicators of improved mental health as well as higher physical functioning [Jokela *et al.*, 2010]. The use of antidepressant medication among Finnish public-sector employees reportedly decreased significantly after retirement, even among those who retired for mental health reasons [Oksanen *et al.*, 2011]. On the other hand, German retirees who had experienced repeated unemployment during their working life showed significantly more anxiety and depression compared to retirees without such episodes. Those with higher current household income were found to be less affected [Zenger *et al.*, 2011]. Interestingly, in a study from the U.S., after adjusting for sociodemographic covariates, employed persons over age 65 had a significantly lower prevalence of depression, compared to employed persons age 65 and lower. However, those over age 65 who faced job strain, effort reward imbalance and were dissatisfied with their work had increased depressive symptoms [Mezuk *et al.*, 2011]. In another study from the U.S., among those who during late midlife reported that work stress interfered with family, retirement was associated with fewer depressive symptoms [Coursolle *et al.*, 2010]. A cross-sectional study of a nationally representative sample of over 12 000 retirees indicated that those with so-called "career bridge employment" had better mental health than those with full retirement. The authors [Zhan *et al.*, 2009] conclude that engaging in bridge employment is likely to be beneficial for overall health.

> To summarize this Chapter, a large body of evidence has accumulated over several decades indicating that the work environment can indeed impact upon mental health and more broadly upon psychosomatic health. The mechanisms involved are explored in the next Chapter. At the same time, the adverse consequences of unemployment and job insecurity underscore the importance of stable work for psychological well being. Efforts aimed at promoting return to work are thus fully justified from the vantage point of neuropsychiatry.

Chapter 3

Work Stress Mechanisms and Mental Health: A Focused Overview

In the previous chapter, we provided a short review of the evidence linking work stressors to adverse health outcomes, with a focus upon mental health. We will direct our attention in this chapter to some mechanisms by which these associations may occur. Our primary framework will be how the human central nervous system processes information, makes decisions and, on that basis, carries out actions. We will examine the affinities and the aversions of the human being at work and describe the burden of work processes upon the nervous system and how this burden can impact upon health. In the latter portion of the chapter, we examine these processes in more direct relation to psychiatric and neurological disorders.

Before proceeding further along these specific lines, we will briefly discuss gender, which has an important bearing upon these mechanisms in a wide context, with fundamental implications for the entire area.

3.1 Gender, Work Stressors and Health: A Richer Conceptualization

In Chapter 2, we repeatedly observed different patterns of associations between work stressors and health among men and women. Gender is recognized as a key effect modifier of the relation between the work environment and health outcomes [Belkić, Landsbergis *et al.*, 2004] [Messing 2000]. As gender-related issues have been incorporated into work stressor models, these models have become much richer and more meaningful.

Brooker and Eakin [2001] note that power and control are frequently included in models of work stress,

> "...but they tend to be narrowly conceptualized. Often the research presents a series of empirical findings, rather than an integrated conceptual model which clearly specifies the pathways by which individual work experiences are linked to health and to the broader social context" (p.97).

These authors point out that the Job Strain Model, for example, has viewed the psychosocial work environment as analogous to the physical work environment, with an emphasis on exposures. However, the cognitive or symbolic significance of physical entities and events at work can also impact upon health. This contextual meaning may be closely related to issues of power.

A salient illustration is working in a small, crowded workspace, which can be viewed as a physical stressor, by its effect upon air quality, noise levels, mobility, etc. However, this cramped workspace can also convey a message of low status and prestige and thereby can influence self-esteem and dignity, as well. While the physical stressors can obviously affect health, so can these symbolic factors.

Numerous familiar scenarios can be further evoked, whereby gender and power relations profoundly affect experience and thereby health. To name a few: the all too often demeaning experience of clerical workers (frequently female) *vis-à-vis* their bosses (often male, although this is changing); sexual harassment, *inter alia.* These situations arise in direct relation to gender and power relations.

As inferred, poor self-esteem is a frequent concomitant of these experiences, and may be related not only to the fact that the job is routine and lacks autonomy, but also to poor social relations with inadequate respect [Brooker 2001]. Empirical studies have indeed shown an association between low self-esteem and depression [Brown & Moran 1997]. Unhealthy behaviors such as smoking and alcohol consumption can be consequences of poor self-esteem, as well [Corbin *et al.*, 1996] [Walitzer & Sher 1996].

Concordantly, emotional or symbolic rewards, i.e. gratification and sense of meaning, may compensate to some extent for the objective difficulties of occupations such as teaching, the health professions and social work. It has been well established that there is a hierarchical distribution of these emotional rewards, favoring those with more power and control within the work organization [Belkić & Savić 2000].

It is also important to consider the gender context of various occupations: e.g. are they male- or female-dominated? In the earlier cited study of accountants and nurses of both genders [Evans & Steptoe 2002], it was suggested:

> "when men and women occupy jobs in which they are in the cultural and numerical minority, there may be adverse health effects that are gender-specific" (p. 481).

Moreover, we noted that the active learning hypothesis of the Job Strain Model in relation to sickness absence was not operative for women with large families. Namely, heavy job demands, irrespective of levels of decision-making latitude, were associated with more sick leave for women

[Evans & Steptoe 2002]. It has also been found that associations between self-reported working conditions and health may be underestimated among women, since their actual control is over-estimated and hindrances underestimated [Waldenström & Härenstam 2008]. This complexity and multiple roles illustrate why the work-related risks are often "hard-to-pin-down" among women [Messing 2000]. With expansion of our knowledge about the relations among work, gender and health, further new directions are suggested, with a focus upon health rather than distress [Nelson *et al.*, 2002].

> At this juncture it is well to emphasize that, traditionally, women have borne a major burden outside the arena of paid working life: responsibility for home and family. For many reasons, including and perhaps especially due to its unpaid nature, this work has often been "invisible" or "silent", notwithstanding the demands upon cognitive and emotional resources [Belkić & Savić 2000] [Hochschild & Machung 1989]. The "silent" burden of work will be an important theme explored in this Chapter, and later on throughout this book as well.

3.2 Econeurologic Mechanisms: Mental Burden of Work Processes

Stunning progress has been made in our understanding of how the human being, via the central nervous system (CNS) handles information, transforming it into output of value and meaning. We now address the question: How can that knowledge be harnessed to inform us in our quest to organize work so that it becomes in better harmony with human needs and capacities?

Previously, we had focused heavily upon the cardiovascular system and thereby formulated the concept of econeurocardiology, the biological paradigm by which environmental factors are processed by the central nervous system, and which can result in pathophysiologic changes that increase risk of adverse cardiac events [Belkić, Schnall, *et al.*, 2000][Wolf & Belkić 2000]. The causal webs linking mentally stressful activity, the central nervous system and CVD outcomes have been very well documented, as reviewed in, e.g. [Belkić, Schwartz *et al.*, 2000] [Eliot 1974] [Folkow 1994] [Henry 1994] [Kulbertus & Frank 1988] [Lown 1990] [Natelson 1985] [Rozanski *et al.*, 1999] [Schneiderman 1978] [Wolf 1995]. Via the concept of econeurocardiology, we thereby postulated that the more insight gained into what mental burden actually means, and the better we implemented that knowledge to humanize work, the better the cardiovascular system could be protected [Belkić & Savić 2000]. The topic of "econeurocardiology" will be revisited in the last section of this Chapter.

We have expanded that integrative, "holistic" approach to incorporate a broader set of health outcomes, and herein focus more heavily upon mental health.

3.2.1 *A deeper understanding of psychological demands*

As a starting point, we will take one of the dimensions of the Job Strain Model: psychological demands and will delve more deeply into its meaning. Indeed, it will be demonstrated that we can go much further than asking whether one "works hard" and "works fast." Rather, we seek to analyze work in terms of the time dimension and allocation of mental resources.

Thus, we aim to address in a more concrete way, the very question of "how fast is too fast?" or "how hard is too hard?" Approaches to quantifying the mental burden of work using more objective means can help overcome many of the difficulties inherent in self-report methods [Greiner *et al.*, 1998] [Kristensen 1996] [Sackett 1979] [Schnall, Landsbergis & Baker 1994].

These insights complement the worker's perceptions of his or her tasks. Through an interactive participatory approach, guidance is thereby obtained for formulating and implementing intervention strategies.

3.2.1.1 *Mental chronometry: the time dimension of information processing*

The time dimension is critical to our understanding of psychological demands. Thus, we review how information is handled along the time axis.

This process is illustrated in Fig. 3.1, as derived from Ref. [Ivanitsky 1980], where it is seen that the incoming signal is assessed first with respect to its physical attributes, and later for its meaning to the individual. On that basis, a decision is made, which may result in some action.

From this view along the time axis, we can see that about a tenth of a second (≈ 100 milliseconds) is needed to register the sensory aspects of the signal.

This is recorded in the primary cortex, and on the signal-averaged electroencephalogram, a wave at about 100 milliseconds can be observed. During this time, the dominant process is perception.

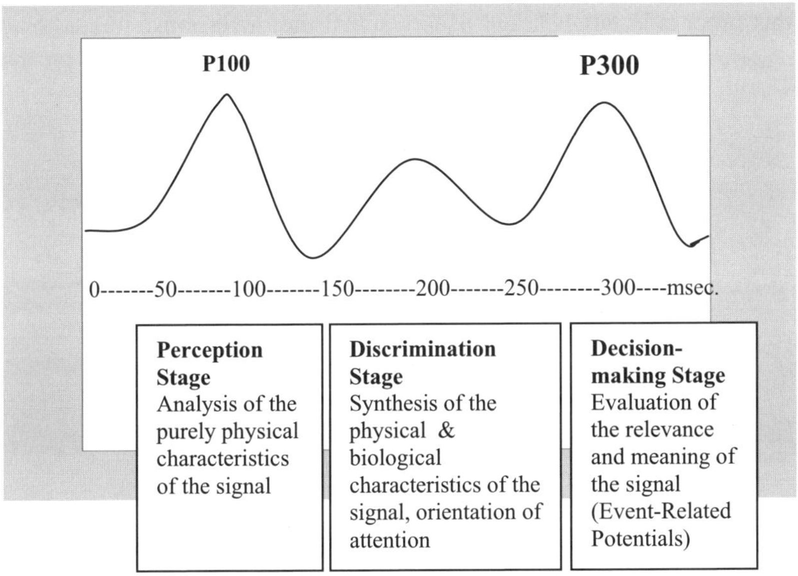

Figure 3.1 The time line of information processing by the central nervous system, as reflected in a schematic representation of the evoked potential curve, with prominent positive waves (pointing upward) at approximately 100 milliseconds (msec) and 300 msec, reflecting the P100 and P300, respectively.

An example of a visual evoked potential recording from our laboratory in Belgrade in shown in Fig. 3.2.

At least twice as long thereafter[1], i.e. about a third of a second (≈ 300 milliseconds) after the signal appears is usually the minimum time needed to be able to make a decision about the meaning of the stimulus that has been received by the CNS. At that time, the P300 wave, a positively oriented averaged electrocortical potential, may be seen. The P300 wave is most frequently recorded when attention is selectively focused upon a rarely occurring signal, which has some significance for the person [Sutton & Ruchkin 1984]. The significance is often task related, namely the signal indicates that some kind of cognitive decision and/or action is needed [Ritter *et al.*, 1968]. It should be emphasized that the P300 mainly reflects recognition of specific, relevant stimuli and classification of their meaning

[1]An intervening period after the stage of perception and before the appearance of the Event-Related Potentials, has been termed the "discrimination" phase, reflecting processes such as orientation of attention, recognition of a change in the flow of sensory stimuli, etc. [Ivanitsky 1980] [Kügler *et al.*, 1993] [Mulder & Wijers 1991] [Näätänen & Alho 1995].

and this process is independent of any actual motor response [Donchin *et al.*, 1984] [Savić & Belkić 1998]. (See Section 3.2.1.3 for further elaboration on this point).

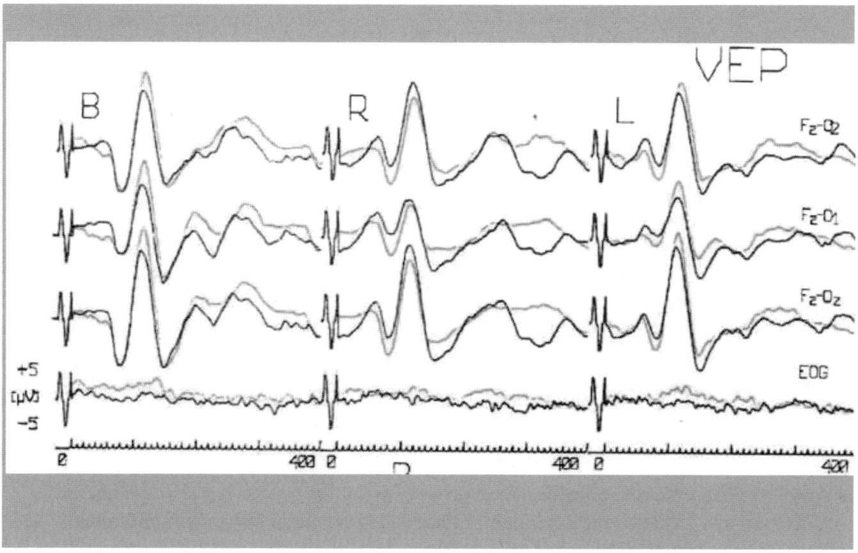

Figure 3.2 Visual evoked potential (VEP). Recording from our Laboratory for Clinical Neurophysiology and Psychophysiology at the Institute of Mental Health, Belgrade.

Channels from the top: #1-3 EEG channels Fz-O2, Fz-O1, Fz-Oz, #4 Electrooculogram (EOG), #5 indicates time in milliseconds.

An example of a P300 event-related potential generated by signals in the auditory modality, as recorded from our laboratory in Belgrade in shown in Fig. 3.3. The P300 exemplifies the so-called "Event-Related" or Cognitive potentials, as described in e.g. [Chiappa 1989] [Coles *et al.*, 1990] [Cooper *et al.*, 1980] [Savić & Belkić 1998], and as first discovered by Sutton and colleagues [Sutton *et al.*, 1965]. Examination of these Event-Related Potentials provides insight into the higher nervous processing resources required by a given task. These can be an indicator of "mental chronometry" [McCarthy & Donchin 1981] whereby brain activity is assessed *over time* as it processes information, makes decisions and lays the basis for task execution. Using concepts from cognitive ergonomics, Event-Related Potentials (ERP) can help us quantify mental burden using the time dimension. Thus, for example, the latency of the P300 reflects the time required to evaluate and correctly categorize a signal.

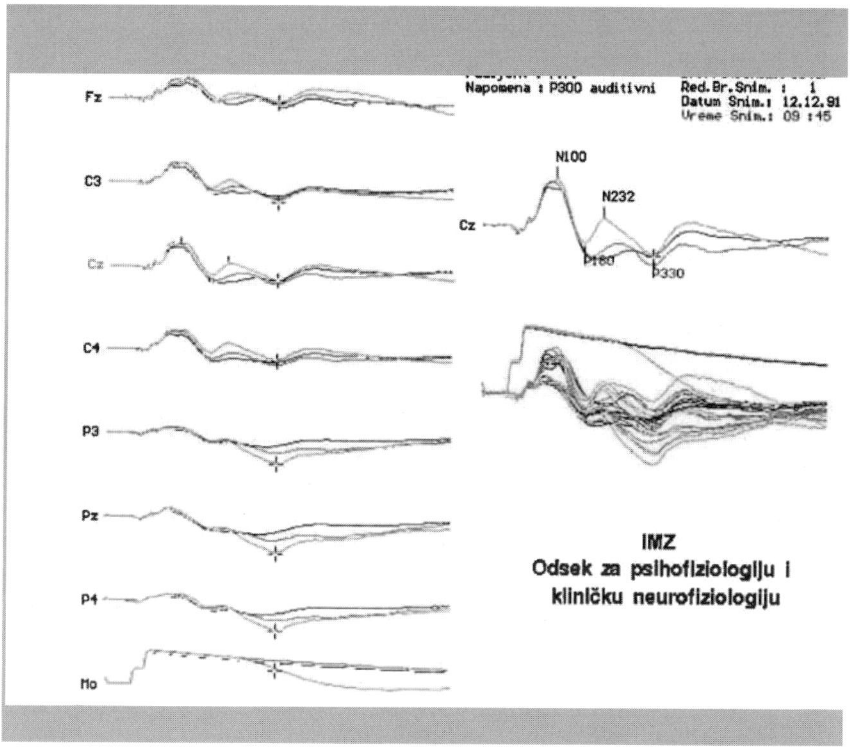

Figure 3.3 P300 event-related potential (auditory modality) and earlier components. Recording from our Laboratory for Clinical Neurophysiology and Psychophysiology at the Institute of Mental Health, Belgrade.

Individual EEG channels shown on left panel, upper portion of right panel shows channel Cz with the main evoked potentials marked (note that positive waves are shown below the x-axis, and negative waves above). The lower part of the right panel shows all the EEG channels superimposed.

When signal detection becomes more complex or for visual stimuli, e.g. when contrast is low, there is a prolongation of the P300 for relevant stimuli [Walton *et al.*, 1987], as illustrated in Fig. 3.4.

As the incoming information becomes more complex, the decision-making process is rendered more difficult (and more time consuming) and, as a consequence, the time required to correctly respond is prolonged. In other words, as the incoming information exacts a greater demand upon the brain's processing resources, the time needed to respond correctly, e.g. reaction time (RT) takes longer. The latter has been well-known for over a century, from the classical observations by Merkel [1885], who demonstrated that as the number of alternatives increases, there is a striking rise in the mean RT, from 200 msec with one signal, to over 300 msec with two equiprobable alternatives and over 600 msec when one must choose among 9 alternatives.

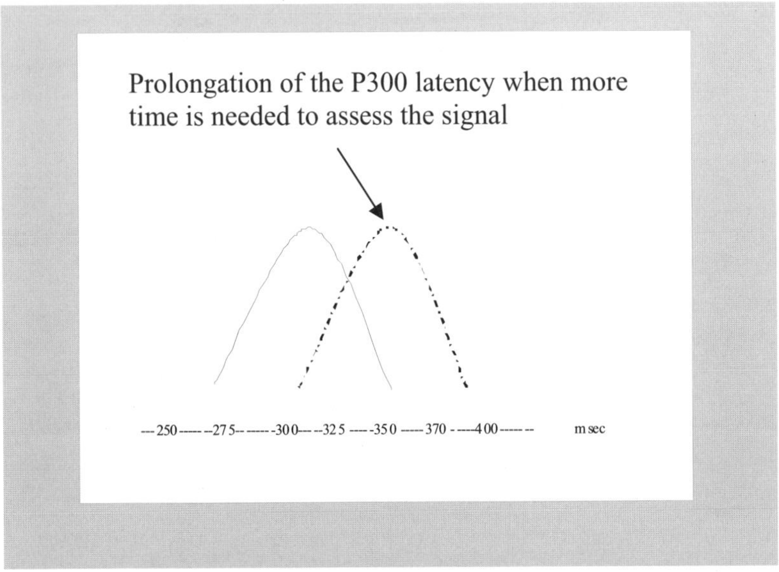

Figure 3.4 Prolongation of the P300 latency as occurs when more time is needed to assess the signal, as schematically illustrated by the chained curve with peak latency of ~ 350 msec, compared to the full curve with a peak latency of ~ 300 msec.

- Another view of "working fast": Levels of information transmission

The neurophysiological principles that we have just presented with respect to the time dimension of mental processes cohere very well with the cognitive ergonomic view of the main phases involved in human work. As shown in Panel 3.1, this has been formulated by Welford [1960] in terms of "levels of information transmission."

When people themselves report working fast, they mainly look at the task performance level, rather than the first two levels (sensory input and decision-making), that are often "invisible."

Thus, for example, we ask the question: is a city bus driver stuck in heavy traffic working fast?

Levels of Information Transmission

- Sensory Input
- Central decision-making:
  Information Processing
- Effecter output:
  Task Performance

Panel 3.1 Derived from Ref. [Welford 1960].

Since the driver is proceeding at a "snail's pace," accomplishment of the task of getting from point A to point B is exceedingly slow. Yet, the rapid inflow of enormous amounts of sensory information and the need for extremely rapid and continuous decision-making indicate that despite making very little progress towards the goal, the driver's central nervous system is indeed working fast and hard. This other view of "working fast" as part of psychological job demands has been well documented in our studies of professional drivers [Belkić, Savić *et al.*, 1992] [Belkić, Savić *et al.*, 1994] Belkić *et al.*, 1996][Emdad *et al.*, 1997] [Savić & Belkić 1995] and is further reviewed in Chapter 5. Fundamentally, then, in order to adequately assess the meaning of "working fast," it is vital to consider all three levels of information transmission, and to do so in as much detail as possible.

- Counter-productivity of speed-up from a neurophysiologic standpoint

From the neurophysiological vantage point, external time pressure such as forced speed–up is counterproductive and potentially dangerous. This is demonstrated via study of the subcomponents of the P300 event related potential. One subcomponent of the P300 is associated with evaluation of the stimulus, and is independent of the actual motor response. However, another subcomponent of the P300 has also been identified with a different cortical localization and that is related to choice reaction time. It appears that these two components are, in fact, independent of each other, as illustrated in a choice reaction time paradigm performed under time pressure [Hohnsbein *et al.*, 1995]. As summarized in Fig. 3.5, it was found that under time pressure the choice reaction subcomponent of the P300 shortened, but the stimulus assessment time remained unchanged. Consequently, the number of performance errors increased. What happened is that the persons were obliged to make quick decisions in order to react to stimuli that had not been adequately evaluated, since the brain had not been given sufficient time to do so!

That study was aimed at gaining a deeper insight into the neurophysiologic concomitants of various aspects of mental workload [Hohnsbein *et al.*, 1995]. In particular, it helps illuminate the brain mechanisms that may mediate the compromise of safe performance, including the observed increase in accident rate when high levels of extrinsic time pressure are imposed [Gardell *et al.*, 1983] [Green *et al.*, 1991] [Greiner *et al.*, 1998].

- Further considerations about the time dimension and work processes

Accurate performance is affected by other time-related factors besides the actual speed of the incoming signals. The dynamics of incoming signal flow must be more fully examined. Not only overly fast, but also extremely slow flow rate, especially over long periods are associated with performance errors. In other words, these are not linear associations but instead, conform to the well-known "U" shaped-curve, with best performance associated with moderate conditions. Deterioration in performance, plus heightened catecholamine excretion occur with not only with over-stimulation but also under-stimulation [Frankenhaeuser & Gardell 1976] [Hebb 1960]. These principles have been corroborated in work scenarios. For example, during a simulated flight paradigm, accurate and prompt detection of a rare event worsened as time progressed on the task, during highly complex task performance but also when carrying out a very simple visual task [Molloy & Parasuraman1996].

Low flow of incoming signals that are very often also homogeneous creates underload for workers in some branches of automatic production, control panel monitoring and for long-route truck drivers. Under these conditions, with no new information for protracted periods of time, a high level of vigilance must be maintained to detect infrequently occurring signals. Task alternation and other counter-measures are needed to protect the health and safety of these workers [Braby *et al.*, 1993] [Levi 1981].

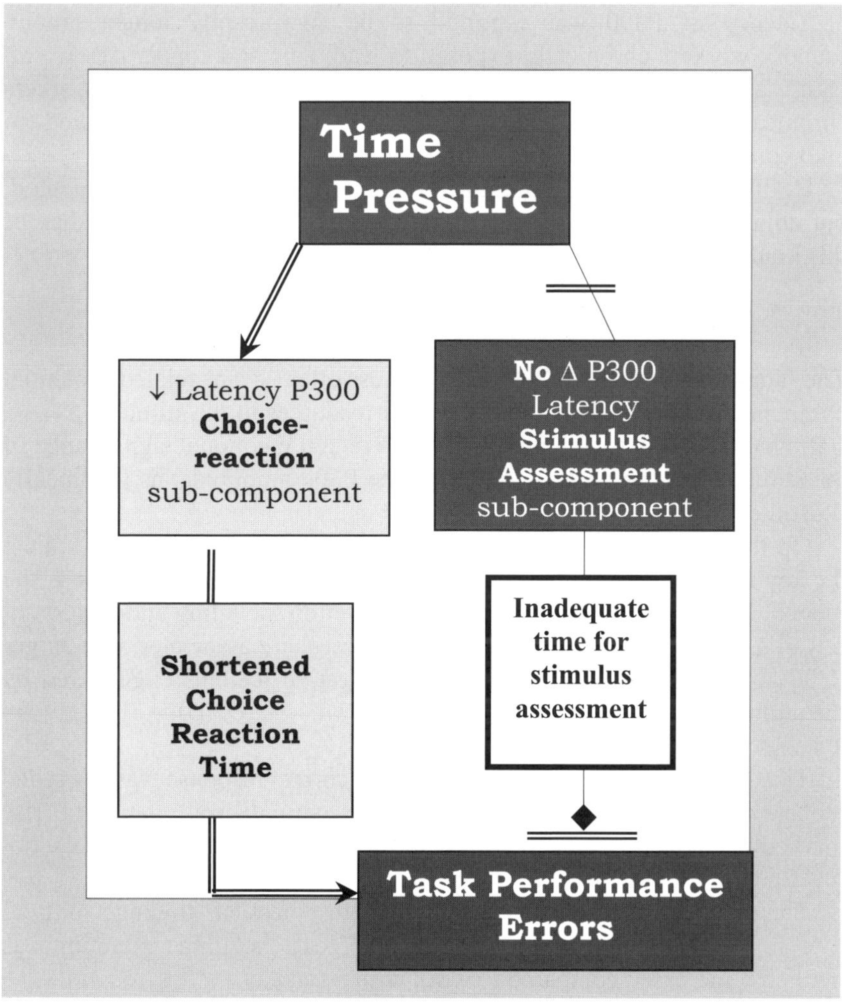

Figure 3.5 The impact of time pressure upon P300 subcomponents and choice reaction time performance, based upon the results of [Hohnsbein *et al.*, 1995].

Noxious physical or chemical exposures can also affect mental chronometry, reflected by event-related potential latency. During a simulated aircraft-landing paradigm, e.g., adding hypoxia and turbulence leads to a prolongation of the P300 latency [Kramer *et al.*, 1987]. Exposure to noise plus lack of sleep are also associated with increased P300 latency [Gunter *et al.*, 1987] [Polich & Kok 1995].

Latency of P300 was reported to be significantly longer among foundry workers chronically exposed to lead, zinc and copper [Murata *et al.*, 1993], and non-significantly longer among steel smelter workers chronically exposed to manganese [Wennberg *et al.*, 1991] compared to unexposed referents.

Event-related potentials are noted to be a sensitive and reliable method, but adjustment for confounders is needed in epidemiological studies of this kind [Araki & Murata 1993].

3.2.1.2 *Allocation of mental resources and P300 amplitude*

The amplitude of the P300 as well as other event-related potential components reflects allocation of mental resources to the stimulus [Donchin *et al.*, 1984]. Overall, the greater the cognitive and emotional significance of the stimulus for the person, the larger the P300 amplitude, as graphically illustrated in Fig. 3.6.

On the basis of a large body of empirical laboratory research, among the key factors affecting P300 amplitude are: the relevance of the task, the mental demands required by the task, motivation including anticipation of rewards, probability of appearance (rare stimuli are associated with larger P300 amplitude) as well as positive or negative feelings engendered by the stimulus [Begleiter *et al.*, 1983] [Duncan-Johnson & Donchin 1977] [Johnston *et al.*, 1987] [Ullsperger *et al.*, 1988].

Thus, for example, when each rapid and correct response was rewarded monetarily, the P300 amplitude to target stimuli was found to rise markedly compared to the paradigm in which there was no material reward associated with task performance [Begleiter *et al.*, 1983].

This finding is broadly coherent with the classical findings of Levi [1972] regarding piece-rate work during which catecholamine excretion was markedly increased compared to work with fixed pay.

When the complexity of a reaction-time task was increased, the P300 amplitude was found to rise accordingly. The task was to respond to certain digits within a series of numbers of increasing length)

In this paradigm, subjective assessment of task difficulty directly reflected the length of the numerical series [Ullsperger *et al.*, 1988].

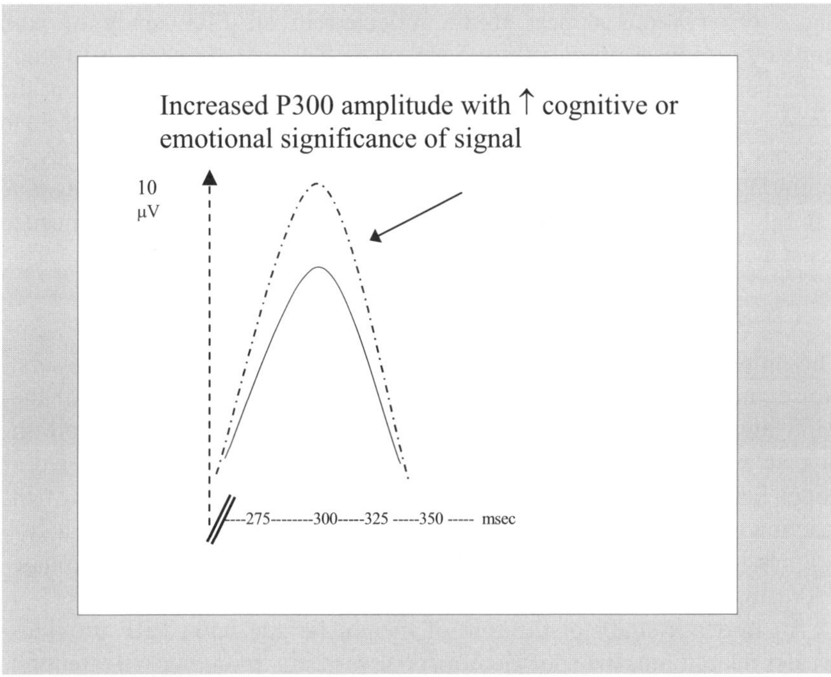

Figure 3.6 Increased P300 amplitude as occurs with heightened cognitive or emotional significance of the signal.

The emotional content of stimuli was assessed in another study [Johnston *et al.,* 1987]. Neutral stimuli were slides of unknown faces, emotionally negative stimuli were grotesque dermatological pathology, and pictures of babies were the positive stimuli. Both negative and positive slides elicited larger P300 amplitudes compared to neutral stimuli.

As noted, with greater complexity of a primary task, the P300 amplitude generally rises [McCallum *et al.*, 1988] [Sirevaag *et al.*, 1984] [Ullsperger *et al.*, 1988]. However, when there is more than one task to be performed, the P300 amplitude to the subsidiary task becomes attenuated as the primary task increases in difficulty. These findings indicate that processing resources are withdrawn from the lower priority task, as the primary task requires more mental energy [Israel *et al.,* 1980] [Sirevaag *et al.,* 1984]. As competing demands are made upon mental resources, fewer resources may be available for a given task. In addition, uncertainty may arise when the load upon memory increases [Kok & Kramer 1997].

These observations appear to be reflected in an ERP study of pain empathy responses among physicians [Decety *et al.*, 2010]. In contrast to study participants without medical or paramedical experience or education, the physicians showed no P300 nor early evoked potential responses to pictures displaying needle-pricks to the body. Thus, physicians may be inhibiting their perception of pain in others in order to avoid negative arousal. Thereby, cognitive resources are freed up to provide needed assistance to their patients.

- Exacerbating stressors and ERP amplitude

The amplitude of the P300 is also affected by exacerbating stressors. Noise and sleep deprivation both are associated with diminution of the P300 amplitude [Gunter *et al.*, 1987] [Polich & Kok 1995]. We have found an inverse relation among professional drivers between number of work hours behind the wheel and the P300 amplitude to a visual odd-ball reaction time task. We interpreted this finding as related to fatigue [Belkić *et al.*, 1996] [Emdad *et al.*, 1996] [Savić & Belkić 1998], which is reported to attenuate P300 amplitude, as well as to prolong its latency [Polich & Kok 1995].

An in-depth study of the role of mental fatigue upon ERP provides greater insight into the specific effects of working upon a visual attention task for a long period of time (3 hours) without a break [Boksem *et al.*, 2005]. The study was motivated by the observation that lapses of attention frequently occurred with prolonged performance of a visual task such as flight simulation for pilots. The participants were 8 male and 14 female healthy university students. Besides increased subjective fatigue rating, prolonged reaction time and performance errors, the difference between N2b amplitude to relevant versus irrelevant stimuli diminished with time on the task. The authors interpret these findings as indicating:

> "a dissociation in the effects of mental fatigue on goal-directed (top-down) and stimulus-driven (bottom-up) attention: mental fatigue results in a reduction in goal-directed attention, leaving subjects performing in a more stimulus driven fashion" (p. 107).

3.2.1.3 *Work processes as reflected in electroencephalographic activity*

Normally, when a person is awake and relaxed with eyes closed, the predominant electroencephalographic (EEG) activity is between 7.5 – 8.0 Hz and 12.5 –13.0 Hz. This is termed alpha rhythm (Fig. 3.7, top panel). When the eyes are opened, the alpha rhythm is normally blocked such that the EEG becomes desynchronized (Fig. 3.7, bottom panel). This occurs as the visual impulses from the retina pass through the reticular activating system, the cortex becomes activated in preparation for handling the visual signals [Moruzzi & Magoun 1949].

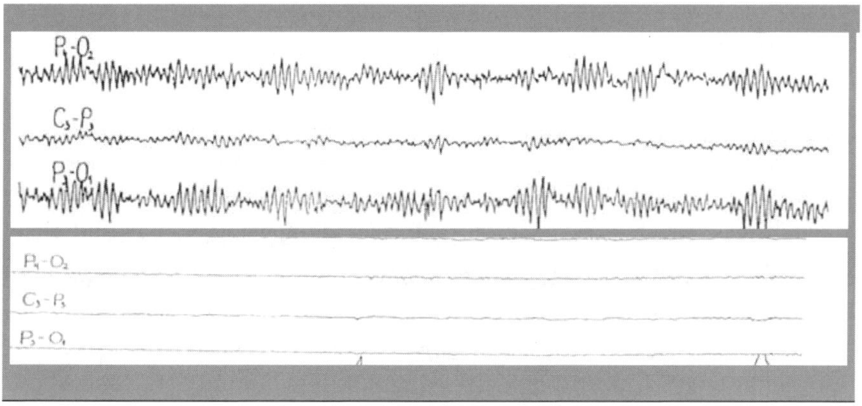

Figure 3.7 Well-expressed alpha activity on the electroencephalogram (EEG) (top panel). With eye-opening, the EEG becomes desynchronized (bottom panel). Recording from our Laboratory for Clinical Neurophysiology and Psychophysiology the Institute of Mental Health, Belgrade.

Electroencephalographic desynchronization can also occur with strong sensory stimuli of any modality, as well as with higher cognitive activity and/or with anxiety. With cognitive loading, blocking of the alpha rhythm has been termed "event-related desynchronization" [Pfurtscheller *et al.*, 1994] [Van Winsum *et al.*, 1984].

On the other hand, EEG recordings during night work have shown increased levels of alpha activity as well as theta activity (between 4Hz and 8 Hz), together with slow rolling eye movements. These physiological findings are associated with the subjective experience of sleepiness [Åkerstedt *et al.*, 2007]. The implications of these findings with respect to accident risk/safety are strongly emphasized [Åkerstedt *et al.*, 2005].

The peak frequency in the alpha region has been proposed as an index of "cognitive preparedness" [Angelakis *et al.*, 2004]. A decrease in the alpha peak frequency has been associated with subjective ratings of fatigue and poorer performance on memory tasks [Klimesh 1999].

In a higher frequency range above alpha, between 12.5 –14.0 Hz and 20 Hz, beta activity is recorded. As the mental workload increases, the EEG activity within the beta band is reported to increase in the occipital region

[Kurimori & Kakizaki 1995]. Beta rhythm is considered to be of cortical origin and may therefore also reflect cortical perfusion [van Luitelaar *et al.*, 2010].

In a lower frequency range below alpha, the theta rhythm between 3.5 Hz and 7.5 Hz is recorded. This theta activity is typically seen in the frontal midline region with performance of various mental tasks and with learning [Basar *et al.*, 2001] [Inaga 1998] [Halford 2003] [Lang *et al.*, 1987] [Yamamoto & Matsuoka 1990].

With increased attention, arousal and/or time pressure during task performance, frontal midline theta activity is reportedly increased [Inaga 1998][Yamamoto & Matsuoka 1990][Slobounov *et al.*, 2000]. Midline frontal theta activity also appears to be associated with positive emotional state during meditation [Aftanas & Golocheikine 2001] and may spontaneously wax and wane with a short periodicity [Halford 2003].

- EEG changes during normal and disturbed sleep: relation to shift work

Polysomnographic recordings are generally obtained from a small set of EEG electrodes, electroocculogram (EOG) electrodes at the outer canthi of the eyes, and submental electromyogram (EMG), as well as respiration and electrocardiogram.

The normal stages are as follows: Stage 1 involves a transition from alpha activity to theta activity on the EEG, with slow, rolling eye movements and a diminished EMG tone. During stage 2 sleep, which comprises about half of all normal sleep time, theta activity predominates with frequent sleep spindles, K complexes and some slow waves (< 4 Hz). Deep (slow wave) sleep occurs during Stages 3 and 4, with more slow waves and high amplitude (>75 μV) EEG activity. Stages 1 to 4 comprise non-REM (rapid eye movement) sleep. The REM stage is characterized by low amplitude EEG activity, decreased muscle tone, and as the name indicates, rapid eye movements (Fig. 3.8). These stages normal occur in cycles of about 1.5 hours in duration, with slow wave sleep primarily occurring during the 1st two cycles [Ercegovac 1971] [Ercegovac & Savić 1982] [Åkerstedt *et al.*, 2007].

Polysomnographically recorded sleep after night work and before morning work is reportedly diminished by approximately 2 hours. Primarily Stage 2 and REM sleep are affected. A similar pattern is seen with very early morning shift work [Åkerstedt 2003]. These physiological findings corroborate the well-established sleep/wake problem in shift workers [Åkerstedt *et al.*, 2007].

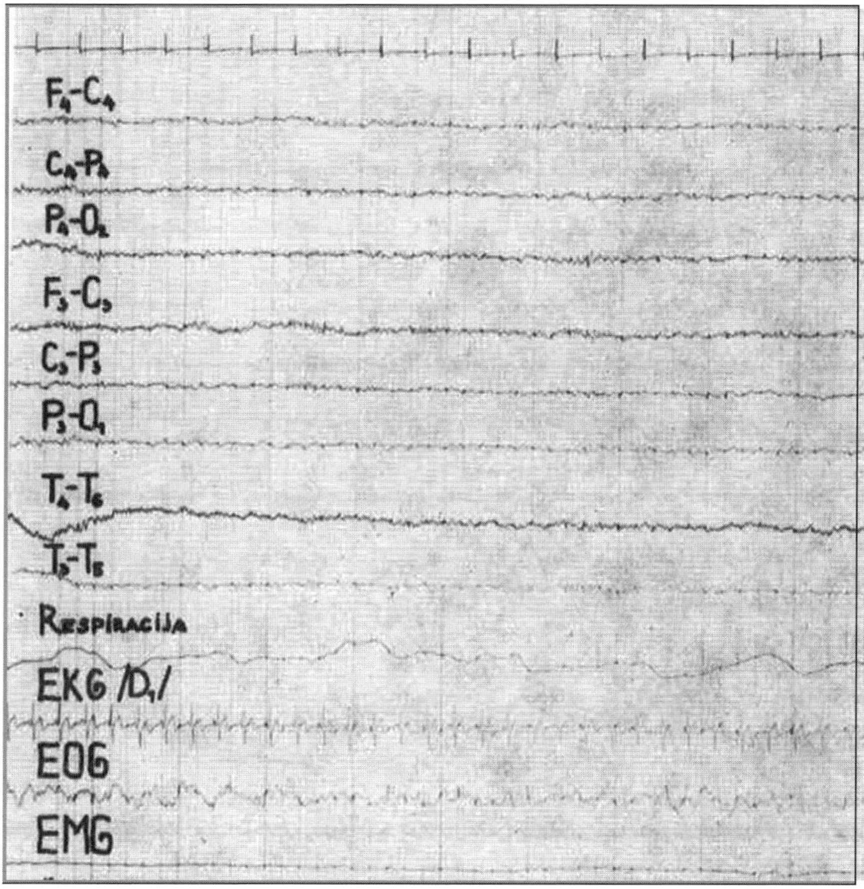

Figure 3.8 Polysomnography during normal REM sleep. Recording from our Laboratory for Clinical Neurophysiology and Psychophysiology at the Institute of Mental Health, Belgrade.

- Quantitative electroencephalographic analysis (qEEG)

Rich information has traditionally been gleaned through visual inspection of the EEG, especially when performed by experienced clinicians. However, for quantitative comparisons, power spectral analysis of the EEG is needed. The standard method for transforming the EEG time signal into the frequency domain has been through the fast Fourier transform (FFT). The FFT is a linear, non-parametric method which can be used to generate a total shape spectrum, but not the component spectrum. Various fitting algorithms are then applied to derive the quantitative information about the actual strength of the components in the frequency bands of interest [Cooper *et al.*, 1980] [Halford 2003] [Prichep 2005]. In sleep analysis, e.g., the advantages of non-linear EEG analysis have been underscored [Ehlers *et al.*, 1991].

More advanced non-linear, parametric signal processing methods can also be applied to acquire this quantitative spectral information with greater certainty, without fitting. These are described in our textbook, with an in-depth explication of the fast Padé transform (FPT) [Belkić & Belkić 2010]. These advanced signal processing methods appear to be particularly appropriate for assessing physiological responses to external perturbations as well as for longer term recordings. As we have suggested:

> "These mathematical advances can help improve clinical decision-making vis-à-vis the dynamic relationship between exposure to a complex work environment with its moment-to-moment as well as longer term changes, on the one hand, and an equally or even more complex set of [physiological] responses, on the other" [Belkić & Belkić 2002a] [Belkić & Belkić 2002b].

3.2.1.4 *Attentional demands of knowledge-based versus skill-based work*

We will now discuss a key distinction with respect to psychological demands, namely, between "automatic" (skill-based) and "controlled" (knowledge-based) work processes. The latter obligatorily uses conscious attentional resources and requires planning [Gaillard 1993]. This type of work is performed *in series*, i.e. one at a time, and consequently there are major limitations as to how much of this type of work can be performed. Some salient examples of knowledge-based work include: complex human interactions, using a new apparatus, emergency operations, handling apparatus failure and dealing with irregularities.

This distinction is very important in analyzing the demands faced e.g. by air traffic controllers [Kalsbeek 1971]. When new, non-routine decisions are required due to unforeseen events, the ATC must consciously intervene, thereby substantially rearranging the "brain control program". According to Levi [1981], work demanding continuous conscious attention should only be performed for very limited periods of time.

There is less limitation to the human capacity for automatic "skill-based" work. This type of work is characterized by rapid, smooth, learned, highly integrated patterns, and, in principle, two or more of these processes could be handled simultaneously [Gaillard 1993] [Neerincx & Griffioen 1996].

Of key importance is the ratio between knowledge-based and skill based activity. Within that framework, the critical dimension is time. Knowledge-based work is extremely sensitive to time limitations. It has been suggested that when a large number of actions need to be carried out within a given time period, the number of knowledge-based processes should be kept to a minimum. On the other hand, a long period of exclusively skill-based processing will lead to underload.

> These insights have been used in practice, for example to better harmonize the tasks of railway traffic controllers. Both overload, as well as underload were thereby minimized [Neerincx & Griffioen 1996].

3.2.1.5 *The concept of energy regulation and the job-strain model*

The concept of "energy regulation" has also been integrated into the levels of information transmission, providing insight into the interaction between the demand and control dimensions [Gaillard 1993]. The need for energy grows as mental demands increase. This energy is generated from arousal mechanisms, some of which are involuntary and others that require conscious mobilization of mental resources.

However, these human cognitive energy reserves have their limits. As a survival strategy, the human being continuously monitors the outcome of his or her efforts, and on the basis of that assessment, exerts cognitive control over the work process. Of critical importance is to obtain feedback and to have sufficient decision-making latitude. Thereby, one is able to decide whether the outcome corresponds to one's goals and intentions. If not, adjustments can be made.

Thus, the concept of energy regulation according to principles of human cognitive function coheres with the Job Strain Model. High psychological workload does not necessarily lead to job strain. It is the lack of decision-making latitude combined with heavy psychological demands that create strain conditions. With sufficient decision-latitude, or control, one can modulate even a fairly onerous, though not overwhelming, psychological workload to meets one's moment-to-moment needs, capacities and goals [Gaillard 1993] [Karasek & Theorell 1990].

Now, in this light, we should revisit Fig. 3.5, concerning the neurophysiologic consequences of time pressure. It becomes clear that the "time" dimension is a critical part of control. In other words, excessive time pressure is not only a demand, but it also undermines control, and is fundamentally incompatible with the way our nervous system should be working [Belkić 2003].

3.2.2 *Emotional dimensions of work*

3.2.2.1 *Emotional burden versus emotional reward of work*

Human labor can potentially yield emotional rewards. Unfortunately, it can also take a heavy emotional toll. As noted, the emotional gratification and a sense of purpose and meaning may compensate for the objective difficulties of such professions as teaching, social work, the health professions, etc. We also noted that there has tended to be a hierarchical distribution of these emotional (as well as economic) rewards, favoring those in the upper echelons, who have more power and control within the work organization. However, under *ideal* conditions, new technologies could provide a more egalitarian distribution of these non-material rewards, related to collaboration and sharing of information [Basini & Hurley 1994]. Karasek and Theorell [1990] note that new production technologies if placed in workers' hands could help them receive direct feedback from the public concerning their contribution. A sense of meaningfulness in work could result, as well as providing new challenges for customizing services and products to meet the public's needs.

The "invisible" or unpaid work performed at home, and most often by women, may also be emotionally gratifying. However, as discussed, this work can also be burdensome, not only physically, but also emotionally. In particular, much energy is needed to exhibit the emotional tone which is demanded by a certain situation, and, as a consequence, it is often necessary to avoid expressing one's true feelings [Hochschild & Machung1989].

These emotional demands are particularly heavy with the double burden of performing paid as well as unpaid work, as is the situation for an ever-increasing number of working people, especially women. The psychological costs of this double burden have been repeatedly demonstrated. In chapter 2, we noted, e.g. that among Finnish municipal employees, women with large households had more sick leave episodes in association with job demands, irrespective of the levels of decision-making latitude, clearly reflecting this double burden [Vahtera & Pentti 1996]. Moreover, it was seen that women in active jobs took less sick leave insofar as they had support from their spouses and/or had a strong sense of coherence. Thus, women in active jobs may be protected against role conflict insofar as they receive adequate support from their husbands and that their sense of coherence is high.

3.2.2.2. *Sensitization: Repeated work exposure to fear-inducing stimuli*

The emotional burden of work can also become heavy when it entails the risk of accidents or other negative outcomes. With repeated exposure to fear-inducing stimuli, sensitization can develop, with heightened behavioral and/or physiological responsiveness. The brain mechanisms for this process are described as follows:

> "Once a fear- or anxiety-inducing sensory stimulus is related through the thalamus into neural circuits involving the cortex, hippocampus, and the amygdala, relevant memory traces of past traumatic experiences are stimulated. It is likely that the potency of the cognitive and somatic response to the stimuli will be strongly correlated with prior experiences due to the strengthening of neural connections within the circuit. These functional neuroanatomical relationships can explain how a single stimulus such as a sight or sound can elicit a specific memory...if the sight or sound was associated with a particular traumatic event, a cascade of anxiety- and fear-related symptoms will ensue" [Charney *et al.*, 1995] (p. 281).

Stimuli can be sensitizing or acquire an "aversive potential" due to their *symbolic* association with disastrous events. In other words, the individual need not have actually experienced the disaster. The nervous system selectively focuses attention to potentially threatening stimuli; neocortical pathways have been identified in animals, which respond preferentially to such threatening stimuli. Such pathways are vital for survival.

Selective attention to threatening visual stimuli such as snakes, spiders or angry faces has been observed in healthy persons even when these stimuli are subliminally presented [Öhman 1986]. Threatening visual signals are especially important, because of their primary consumption of attentional resources [Singleton 1974]. Their intimate neuroanatomical connections, via the midbrain reticular formation, with cortical arousal, as well as with critical outflow tracts have been emphasized in relation to stress-mediated disease [Belkić, Savić, Theorell, *et al.*, 1994].

3.2.2.3 *Threat-avoidant vigilant activity (TAV)*

It can thus be seen that a critical element of mental stress is the intervening variable of threat, in other words one anticipates the possibility of encountering harm of some sort [Lazarus 1967]. When the potential consequences of one's actions can include disaster, work becomes a "threat-avoidant" activity whose primary goal is self-protection. This inevitably becomes associated with negative emotions and often with deleterious mental health outcomes, as well.

Threat avoidant vigilance entails the need to very carefully process incoming information, continuously maintaining a high level vigilance, in order to be prepared to rapidly and appropriately respond at any moment. Even the shortest lapse of attention, the smallest error in assessment or judgment or a slight delay in responding could have serious or even fatal consequences.

Threat-avoidant vigilance or "disaster potential" [Fuller 1984] [Belkić, Savić *et al.*, 1992] was originally formulated in relation to driving activity in general [Fuller 1984]. Clearly, when a driver sits behind the wheel, he or she must constantly be vigilant in order to avoid a traffic accident. This is a heavy burden on the nervous system.

We have applied this concept of threat avoidant vigilance to specific occupational groups such as professional drivers, as well as air-traffic control, sea-piloting, and health professionals, *inter alia* [Belkić 1989] [Belkić, Savić *et al.*, 1992] [Belkić 2003][Belkić & Savić 2008].

As reviewed in chapter 2, many of these occupations are at increased risk for adverse mental health outcomes, as well as other stress-related disorders.

- Electrocortical responses associated with threat-avoidance vigilance

Evaluation of higher cortical responses to stimuli that in some way are linked to threat avoidant vigilance provides a means of modeling the stress response among occupational groups such as professional drivers. The contingent negative variation (CNV) is especially suitable for modeling these responses.

The CNV is a slow negative potential, which characteristically appears with anticipation and expectancy [Grey Walter *et al.*, 1964]. The paradigms used for CNV provide rich and nuanced insights into the function of the human nervous system.

These emerge because the electrocortical responses to two or more inter-related stimuli are examined. Moreover, a post-imperative cortical negativity can also be evaluated. This reflects a delay in resolution, seen characteristically with distraction [Tecce & Cattanach 1987].

An example of a CNV recording from our laboratory in Belgrade is shown in Fig. 3.9.

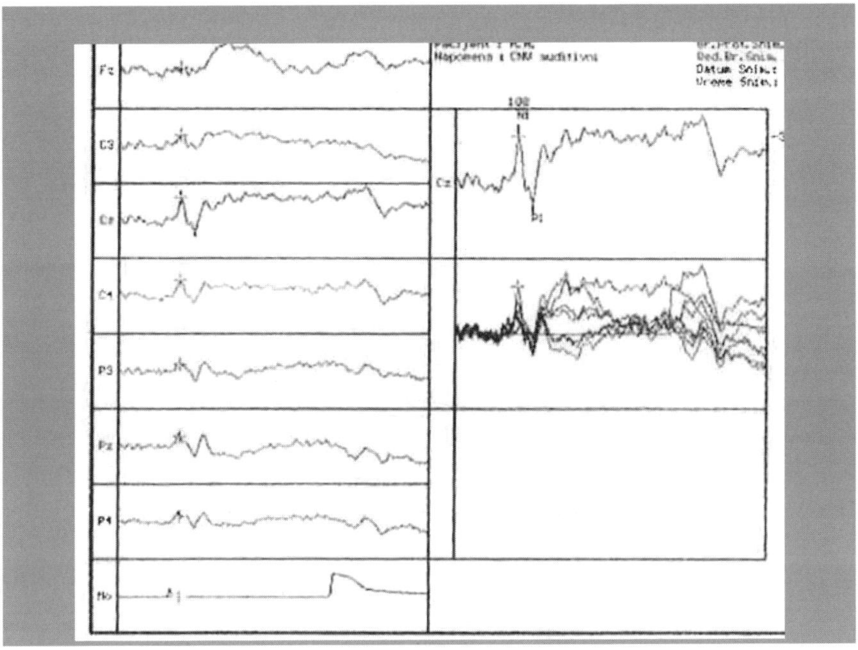

Figure 3.9 Contingent negative variation (auditory modality). Recording from our Laboratory for Clinical Neurophysiology and Psychophysiology at the Institute of Mental Health, Belgrade.

Individual EEG channels shown on left panel, upper portion of right panel shows channel Cz with early evoked potentials marked (note that positive waves are shown below the x-axis, and negative waves above). The middle right panel shows all the EEG channels superimposed.

We developed CNV paradigms with visual stimuli that were first tacitly and then explicitly linked to traffic accident avoidance. In both of these paradigms, urban mass transit drivers showed large CNV responses when anticipating the appearance of the imperative signals [Belkić, Savić *et al.*, 1992]. We interpreted these findings as reflecting increased sensitivity to cognitively relevant visual stimuli among professional drivers.

Some of these findings are illustrated in Fig. 3.10. Among the drivers a large electronegative response is seen associated with the warning stimulus (CNV1) and immediately prior to the appearance of the imperative stimulus (CNV2).

Among the referents, none of whom had any driving experience whatsoever (not even amateur), the CNV responses were significantly less pronounced. All the participants in the CNV paradigm were completely healthy employed men, between the ages of 25 and 40.

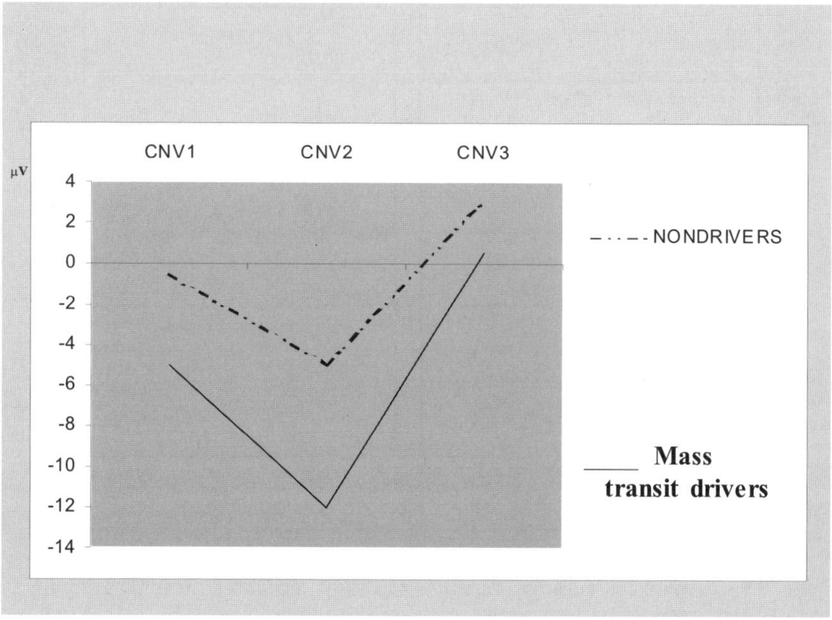

Figure 3.10 Comparison of mean CNV values recorded in channel Cz among 15 city mass transit drivers and 9 non-driver referents to the GO portion of the CNV paradigm which explicitly mimicked traffic conditions [Belkić, Savić *et al.*, 1992].

In our subsequent work we used conceptually similar paradigms but with odd-ball stimuli. We found augmented selective attention (heightened N2 amplitude)[2] to target visual stimuli among professional drivers with borderline and essential hypertension, compared to those who were normotensive. These findings suggested that drivers with hypertension had an excessive expenditure of higher cortical resources when performing threat avoidant vigilant activity. In contrast, the professional drivers with ischemic heart disease showed attenuated selective attentional responses suggesting exhaustion [Belkić *et al.*, 1996][Emdad *et al.*, 1996].

Further insights into how driving as a threat-avoidant vigilant activity burdens higher central nervous system resources are gleaned from a study

---

[2] The N2 component is a negative wave with a latency of ≈ 190 ± 360 msec. It precedes the P300 wave, and also reflects selective attention.

of amateur drivers [Martin *et al.*, 1992]. Differentially greater P300 amplitude and longer latency were found to slides of imminent traffic accidents compared to those showing safe scenes. The time needed to assess these stimuli was prolonged in relation to the threat involved. Yet, reaction times were shortened, actually preceding the P300 in the threatening situation. The subjects speeded-up their motor response to such an extent that information processing was still on-going. Even under conditions of high signal probability (0.5), a prominent P300 appeared in response to the accident slides. (Recall, that P300 typically is seen with relatively rare events), indicating very high selective attention to threatening visual stimuli. These findings are illustrated in Fig. 3.11.

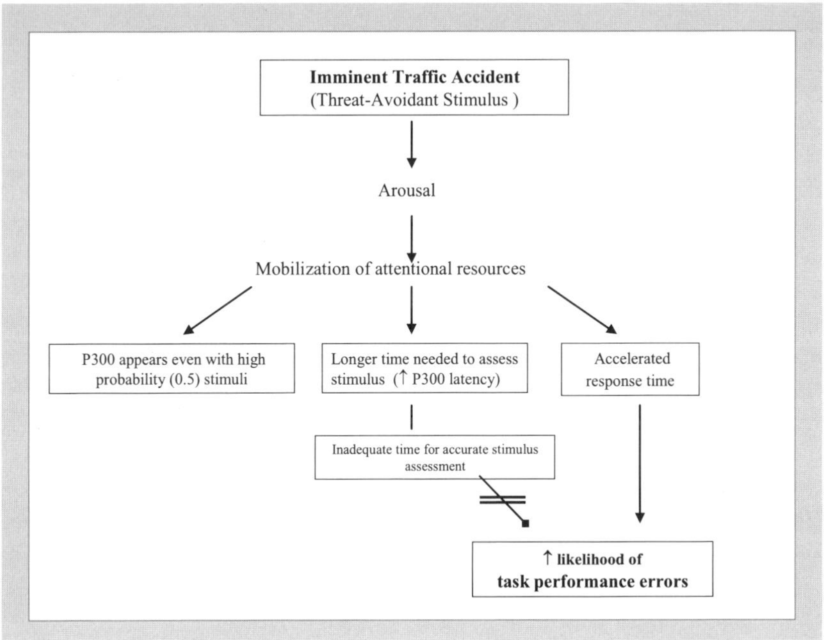

Figure 3.11 Pattern of P300 and reaction time in response to threat avoidant stimuli (imminent traffic accident) based upon the results of [Martin *et al.*, 1992].

The response pattern summarized in Fig. 3.11 was predicted by Fuller [1984], who noted that when threatening stimuli appear suddenly and unexpectedly, the driver is left with limited time to respond safely. The P300 findings of Martin and colleagues [1992] are also consistent with those of Hohnsbein and colleagues [1995], as illustrated in Fig. 3.5, indicating that under time-pressure, response selection time is speeded up, whereas stimulus assessment time remains unchanged, and thereby, the chances for error are greater.

Thus, control in relation to time becomes an even greater necessity in the face of threat avoidant vigilance. In order to handle these heavy demands of the driving situation and other situations requiring TAV, there must be sufficient time to make "anticipatory avoidance response," to recognize the precursors of the potentially disastrous stimulus and take appropriate measures (Panel 3.2). For example, in traffic this would include slowing down at a blind intersection so as to circumvent a potential collision with an unseen, approaching vehicle [Fuller 1984].

Anticipatory Avoidance Responses

Taking control over threat avoidant demands requires sufficient time to make "anticipatory avoidance responses":

To recognize the precursors to a potentially disastrous situation and to take appropriate measures.

For example:

In traffic: slowing down at a blind intersection to avoid a potential collision with an unseen, approaching vehicle.

Panel 3.2 Derived from Ref. [Fuller 1984].

These anticipatory avoidance responses are essential to health and safety, but they consume a large share of these workers' already overburdened attentional resources. Our semi-structured interviews with workers whose jobs entail a high degree of TAV have revealed that this aspect is among the most difficult part of their work [Belkić 1995] [Belkić *et al.*, 1996]. Furthermore, as corroboration to the neurophysiologic observations, progressive sensitization and *not adaptation* appears to be occurring, since this feature was significantly more often cited as the major burden of work with greater number of years on the job.

Seen in this light, unrealistic pressures to stay on schedule could very well be the straw that breaks the camel's back, both in terms of accident risk and to the health of the worker. In order to avoid such situations, compensatory allowance, especially with respect to increased time allocation, must be included into the work planning "equation."

The recovery process, recognized to be vital to worker health in general also needs to be more fully evaluated in face of the heavy burden on the nervous system arising from threat avoidant vigilant activity.

3.3 Burden upon Mental Resources and the Recovery Process

The burden upon mental resources must be viewed not only in relation to performance, but also with respect to its after-effects such as fatigue and impact upon overall health [Hockey 1997]. In particular, it is emphasized that in order to continue to perform under highly stressful conditions, extra resources need to be mobilized, and this has behavioral and physiological consequences [Belkić 2003][Hockey 1997][Savić & Belkić 1995]. There is most frequently a residuum seen after the work is over. This can be reflected in a broad spectrum of manifestations, including inability to unwind, difficulty in subsequent performance of mental tasks, reluctance to engage in social activity notably that which is altruistic, as well as delayed return to baseline of physiological markers such as catecholamine levels [Cohen 1980] [Evans *et al.*, 1989] [Frankenhaeuser & Johansson 1986] [Greiner *et al.*, 1997][Johansson & Aronsson1984] [Razmjou 1996].

The timing and duration of work hours become especially important in this context. In chapter 2 we saw that long work hours and night shift work were associated with numerous untoward consequences. Recall, in particular, that work requiring a high level of mobilization of attentional resources, i.e. knowledge-based work should not be performed for protracted periods of time. The data we presented on attenuation of P300 amplitude among professional drivers who worked long hours behind the wheel provides insight into the neurophysiological costs of prolonged exposure to threat avoidant vigilant activity. Our postulation that this finding was associated with fatigue is supported by an in-depth examination of the causes of driver fatigue [Brown 1994]. Among these causes were: long periods behind the wheel, inadequate time for rest and continuous sleep related to scheduling of work rest and sleep periods within each 24-hour cycle.

Increasing attention has been paid to the role of recovery as an explanatory mechanism in the relation between stressful work and adverse health outcomes [Geurts & Sonnentag 2006]. The Effort-Recovery Model [Meijman & Mulder 1998] posits that the physiological reactions associated with heavy expenditure of energy at work can develop into a chronic burden if there is prolonged exposure and inadequate recovery. The key to recovery is considered to be a return to baseline of psychophysiological systems during the period after work, when these demands are not present. This is termed "unwinding." Insofar as this unwinding does not lead to full recovery, the worker remains in a "sub-optimal state" and must mobilize special effort to perform at work. Over time, if this process continues, chronic fatigue, anxiety, sleep disorders, *inter alia*, can ensue. Findings concordant with this model have been reported among Dutch professional drivers. Need for recovery was found have a significant multivariate association with complaints of fatigue, emotional exhaustion and psychosomatic complaints [Sluiter *et al.*, 1999].

The "Allostatic Load Theory" [McEwen 1998] more explicitly links biological systems: the autonomic nervous system, the hypothalamic pituitary adrenal axis and other neuroendocrine axes as well as the immune system to the recovery process. These systems are critical to the "ability to achieve stability through change" which is termed "allostasis" (p. 171). In a study of women working in the health sector, poor recovery from work was associated with several of these physiological markers of heavy allostatic load [von Thiele *et al.*, 2006]. Namely, elevated heart rate and blood pressure, serum lipid and prolactin levels were found among those with fatigue and sleep problems compared to the women who had a more favorable pattern of recovery. Allostatic load appears to be prognostically important. In a 7-year longitudinal study mortality and physical functioning were significantly predicted by allostatic load[3] among over 4 000 men and women aged 70 to 79 [Seeman *et al.*, 2001].

3.3.1 *The role of cognitive appraisal*

According to the classical definition of coping, cognitive or behavioral techniques are employed in attempts to reduce the impact of stressors [Lazarus & Folkman 1984]. Coping clearly plays an essential role in the recovery process.

---

[3] The components of allostatic load were: highest quartile of systolic and diastolic blood pressure, waist-hip ratio, total cholesterol to high density lipoprotein (HDL) component, glycosylated hemoglobin, cortisol and catecholamine excretion, and lowest quartile of serum HDL cholesterol and dehydroepiandrosterone sulfate.

Coping can act as a mediator as well as a moderator of the relation between stressors and the stress response. Among the plethora of potential coping methods, Kozlowski [1998] emphasizes the key importance of social support. He also points out that interventions aimed at improving the work environment on an individual or organizational level can be considered part of the coping process, as well.

Antonovsky [1991] views this complex process across the life trajectory. Through his "Sense of Coherence" formulation, he emphasizes the need for a "global orientation that expresses…a pervasive, enduring though dynamic feeling of confidence that one's internal and external environments are predictable and that there is a high probability that things will work out as well as can be reasonably reasonably expected" (p. 184). As noted, a strong sense of coherence was found, e.g., to be a buffer against sick leave among women working in active jobs [Vahtera & Pentti 1996].

When coping options are not available or ineffective, when the individual lacks a sufficient armamentarium of coping techniques, when ruminative thoughts about the stressors persist, *inter alia*, the process of recovery can be severely impaired [Geurts & Sonnentag 2006]. Substantial investigation has been devoted to the "defeat reaction," which is closely linked to the concept of "learned helplessness."

Defeat reactions tend to activate the hypothalamic pituitary adrenal axis, with release of glucocorticoids. This type of reaction can be activated by extreme fear, hopelessness or exhaustion [Schwartz et al. 2000]. The defeat reaction is classically associated with depression.

Social support is viewed as a critical means to help such individuals.

> "The group's power to sustain the victim's hope and in so doing to induce him [or her] to continue to make an effort is the reason social support proves to be of great practical value" (p. 377)[Henry 1992].

We will now examine these neurophysiological processes in more direct relation to psychiatric and neurological disorders. Our main focus will be upon event-related potentials, ERP and quantitative electroencephalography, qEEG, which, as outlined in the first part of this Chapter, provide a unique window into cognitive and emotional activity of the human nervous system.

3.4 Event-related Potentials, Quantitative EEG and Neuropsychiatry

Event-related potentials and quantitative EEG analysis obviously do not substitute for clinical diagnosis of neuropsychiatric disorders. Nevertheless, they can be used to help corroborate some diagnoses, since there are some patterns which are quite characteristic of certain entities, even though there is much overlap and lack of specificity. The main reason for applying these neurophysiological methods in relation to neurologic and mental health disorders is that these methods reflect the functioning of the central nervous system. The relative objectivity of these methods can be helpful in gaining a better understanding of the etiology of these disorders [Zubin *et al.*, 1986]. They may serve as an adjunct to the clinical classification of psychiatric disorders [John & Prichep 2006], and could be particularly helpful because of the lack of ethnic or cultural bias, accurately identifying healthy, normally-functioning persons in a large number of countries [Prichep 2005]. Despite differences in recording paradigms, it has been noted that the findings are fairly consistent [Barrett *et al.*, 1986]. Moreover, ERPs can provide

> "a level of temporal precision and resolution currently unavailable from other methods of measuring neural activity, e.g. functional magnetic resonance imaging (fMRI) and positron emission tomography (PET)" (p. 123) [Karl *et al.*, 2006].

At the same time, it should be noted that the cognitive demands of the ERP task are considered to be of importance in evaluating responses among patients with mental health disorders [Bruder 1992].

Besides their role in diagnostics, ERP and qEEG have also been used to assess prognosis and for monitoring the recovery process. It is here that these methods have been especially helpful since within-patient comparisons over time are free from inter-individual variations [Savić & Belkić 1998]. Work-related interventions could conceivably be followed along the same lines.

In the present context, it should be recalled that event-related potentials can reflect various aspects of the burden of work processes upon mental resources, as reviewed earlier in this chapter. To our knowledge, however, there have not yet been any systematic studies of how the ERP and qEEG patterns associated with work processes might be of relevance to specific mental health disorders. Nevertheless, there are some striking similarities. Also, our own clinical experience suggests that indeed work stressors impacting upon neurophysiological function as seen in event-related potentials and qEEG, have played a role in the mental health processes under examination. Some of these observations will be presented in Part II of this book in conjunction with the clinical cases studies.

3.4.1 *Anxiety*

Anxiety has been considered as a cognitive process, with expectancy as a major component. Anxiety is said to occur when a person cannot accurately anticipate and control stimuli that are perceived as being stressful [Proulx & Picton 1984]. Concordant with the fact that the contingent negative variation is associated with expectancy, a number of studies indicate that patients with high levels of anxiety show smaller CNV compared to non-anxious persons, and that the CNV become more attenuated with distraction among anxious persons.

A CNV study [Proulx & Picton 1984] of 30 women with high, average and low Spielberger Trait Anxiety scores provides a more nuanced view of the relation between CNV, expectancy and involvement in a task. It was found that the women with high trait anxiety did not establish the expectancy as rapidly as did those with low trait anxiety. However, once the women with high anxiety learned the stimulus associations of the paradigm, they showed significantly higher CNV amplitudes compared to the women with low anxiety. These authors therefore suggested:

> "once expectancies have been established anxious [persons] may actually become more involved in the task than necessary" (p. 619).

Thus, persons with high anxiety may have more difficulty in efficiently directing mental effort to the task at hand.

Healthy male volunteers (army soldiers) with high Spielberger trait anxiety showed significantly greater GO:NOGO differentiation to a neutral CNV paradigm compared to one that was explicitly said to test their intelligence. State anxiety, but not reaction time, also increased with the intelligence-testing paradigm. It was suggested that persons with high anxiety were disrupted by the anticipation of failure [Glanzman & Froehlich 1992]. We might also suggest that gender differences with respect to trait anxiety contributed to the somewhat different CNV findings of Proulx and Picton [1984] and of Glanzman & Froehlich [1992], although admittedly the study designs are substantially different, as well.

In comparison to those with low anxiety, healthy university students of both genders with high Spielberger Trait Anxiety showed significantly greater mean amplitude of the P400 when performing visual semantic matching tasks that included threatening, neutral as well as positive content [Weinstein 1995]. The authors point out that their study by design "specifically activates cognitions that are congruous with anxiety" (p. 857). They conclude that these healthy, young individuals with high-anxiety trait (i.e. not clinically anxious) showed enhanced processing of threatening information compared to otherwise similar individuals with low trait anxiety. In a study which included twelve patients with clinically diagnosed anxiety disorders and twenty-four apparently healthy referents with high and low state anxiety, the patients showed the highest P300 amplitude to frequent auditory stimuli [Chattopadhyay *et al.*, 1980]. However, another study showed no significant differences in auditory event-related potentials comparing twelve patients who met the diagnostic criteria for generalized anxiety disorder and twelve age-matched healthy referents [Drake *et al.*, 1991].

It has been suggested that there may be changes in auditory processing in generalized anxiety disorder, concordant with "concepts integrating the exteroceptive sensory systems into the functional neuroanatomy of anxiety and fear" (p. 106) [Clark *et al.*, 2009]. A study of twelve outpatients meeting DSM-III criteria for generalized anxiety disorder compared with apparently healthy students revealed that the patients were slower than non-anxious controls in color naming of both threat words and positive words. Whereas it is seen that selective attention to emotional material is a normal response, it is suggested that anxiety disorders may be related to a more specific and persistent type of selective attention to threat [Martin *et al.*, 1991].

Among the salient findings in the sparse literature on qEEG in anxiety, are that frontal midline theta activity appears to be attenuated. With pharmacological treatment, theta activity is reported to increase among patients with anxiety disorder [Halford 2003][Suetsugi *et al.*, 1998] [Suetsugi *et al.*, 2000].

3.4.1.1 *Panic disorders*

The responses to several choice-reaction CNV paradigms of fifteen un-medicated patients of both genders with panic disorder according to DSM-III criteria with or without agoraphobia have been compared to fifteen healthy volunteer referents [Korunka *et al.*, 1993]. There were no statistically significant differences between the two groups with regard to amplitude of P300 or CNV. The warning stimuli (S1) for the two different options were described as "readily distinguishable tones." It may be, however, that the tasks were not sufficiently difficult to elicit significant between-group differences, as per the above-noted observation of Bruder [1992].

The small groups not fully matched for gender should also be noted. Another study of patients with panic disorder did reveal heightened P3a responses to stimulus change [Clark *et al.*, 1996]. This finding was considered to reflect impaired inhibition of irrelevant stimuli [Karl *et al.*, 2005].

3.4.1.2 *Specific phobias*

Specific phobias are particularly amenable to examination with event-related potentials. This is seen in a study [Dubrovsky *et al.*, 1978] of fourteen female patients with long-standing, specific phobias to e.g. dogs, snakes or spiders. These phobias were sufficiently severe to impact upon social life. At baseline prior to therapy, the mean CNV amplitude and duration of post-imperative negativity were significantly greater in CNV paradigms in which the specific phobogenic stimuli were the imperative stimuli compared to CNV paradigms with non-disturbing imperative stimuli. Reaction time was also more rapid in the phobogenic paradigm.

Six of the patients subsequently underwent behavior modification therapy, which reduced their phobic anxiety and avoidance scores, concordant with psychiatric evaluation and self-assessment. After therapy, the amplitude of CNV to the previously phobogenic stimuli was significantly reduced and the duration of post-imperative negativity significantly shortened in comparison to the results prior to therapy. The electrocortical responses for the non-disturbing CNV paradigm were essentially unchanged. The authors emphasize that these results shed new light on phobic neuroses and the processes involved in behavioral therapy. They note enhancement of attentional processes that facilitate the selection of relevant stimuli from the environment. Furthermore, the process of desensitisation therapy involves the establishment of a "functional connection between the relaxed condition and the phobogenic stimuli" (p. 538), and this may be associated with "a new association presumably in the limbic structures involved in these emotional states," and these could modulate the frontal regions where CNV's are mainly generated. We would add the comment, that the heightened CNV responses among professional drivers to threat-avoidant stimuli [Belkić, Savić *et al.*, 1992] raise some interesting parallels with the baseline findings of Dubrovsky and colleagues [1978].

Although not statistically significant, somewhat discordant findings are reported in an ERP study of 24 healthy male university students with high or low scores on fear of mutilation (unrelated to Spielberger trait anxiety) [Klorman & Ryan 1980]. The participants with high fear of mutilation tended to show higher early and late CNV to a neutral CNV paradigm compared to that in which the imperative stimulus was a picture of a mutilated body. The participants with low mutilation fear, in contrast, tended to have larger CNV responses to the gruesome slides. Comparing the results of these two studies, it may be that the attentional mechanisms involved in specific phobia are distinct from fear of a broader category of threatening stimuli. Moreover, the differences between studies carried out among patients and studies of healthy individuals should be borne in mind. It should also be noted that a somewhat similar subsequent investigation among university students with presentation of pleasant versus gruesome slides, elicited significantly greater P300 amplitudes among the students with high mutilation fear compared to those with low fear [Yee *et al.*, 1987].

A more recent ERP study among patients with specific phobia to spiders indicated enhanced P300 and P400 components and more rapid reaction times to an emotional Stroop task involving spiders compared to responses to pleasant stimuli (flowers) [Kolassa *et al.*, 2006].

3.4.2 *Post-traumatic stress disorder*

As obviously indicated by the name, exposure to traumatic experiences can lead to the development of PTSD (Appendix A, Section 1).
Manifestations of this disorder frequently include attentional dysfunction, with difficulty in inhibiting distracting signals. Information processing can be affected, with increased response to stimuli reminiscent of the traumatic events. Persons with PTSD show an attentional bias toward trauma-related stimuli [Buckley *et al.*, 2000].

Event-related potentials have been very useful in examining "the neuroelectric correlates of hypothesized alterations in information processing in persons with post-traumatic stress disorder" (p. 123) [Karl *et al.*, 2006]. An early study compared eighteen patients with PTSD and 20 healthy referents matched for age, gender, years of education and scores on the national adult reading test [McFarlane *et al.*, 1993]. Besides specific indices of PTSD (including avoidance and intrusion on the Impact of Events scales), scores for Zung Depression, GHQ, as well as state and trait-anxiety were all significantly higher among the patients. An auditory ERP paradigm, with a background of neutral distracter tones was used. The patients showed significantly attenuated P300 amplitudes, and unlike the referents, the P300 responses to the distracter tones did not differ significantly from those to target stimuli. While the two groups did not differ in accuracy of task performance, the patients showed significantly slowed reaction time to the target stimuli. These findings are considered to indicate that the patients with PTSD had abnormal high-order processing of attended stimuli, with impaired discrimination of stimuli, which delayed assessment of stimulus relevance [MacFarlane *et al.*, 1993]. Meta-analysis of ERP studies with neutral P300 paradigms indicates, concordantly, that persons with PTSD show diminished P300 amplitudes to neutral targets (P3b) and neutral distracters (P3a) compared to referents who do not have PTSD but who were exposed to trauma [Karl *et al.*, 2006].

Event-related potential responses among persons with PTSD appear to be related to the context of the stimuli. In contrast to the above-described findings for neutral ERP paradigms, when the distracters were associated with the trauma, patients with PTSD showed heightened P3a amplitudes to the distracters. They also displayed increased P3b amplitudes to neutral targets in the trauma-related context. These findings may reflect impaired inhibition of irrelevant stimuli, as was the case for patients with panic disorder. However, among patients with PTSD this impairment appears to be associated with trauma-related stimuli [Karl *et al.*, 2006].

There is some evidence for a gender-specific pattern in P200 responses among persons with PTSD. Male combat veterans with PTSD consistently showed a P200 reducing response[4] [Karl *et al.*, 2006]. However, a study of female combat nurses revealed that an augmenting P200 response was associated with PTSD severity [Metzger *et al.*, 2002].

Among the more consistent qEEG findings in persons with PTSD are increased beta and decreased alpha activity. There may be a correlation between abnormalities of alpha activity and severity of PTSD symptoms [Clark *et al.*, 2009].

3.4.3 *Depression, burnout and related disturbances*

In depression or dysphoria there is some evidence of lowered P300 amplitude and prolonged latency [Himani *et al.*, 1999] [Josiassen *et al.*, 1986] [Karaaslan *et al.*, 2003]. However, the data are quite inconsistent [Halford 2003] [Houston *et al.*, 2004]. Halford [2003] states that "it is difficult to draw conclusions about P300 abnormalities in depression because of the heterogeneity of patient groups studied, including melancholic depression, geriatric depression,

---

[4] Augmenting is defined as increasing amplitude with increased intensity, reducing as decreasing amplitude with increasing intensity. These responses are considered to reflect gating mechanisms that regulate cortical sensory input. Augmenting may indicate that the cortex seeks out increases in stimulus intensity, while reducing may represent a shutting out of increased stimulation [Karl *et al.*, 2006].

depression with silent cerebral infarction, and medically and non-medically treated depression" (p.379).

The data are similarly inconsistent concerning depression and CNV, with some studies indicating attenuation [Ashton *et al.*, 1988] [Claverie 1984] [Giedke & Bolz 1980] [Tecce & Cattanach 1987], whereas others do not [Elton 1984] [Knott & Lapierre 1987]. However, the severity of depression, including suicidal behavior, does appear to be reflected in greater attenuation of the CNV [Ashton *et al.*, 1994] [Hansenne *et al.*, 1996] [Papart *et al.*, 1990]. In a study of twenty patients hospitalized for depression all of whom met the DSM-III-R criteria for major depressive disorder, those with a history of attempted suicide showed a significantly lower P200, P300 and CNV compared to those without previous suicide attempts [Hansenne *et al.*, 1996]. In addition, the amplitude of the P300 was inversely related to suicide risk and hopelessness, as assessed by questionnaire, although severity of depression, *per se* did not significantly affect P300 amplitude.

Among the most consistent qEEG findings in depression is frontal asymmetry in the alpha band expressed by increased alpha power in the left frontal areas in comparison with the right frontal areas [Grin-Yatsenko *et al.*, 2009]. Abnormal frontal midline theta activity has also been reported in quite a few studies in which qEEG was performed among patients with depression [Halford 2003].

3.4.3.1 *Anhedonia*

The relation between anhedonia and ERP responses has been examined in a few studies of university students. Compared to referents, those with high anhedonia scores showed lower amplitudes of CNV and P300 [Miller *et al.*, 1984] [Simons 1982]. The attenuation was particularly pronounced for hedonic stimuli among the female participants with high anhedonia scores.

3.4.3.2 *Burnout*

There have been a few attempts to identify characteristic neurophysiological features of burnout syndrome [Åkerstedt *et al.*, 2007] [van Luitelaar *et al.*, 2010]. One of these studies [van Luitelaar 2010] examined thirteen patients diagnosed with burnout syndrome, which by definition is work-related, and "who could not be diagnosed as depressed." Compared to healthy controls, the patients with burnout showed significantly lower P300 amplitude, but not latency. Moreover, only the patients with burnout exhibited two P300 components. The authors hypothesize that the patients with burnout might be "processing the stimuli in a controlled rather then automated manner" (p. 216).

The qEEG findings from the thirteen patients with burnout were distinct from those typically seen in patients with depression. Namely, there was no difference between patients with burnout and controls regarding EEG asymmetry. In other words, no frontal asymmetry was observed in the patients with burnout. The patients with burnout showed a significantly lower alpha peak frequency compared to the controls, consistent with fatigue, as well as a decrease in beta power [van Luitelaar *et al.*, 2010].

- Sleep disturbances in burnout and depression

A polysomnographic study [Ekstedt *et al.*, 2006] of twenty-seven patients with burnout compared to matched controls, revealed a lower delta power (0.5 Hz to 4.5 Hz) density in the patients compared to the referents. Even though the patients with burnout slept as long as the controls; their sleep pattern was disturbed with lower sleep efficiency, longer sleep latency as well as less slow wave sleep, more stage 1 sleep, more time awake and a higher number of arousals. Most indices of subjective sleep quality and ability to recover were also disturbed in the patient group. The authors concluded that suppressed slow wave sleep, poorer sleep efficiency and more fragmentation, together with the subjective reports, indicate an impaired recovery during sleep in patients with burnout. It was suggested that these sleep disturbances may contribute to the fatigue component in the burnout syndrome [Ekstedt *et al.*, 2006][Åkerstedt *et al.*, 2007].

The described polysomnographic changes and sleep disturbances among patients with burnout are quite similar to those described among patients with depression. Namely, qEEG analysis showed decreased delta power throughout the night and decreased slow wave activity during non-REM sleep as well as disinhibition of REM sleep in depressed patients [Kupfer *et al.*, 1986] [Steiger & Kimura 2010]. Impaired sleep is recognized as a major symptom of patients with depression.

3.4.4 *Bipolar disorder*

There is quite consistent evidence of prolonged P300 latency among patients with bipolar disorders compared with healthy referent groups. With remission, P300 latency appears to normalize. On the other hand, the data are conflicting concerning P300 amplitude among patients with bipolar disorders [Fridberg *et al.*, 2009]. Preattentive auditory processing, including reduction in amplitude of mismatch negativity (MMN) are also reported [Jahshan *et al.*, 2012]. It has been suggested that among patients with bipolar disorder, attentional dysfunction may occur due to interfering neuronal processing that is unrelated to the task at hand [Howells *et al.*, 2012]. There also may be an attentional bias among persons with hypomania towards immediate as opposed to delayed rewards [Mason *et al.*, 2012].

Facial affect processing is also reported to be impaired among patients with bipolar disorders. This may be related to hampered complex judgments about faces, associated with prolonged N250 latency and decreased amplitude compared to healthy referents [Wynn *et al.*, 2012].

At rest euthymic patients with bipolar disorder showed significantly decreased theta band and increased beta band power in the frontal and cingulate cortices, compared to referents. When a cue was presented, the patients with bipolar disorder showed a P300-like wave over the frontal cortex, possibly reflecting activation of non-relevant information processing. After cognitive therapy based upon "mindfulness," this P300-wave was attenuated and beta band power was diminished among the patients with bipolar disorder. These findings are interpreted as "improved attentional readiness and attenuated activation of non-relevant information processing during attentional processes" [Howells *et al.*, 2012].

3.4.5 *Psychoses*

The amplitude of the P300, but not the N200 component, is reportedly attenuated among patients with schizophrenia compared to healthy referents [Barrett *et al.*, 1986][Ford *et al.*, 1992]. There are also some data (although not entirely consistent) indicating that the P300 latency is prolonged in schizophrenia [Halford 2003] [Mathalon & Ford 2002]. These findings are interpreted to indicate that with schizophrenia the higher levels of processing information are affected [Zubin *et al.*, 1986]. Frontocentral MMN and P3a amplitudes appear to be attenuated among patients with schizophrenia [Kaur *et al.*, 2012].

Assessment of facial affect is also reported to be impaired among patients with schizophrenia. This appears to be related both to structural encoding of faces reflected in a decreased amplitude and prolonged latency of N170, as well as to hampered complex judgments about faces, associated with prolonged N250 latency and decreased amplitude compared to healthy referents [Wynn *et al.*, 2012].

The CNV paradigm most often used among patients with schizophrenia is one in which conditions of distraction are engendered.

Therein, a dramatic attenuation of CNV amplitude has been observed [Heimberg *et al.*, 1999] [McCallum & Abraham 1973] [Tecce & Cattanach 1987]. Another finding related to CNV that has been quite consistent among patients with schizophrenia is prolonged negativity ("post-imperative negative variation," PINV) which appears to reflect the degree of psychopathology [Dongier 1973], and has been interpreted as an indicator of abnormal attention-arousal mechanisms [Tecce & Cattanach 1987]. In a study of thirty-six hospitalized patients on medication, with clinical diagnoses of psychosis (21 patients), neurosis or personality disorder (15 patients), affect-laden thoughts were associated with attenuated CNV amplitude and incongruity of affect was correlated with larger PINV. Obsessive thoughts were found to be associated with longer PINV [Bachneff & Engelsmann1980].

According to some authors, comparison of the ERP findings among patients with schizophrenia and bipolar disorders suggests some overlap, with possible common pathophysiology [Kaur *et al.*, 2012][Wynn *et al.*, 2012]. Overall, these ERP findings appear to be more severe among patients with psychoses [Jahshan *et al.*, 2012].

3.4.6 *Migraine headache*

Though no consistent structural disturbances have been found, migraine headaches are attributed to CNS dysfunction. Overall, clinical and neurophysiological studies reveal changes in cortical responsivity to external stimuli associated with migraine headaches with and without auras [Ambrosini *et al.*, 2010].

The most consistent finding among patients with migraines is decreased habituation to repeated stimuli, assessed by evoked potentials. Cortical responsivity changes over time, with an increase during the days immediately prior to the attack. During the actual attack, activation of endogenous pain control systems appears to cause increase serotonergic transmission and normalization of cortical responsiveness. Most studies report that during and three days prior to an attack, unilateral decreased alpha activity is seen on qEEG on the side of the attack [Ambrosini 2010].

A photic drive response has also been found among persons with migraines, but this is not specific, since it can also be seen among persons with primary headache disorder as well as healthy referents [Ambrosini 2010]. Quantitative EEG analysis among fifteen patients with migraines has revealed an increased beta band activity in response to flash stimulation [Akben *et al.*, 2011].

Concordantly, both the orienting component of N1 and the P3a were larger in an auditory habituation paradigm among patients with migraines during the interictal period compared to controls. However, these findings normalized among the patients with migraines during headache attacks [Demarquay *et al.*, 2011]. During the interictal period, among patients with migraines there is fairly consistent evidence of decreased P300 amplitude in active oddball paradigms, whereas data are conflicting concerning the latency of P300 [Chen *et al.*, 2007].

Heightened electrocortical negativity in CNV paradigms has been quite consistently reported during asymptomatic periods among persons who suffer from migraine headaches [Besken *et al.*, 1992] [Böcker *et al.*, 1990] [Kropp & Gerber 2005]. This appears to be mediated by complex noradrenergic and dopaminergic mechanisms of arousal and activation related to stress [Böcker *et al.*, 1990][Nagel-Leiby *et al.*, 1990]. It has also been found that between attacks, there is diminished habituation to repeated stimuli. This finding is considered to reflect insufficient control during alerting [Savić & Belkić 1998]. When visual stimuli were highly attended, reaction time was significantly faster and the early components of ERPs differed significantly among migraineurs with aura compared to those without aura and to persons without migraines. This was attributed to "an overactivated central mechanism and an enhanced level of attention" (p. 413) [Woestenburg *et al.*, 1993]. These findings appear to reflect attenuated habituation during the recording session, and are found to be most pronounced on the day prior to the migraine attack. It has been proposed that "pre-emptive" strategies might therefore be employed to diminish the high cortical arousal [Kropp & Gerber 2005]. That such strategies may be effective is indicated by the finding that, in contrast to biofeedback, special behavioral training sessions to promote habituation to aversive stimuli among children with migraines reveal both normalization of CNV habituation and reduction in headache frequency [Sinatchkin *et al.*, 2010].

3.4.7 *Epilepsy*

It has been noted that both migraine headaches and epilepsy are "persistent disorders characterized by recurrent neurological attacks" [Akben *et al.*, 2011]. These two entities are also characterized by cortical hyperexcitability which may be the pathophysiologic link that helps explain some of their similarities and possible comorbidity [Akben *et al.*, 2011][Badawy & Jackson 2012] [Verrotti *et al.*, 2011]. However, in contrast to patients with migraine, fourteen patients with epilepsy in response to flash stimulation showed little or no increase in beta band activity, whereas power in the alpha band was increased without flash stimulation [Akben *et al.*, 2011]. The association between frontal midline theta and epilepsy reported in some early studies [Ciganek 1961] [Mokran *et al.*, 1971] was not confirmed in later investigations [Pellouchard *et al.*, 1999] [Westmoreland & Klass 1986]. Frontal midline theta activity is therefore not considered to be a specific finding in epilepsy [Halford 2003]. The limited published data concerning qEEG and epilepsy is conflicting.

On the other hand, overall, the EEG is considered to be most useful in evaluating patients with suspected epilepsy. The appearance of EEG seizure activity: abnormal, repetitive, rhythmic activity with an abrupt onset and ending is considered to establish the diagnosis of epilepsy [Aminoff 1998]. However, the absence of such findings by no means excludes the presence of epilepsy. During simple or complex partial seizures, e.g. there may be no EEG changes whatsoever. Moreover, it is difficult, if not impossible to record the EEG during clinical events, since these events generally occur unpredictably and may be quite rare. During the interictal period, bursts of abnormal discharges with spikes or sharp waves strongly support the diagnosis of epilepsy, but are not entirely pathognomonic.

Patients with temporal lobe epilepsy reportedly show reduced mismatch negativity responses to speech sounds at the bilateral mastoid sites but not at the fronto-central regions [Hara *et al.*, 2012]. Earlier studies indicate that the latency of the MMN is prolonged among patients with temporal lobe epilepsy and that the abnormalities may differ according to tonal versus phonetic changes [Hara *et al.*, 2012].

Among patients with epilepsy the P300 latency is reported to be prolonged, but the amplitude is often found to be normal, insofar as no psychotic symptoms are present [Ford *et al.*, 2001]. However, more recent investigations indicate that P300 amplitudes may also be attenuated among various groups of patients with epilepsy. In a comparison of patients with generalized epilepsy of the *absence* type and those with complex partial epilepsy, in comparison with healthy referents, both patient groups showed a reduction in the P300 amplitude of a visual paradigm, whereas only the patients with *absence* seizures showed P300 attenuation to the auditory paradigm [Duncan *et al.*, 2009]. A study of ten patients with temporal lobe epilepsy showed significantly lower P300 (P3b) amplitudes in auditory and visual paradigms compared to age and gender matched referents [Bocquillon *et al.*, 2009]. On the basis of these findings, it was concluded that the reduction in P300 amplitude may reflect cortical dysfunction caused either by the epileptic focus or by more complex mechanisms that interfere with normal attentional pathways.

In contrast to these findings, among patients with refractory temporal lobe epilepsy who had undergone anteromedial resection of the medial temporal lobe, the P3a (the so-called novelty P3) response to repeated novel stimuli does not decrease which is an abnormal response. It was therefore concluded that "bilaterally intact hippocampi are necessary for the brain to appreciate that a repetition of a novel sound has occurred, perhaps due to disruptions in ipsilateral hippocampal-prefrontal pathways and/or between the left and right hippocampi" (p. 3474) [Friedman *et al.*, 2011].

Amygdalar damage among patients with medial temporal lobe epilepsy was associated with attenuated early (P1, 100-150 ms) and late (500-600 ms) ERP responses to fearful facial expression. Interestingly, amygdalar damage did not appear to affect the actual perception of the fearful expression (150-250 ms). Thus, there may be several processing stages related to exposure to fearful faces, and only some of these are dependent upon amygdalar function [Rotshtein *et al.*, 2010].

There appears to be very little study of CNV among patients with epilepsy [Halford 2003]. Early case reports indicate that during interictal periods of temporal discharge, the CNV may be attenuated and disorganized [Zapoli *et al.*, 1969], although after posterior spike and wave activity ceased, the CNV activity was reportedly normal [Zapoli *et al.*, 1977]. The need has been emphasized to find the best set of neurophysiologic methods for routine clinical practice for patients with epilepsy [Halford 2003]. Greater integration is needed between event-related potentials and functional imaging within the clinical setting [D'Arcy *et al.*, 2011].

• Comment

We have focused upon what is in fact a small sampling of an enormously complex area of event-related potentials and quantitative EEG in the above-presentation concerning the mental burden of work processes as well as concerning specific neuropsychiatric disorders. The scope of the present book obliges us to only briefly mention such obviously vital topics as e.g. brain localization and neurochemical mechanisms. The interested reader is also referred to the cited references for fuller discussions of methodological issues in ERP research, models and interpretation of specific ERP components and sub-components.

There is a baffling array of paradigms used to model the dynamics of cognitive ergonomics. As mentioned earlier, the actual brain processes occurring in relation to these dynamics can be studied in a number of other ways, including PET, fMRI *inter alia.* The PET scan can reveal both the involvement of various neuroanatomic structures, as well as identifying which neurochemical pathways are activated [Orrison *et al.*, 1995].

Changes in regional blood flow have been registered in relation to specific emotional states associated with various stimuli [Fretska *et al.*, 1999]. Moreover, there have been studies combining these modalities with ERP. For example, among patients who developed PTSD following the Tokyo subway sarin attack lower P300 amplitudes were found together with smaller anterior cingulate cortex volume on MRI, compared to persons who were exposed to the same trauma but did not develop PTSD [Araki *et al.*, 2005]. Combined ERP and fMRI studies have been suggested for observing complementary responses from the same stimulation event, with the aim of improved understanding of the physiological processes underlying brain activation and the functional organization of the brain [Kruggel *et al.*, 2000].

In the final section of this Chapter, we briefly return to a topic mentioned earlier, the relation among the environment, the central nervous system and target organ responses, with emphasis on the cardiovascular system. Recall, this is termed *econeurocardiology*.

3.5 The Environment — Brain — Cardiovascular System: Econeurocardiology

As reviewed in Chapter 2, (Section 2.5.1) there is strong epidemiological evidence of a link between work stressors and cardiovascular disease, including and especially hypertension. In 1985 Benjamin Natelson [1985] introduced the concept of "neurocardiology," as an interdisciplinary area linking the neurosciences and cardiology. He underscored the need to fully appreciate the role of the nervous system in the pathogenesis of cardiac dysfunction. The biological underpinnings of this concept are very rich and multi-faceted, having developed over many decades since Cannon's classic studies [1914] and those from Selye [1976], Henry [Henry 1992], Wolf [1995], Levi [1972], Frankenhaeuser and Johansson [1986], *inter alia*, to the exhaustive clinical treatise of RS Eliot [1974]. In a subsequent publication, Natelson and Chang [1993] emphasize "the role of stress in turning on the neural link that connects the environment to the heart" (p.

293). As noted at the beginning of this Chapter, the associations between mentally stressful activity, the central nervous system and CVD outcomes have been extensively substantiated, as reviewed in e.g. [Belkić, Schwartz *et al.*, 2000] [Eliot 1974] [Folkow 1994] [Henry 1994] [Kulbertus & Frank 1988] [Lown 1990] [Natelson 1985] [Rozanski *et al.*, 1999] [Wolf 1995].

In this concluding section of the present Chapter, we present some of our own clinical research experience in formulating and applying stress models relevant to working populations at high risk of CVD. This has helped spur the conceptual development of econeurocardiology, which can be of practical utility in helping to guide preventive strategies and also for assessing and promoting work fitness [Belkić, Savić, Theorell *et al.*, 1994].

In the early 1980's we began our quest through laboratory evaluation of cardiovascular reactivity to various work-related stressors [Belkić 1984]. The overall aim has been to find non-invasive, sensitive and specific tools that could identify initial and often reversible changes, at a stage when timely intervention would be most effective. We thereby sought to model complex bio-psychosocial relationships with the aim of improving early detection and prevention of disease.

This work was initiated at the Institute of Occupational Medicine, Belgrade University Clinical Center, and was informed by the well-established approach towards occupational pulmonary disease, including a functional diagnostic laboratory together with field investigations, lead by Professor Velimir Potkonjak.

3.5.1 The glare pressor test

We began by evaluating the blood pressure responses of 22 healthy male workers to a large battery of diverse procedures, including several standard mental stress tests, aerobic and isometric stress, sensory stimuli such as 90 dB noise, the cold pressor test, and exposure to impulses of glare from an ordinary car headlight [Belkić 1984].

To our surprise, the blood pressure rise in response to glare was highly significant. In fact, the diastolic response was among the greatest when compared with all the other stressors.

Notably, there was a diastolic blood pressure increase of 30 mm Hg observed in one of the study participants, an amateur driver. This participant later spontaneously told us that he had been in a collision with an oncoming vehicle after having faced glare from a headlight while driving at night on a poorly lit road.

On the basis of these findings, we introduced the "Glare Pressor Test" [5] [Belkić 1986]. In our subsequent study carried out at the Ambulatory Center for Occupational Health in Belgrade [Belkić *et al.*, 1987] the glare pressor test (GPT) with blood pressure measurement and continuous electrocardiogram was applied in professional drivers, amateur drivers, non-drivers who had work exposure to glare from other sources (welding), and non-drivers with no other professional glare exposure. These groups of workers were all undergoing systematic preventive examinations and were offered the possibility to participate in this study. The professional and amateur drivers showed significantly higher diastolic responses to the GPT than did the non-driver referents. The group exposed to welding glare did not differ from the referents in their response to the GPT. The GPT elicited ventricular arrhythmias only in professional drivers who drove at night. These findings seemed to support Fuller's [1984] postulation, suggesting that headlight glare, as a symbolically aversive visual stimulus for the driver, was indeed capable of evoking a powerful autonomic response.

3.5.1.1 *Central arousal and cardiovascular responses to the GPT*

The above-described results suggested that stimuli can be sensitizing or acquire an "aversive potential" based upon their *symbolic* association with disastrous events. It is not essential that one has personally experienced such events. As noted:

- Brain mechanisms exist which focus attention to potentially dangerous phenomena in one's surroundings.
- Visual signals are particularly important, because of their primary consumption of attentional resources [Singleton 1974].
- There are intimate neuroanatomical connections, via the midbrain reticular formation, with cortical arousal, as well as with outflow tracts to the cardiovascular system, that are likely to be involved in stress-mediated cardiovascular disease [Belkić, Savić, *et al.*, 1994].

Adjacent to the Ambulatory Center for Occupational Health in Belgrade was the Institute for Mental Health, where the Laboratory for Neurophysiology and Clinical Psychophysiology had been established, in

---

[5] During this test, light impulses from an ordinary car headlight were delivered at 55-s intervals through a dark cylinder, 1 m in length. A total of five light flashes were presented so that the entire glare pressor test lasted 5 min.

which multichannel electroencephalographic and polygraphic recordings were carried out, such as those illustrated in Fig. 3.12, as well as those shown earlier in this Chapter. This geographic proximity was fortuitous, and rendered logistically feasible our next step in the investigations: applying the Glare Pressor Text with EEG and polygraphic recording in the laboratory.

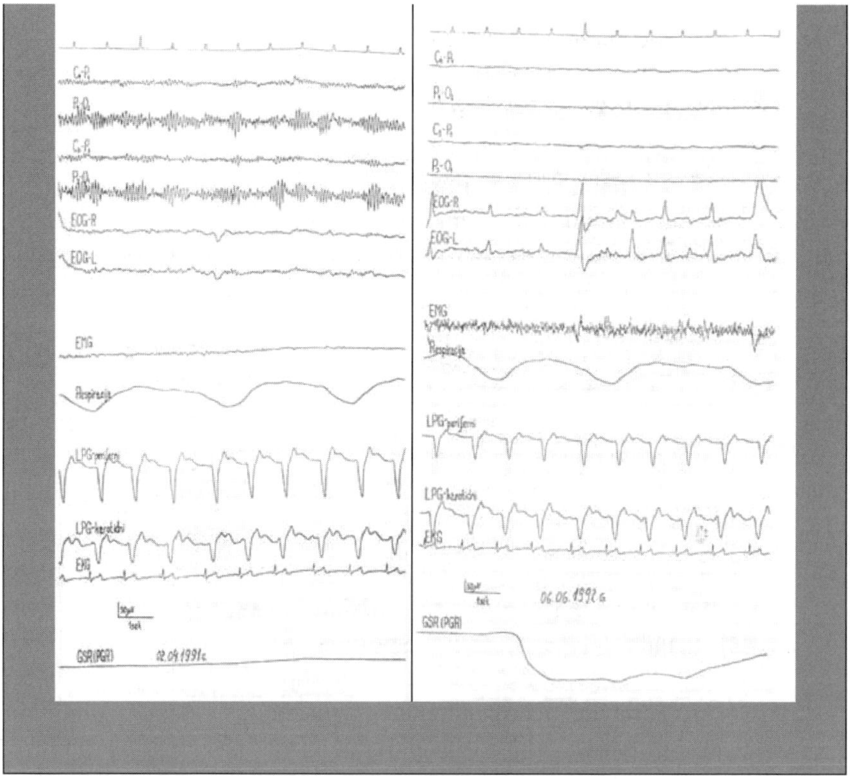

Figure 3.12 EEG and polygraphy, at rest and during arousal. Recording from our Laboratory for Clinical Neurophysiology and Psychophysiology at the Institute of Mental Health, Belgrade.

Left panel: Relaxed with well-expressed alpha activity, minimal muscle tension on electromyography (EMG) and no Galvanic skin response (GSR).
Right panel: Arousal with EEG desynchronization, muscle tension with heightened EMG amplitude, peripheral vasoconstriction with diminished digital pulse amplitude, and pronounced GSR.
Channels from the top: #1 time in seconds, # 2-5 EEG, #6-7 EOG, #8: EMG, #9: Respiration, #10-11: digital & carotid plethysmogram, #12: ECG, #13 GSR.

We examined young, healthy professional drivers with night driving experience, and non-driver referents [Belkić 1989][Belkić, Ercegovac, *et al.*,1992]. Inclusion criteria included normal resting ECG and clinic blood pressure ≤ 140/90 mm Hg, normal cardiopulmonary, neurologic and opthalmologic examination.

The drivers who participated in glare pressor test also wore an ambulatory ECG (Holter monitoring) during work and rest [Belkić 1989][Belkić, Jelić, *et al.*, 1991].

Of the 19 participating drivers, 15 showed persistent blockade of spontaneous alpha activity or complete EEG desynchronization after the first glare impulse, with significant fall in digital pulse amplitude and rise in diastolic BP, reflecting vasoconstriction, which is reported to occur in response to conditional aversive stimuli [Bond 1979].

The electromyogram (EMG) revealed a significant increase in facial muscle tone. Thus the professional drivers exhibited electrocortical, somatic, and autonomic arousal indicative of a defense reaction in response to exposure to an automobile headlight, whereas no significant effects of the glare pressor test were found in the non-drivers.

The response of drivers to the glare pressor test is characteristic of the type A reaction to a specific challenge. Hyperalertness is objectively confirmed by the finding of EEG desynchronization. Tight facial musculature is reflected in the increased amplitude of the EMG. Greater frontal EMG amplitude has been reported in drivers than in persons with passenger status, apparently reflecting "readiness for performing motor activity as well as general tension in cognitive tasks" (p 800) [Zeir 1979].

Most of the drivers recovered their baseline levels of alpha activity and showed milder diastolic blood pressure, as well as digital pulse changes, after the final (fifth) glare impulse. Thus, with repeated exposure to the glare impulses, the drivers seemed to distinguish the laboratory exposure from the real exigencies of driving.

> In two drivers, however, it was the 5th (last) glare stimulus which elicited the most pronounced physiological changes.

- Caṣe studies—in brief

For a long-route truck driver in his early thirties, it was the fifth glare impulse which most rapidly elicited ventricular arrhythmias, together with a marked Galvanic skin response (Figure 3.13 (left panel)). As seen in the right panel of Figure 3.13., ventricular arrhythmias from two foci and "R on T" phenomena were recorded. These arrhythmias occurred during driving.

This driver had worked at his present job for about ten years and reported long work hours (12 hours per day, 6 days per week). He frequently slept in the cabin, since he could not go home after work. His family history was strongly positive for hypertension. He smoked 20 cigarettes per day and was sedentary during his leisure time.

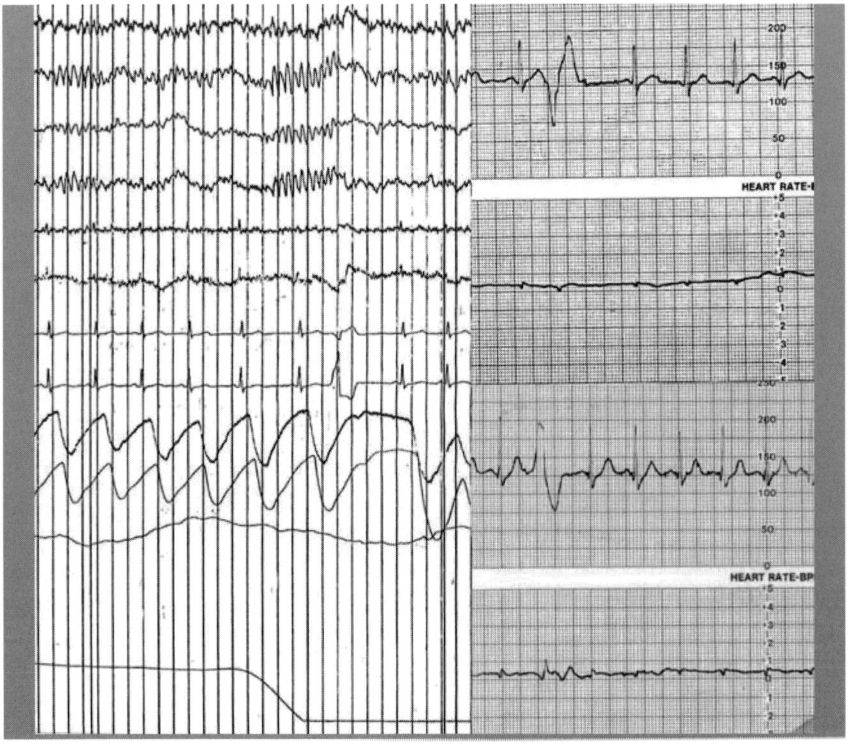

Figure 3.13 Ventricular arrhythmia and Galvanic skin response to the 5th glare impulse of the Glare Pressor Test (left panel). Right panel: "R on T" phenomenon and ventricular arrhythmia from 2 different foci, registered while driving.

Recording from our Laboratory for Clinical Neurophysiology and Psychophysiology at the Institute of Mental Health, Belgrade (Left Panel) and from the Center for Cardiac Pacing and Electrophysiology, University Clinical Center, Belgrade (Right Panel).

Left panel: Channels from the top: # 1-4 EEG, #5-6: EMG, #7-8 ECG, #9-10: digital & carotid plethysmogram, #11: respiration, #12: GSR.

A city bus driver, with marked type A behavior, demonstrated complete EEG desynchronization during the entire GPT and a pronounced rise in blood pressure (especially diastolic) at the final, compared with the 1st glare impulse (Figure 3.14).These responses were considered maladaptive, suggesting hypersensitivity to glare exposure with a breakdown of protective mechanisms. Holter monitoring revealed ventricular extrasystoles in pairs during sleep-wave transition (Figure 3.15).

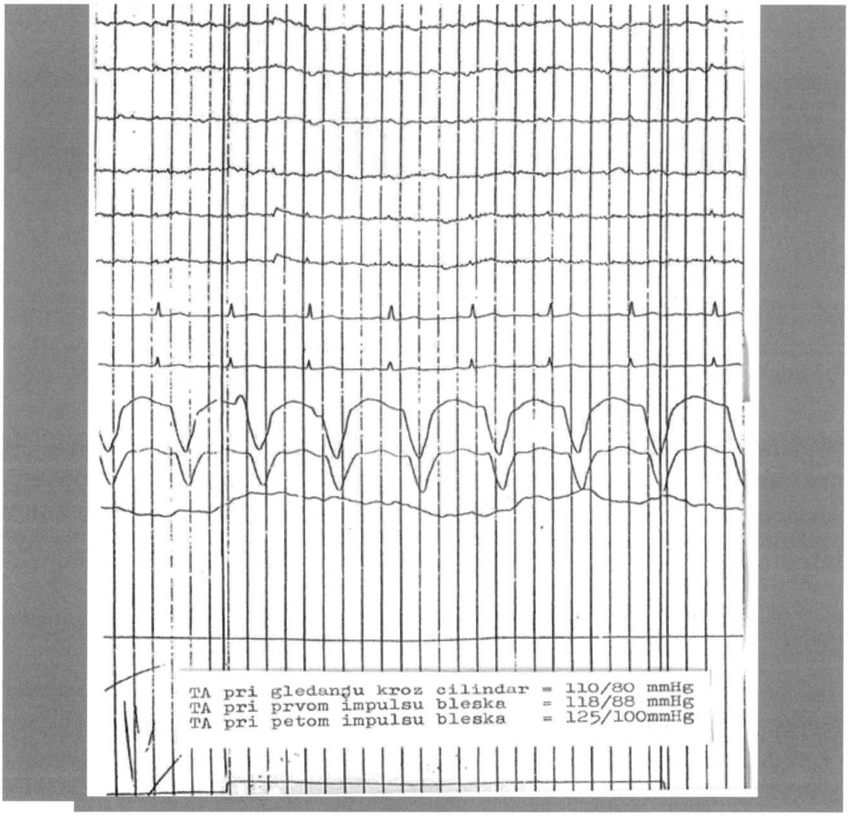

Figure 3.14 Complete EEG desynchronization after the 5th glare impulse of the Glare Pressor Test, with rise in systolic and diastolic blood pressure:

⇒ 110/80 mmHg while peering through the dark cylinder
⇒ 118/88 mmHg at the 1st glare impulse
⇒ 125/100 mmHg at the 5th glare impulse

Recording from our Laboratory for Clinical Neurophysiology and Psychophysiology at the Institute of Mental Health, Belgrade. Channels from the top: Channels from the top: # 1-4 EEG, #5-6: EMG, #7-8 ECG, #9-10: digital & carotid plethysmogram, #11: respiration, #12: GSR.

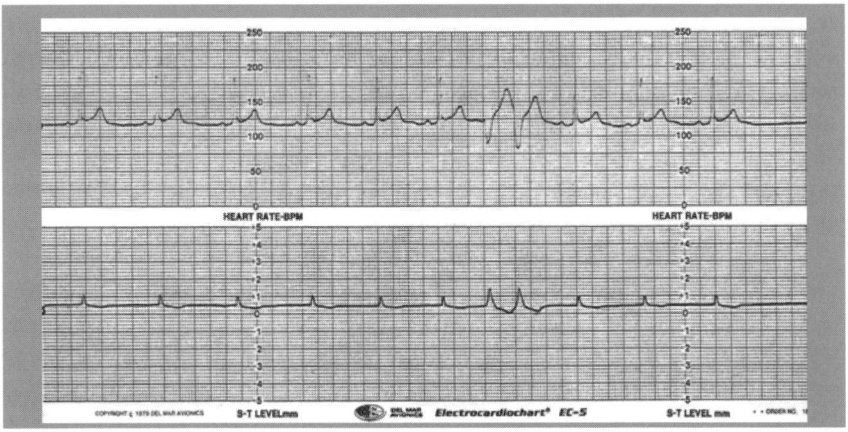

Figure 3.15 Paired ventricular arrhythmias during early morning (sleep-wake transition) on Holter monitoring. Recording from our Center for Cardiac Pacing and Electrophysiology, University Clinical Center, Belgrade.

Both of these drivers, although clinically healthy according to standard screening criteria, including an exercise stress test, showed noteworthy ventricular arrhythmias during Holter monitoring. They also had a very high standard risk factor status and both worked very long hours. Although still apparently healthy, we considered these findings as indicative of increased risk. With the active participation of these drivers, we sought measures to protect their health status as well as work capacity.

3.5.1.2 *The GPT among professional drivers with hypertension and/or ischemic heart disease*

Having demonstrated that young, healthy professional drivers show heightened central nervous system arousal and cardiovascular hyperreactivity to the glare pressor test, in our subsequent study we applied the GPT in four groups of male professional drivers (age 25-52 years): 12 professional drivers with ischemic heart disease, 12 with hypertension, 12 with borderline hypertension, and 34 who were healthy—as well as in 23 healthy, non-professional driver referents [Belkić *et al.*, 1996] [Emdad 1997] [Emdad *et al.*, 1998b]. A threat avoidant ERP paradigm was also part of the clinical research protocol. These studies were carried out at the Karolinska Institute, National Institute for Psychosocial Factors and Health, and at the National Institute for Occupational Health, Stockholm. Our aim in applying the GPT among these groups of drivers was to evaluate sensitization to this night driving stressor in relation to degree of cardiovascular disease severity.

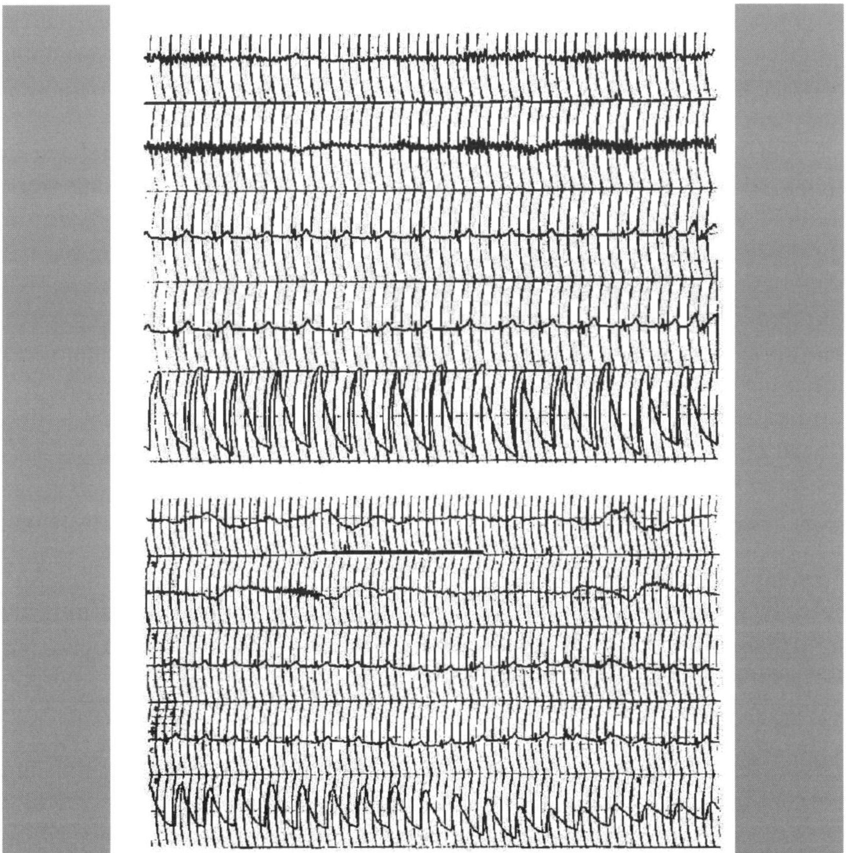

Figure 3.16 EEG and polygraphic recording at rest (top panel) and at the fifth glare impulse of the Glare Pressor Test (bottom panel) in a city bus driver with borderline hypertension. Recording from our laboratory at the Institute for Psychosocial Factors in Medicine, Stockholm.

Top panel: Relaxed readiness with well-expressed alpha activity and high amplitude of digital pulse. Bottom panel: EEG desynchronization and marked peripheral vasoconstriction with diminished digital pulse amplitude immediately after the glare impulse. From Ref. [Emdad, Belkić, Theorell, Cizinsky, Savić, Olsson. (1998) J. Occup. Health Psychol., 3, pp. 147 – 160], reprinted with permission by the American Psychological Association.

Channels from the top: #1: EEG C4-O2, #2: indicates time in seconds, with the thickened black line indicating the glare impulse, # 3 EEG C3-O1, #4-5: ECG leads V5 & V3, respectively #6: Digital plethysmogram.

After glare exposure, the drivers with ischemic heart disease showed the most pronounced alpha blockade, a significant increase in diastolic blood pressure, and, unlike the other groups, a persistent drop in digital pulse volume. The drivers with borderline hypertension reacted initially with a significant rise in diastolic blood pressure and digital vasoconstriction, mainly without central nervous system arousal. The diastolic BP remained constant in normotensive professional drivers above age forty.

The drivers' cardiovascular responses to glare were inversely related to reported stressors and subjective experience. Anxiety trait and long work hours were associated with heightened central arousal to glare in professional drivers. The results suggest that there may be progressive degrees of sensitization to glare exposure among these professional drivers, with the least among those above age 40 who remained normotensive, moderate levels in those with borderline hypertension, and the most severe in drivers with ischemic heart disease. An example of a response to the Glare Pressor Test of a professional driver with borderline hypertension is shown in Fig. 3.16.

3.5.2 *Further directions*

We now briefly mention a particularly salient example concerning the way in which branches of research have developed with respect to heart rate variability. It was cognitive ergonomists who first described the relation between loss of heart rate variability (HRV)[6], and mental burden [Boyce 1974] [Kalsbeek & Ettema 1963] [Kalsbeek 1967] [Luczak & Lauring 1973] [Mulder & van der Meulen 1973]. Although there was also some recognition by clinical researchers before and during that period that attenuated heart rate variability was associated with cardiac dysfunction [Wenckebach & Winterberg1927], and with sudden arrhythmic cardiac death in infants [Hon & Lee 1965] and in adults [Wolf *et al.*,1978], almost two decades elapsed before the clinical importance of heart rate variability became widely appreciated, with the confirmation that HRV is a strong, independent predictor of mortality in patients post-acute myocardial infarction [Task Force European Society of Cardiology 1996]. Assessment of HRV was performed among emergency room physicians during night work, revealing an increase in low (0.04 – 0.15 Hz) to high frequency (0.15 – 0.4 Hz) ratio, compared to periods immediately preceding and after the work shift [Adams *et al.*,1995]. It

[6] This was the high frequency (0.15 to 0.4 Hz) component, or so-called respiratory sinus arrhythmia.

has been suggested that spectral analysis of HRV could be used "to predict optimal work time under a combination of enhanced mental load and other stressors" [Kristal-Boneh *et al.*,1995] (p. 90). As noted, advanced signal processing methods appear to be particularly appropriate for assessing physiological responses to external perturbations as well as for longer term recordings [Belkić & Belkić 2002a]. These methods are being applied to assess heart rate variability among physicians as a heavily burdened occupational group [Belkić, Belkić & Savić 2002].

The econeurocardiologic and econeurologic mechanisms reviewed in this chapter provide a deeper understanding of how work stressors can impact upon health. These insights are vital to a more robust approach to evaluating and preserving work fitness, the topic of the next Chapter.

Chapter 4

Work Fitness and Occupational Rehabilitation: The Current Standard of Care

We now present an overview of the current "standard of care" concerning work fitness and occupational rehabilitation. The standards vary to some extent according to the country and legislative framework. Our focus, though not exclusive, will be on mental health and neuropsychiatric disorders, as the central theme of this book.

4.1 Mental Health Disorders, Work Fitness and Rehabilitation

4.1.1 *General observations*

Mental health disorders are recognized to be a major cause of disability at the workplace [Andersen *et al.*, 2012] [Engström & Janson 2007] [Pro 2005], associated with longer sick leave duration compared to other causes [Flach *et al.*, 2011]. Work fitness and rehabilitation are particularly difficult issues in relation to psychiatric disorders. As emphasized by the U.K. Royal College of Psychiatry, persons with mental health disorders "must contend with fear, ignorance, and prejudice that can pose far greater barriers to employment than the direct effects of mental illness itself" (p. 147)[Teasdale & Deahl 2007]. The stigma associated with psychiatric disorders renders possibilities for employment more difficult than for persons with broadly comparable physical disabilities [Manning & White 1995]. Employees who develop mental health problems are likely to hide these difficulties from their employer. If sick leave is needed, reasons other than mental illness will frequently be given. Especially if the work environment is difficult and demanding:

> "A conspiracy of silence may develop between employer (unwilling or unable to create a psychologically less demanding environment) and employee (reluctant to admit to an inability to cope)" (p. 148) [Teasdale & Deahl 2007].

Persons with mentally or socially restricted work capacity are nearly twice as likely not to be employed after rehabilitation compared to those with somatic work restriction, based upon the results of a 6-year follow-up multi-professional intervention study from Sweden [Jakobsson *et al.*, 2010].

4.1.1.1 *Illness model versus disability model*

Rather than relying upon the usual "illness" model, in order to more effectively handle employment-related issues, it is emphasized that psychiatrists could better communicate with occupational health physicians by focusing upon problems, strengths and weaknesses within the framework of a "disability" model [Teasdale & Deahl 2007].

Feelings of exhaustion, difficulties in concentrating and maintaining attention, problems communicating with others and general social skills frequently hamper work capacity. Motivation and reliability may be affected by mental ill-health. Naturally, posing a risk to oneself or others is a major deterrent to returning to work. On the other hand, despite having a psychiatric diagnosis, many employees perform in a totally satisfactory manner and avoid illness behavior completely [Teasdale & Deahl 2007]. In fact, it is the psychiatric symptoms that are often much more important than the diagnosis itself [Pro 2005].

When assessing fitness for work, particularly with regard to mental health disorders, work history, the demands of the job and the patient's strengths and weaknesses are vital considerations. Motivation and confidence are recognized as important components of work fitness. The broader social milieu at work must also be taken into account, notably the expectations of colleagues and supervisors, the possibility of supervision and available training development programs. More caution is necessary when safety could be affected [Teasdale & Deahl 2007].

Although it is commonly presumed that persons with mental health disorders have unrealistic employment expectations and poorly developed vocational goals, over 80% of people in supported employment programs expressed clear job preferences that were realistic and stable over time [Becker *et al.*, 1998]. Nevertheless, persons with psychiatric disability may have decreased insight concerning realistic hours, wages and requirements [Tse 2002].

4.1.1.2 *Suggested strategies for vocational rehabilitation of persons with mental health disorders*

Despite numerous programs and strategies aimed at helping persons with mental health disorders to return to work (RTW), there is minimal evidence concerning their effectiveness [Teasdale & Deahl 2007]. For example, a stress management program implemented among twenty-four female patients on long-term sick leave for work-related psychological symptoms was effective in ameliorating the symptoms, but not in improving return to work rates [Grossi & Santell 2009].

Important general issues are whether early RTW would promote or hamper recovery. Bolstering self-confidence is crucial. The extent to which the work conditions contributed to the mental health disorder also needs to be assessed. However, in certain settings, such as in the U.S., some authors have stated that it is not "ethically appropriate for the treating clinician to offer conclusions about causation" (p.420)[Steinberg 2011]. In contrast, many Scandinavian and other European authors suggest that RTW interventions should focus not only upon coping strategies of the individual, but also upon the work conditions [Andersen *et al.*, 2012]. Particularly in Scandinavia, coordination among various social and rehabilitation systems is cited as an important component of successful RTW among employees with common mental disorders.

Modified hours, working from home as a temporary solution and task selection to avoid excessive pressure are cited as possible strategies for RTW [Teasdale & Deahl 2007]. For severe mental health disorders, sheltered environments have been used [Norman 2006]. Yet, it is noted that individuals working in such environments rarely progress to actual "open" employment [Teasdale & Deahl 2007]. A telling finding among 233 Swedish female white-collar workers on longer-term sick leave for minor mental disorders is that nearly half of the 69% who returned to work had changed jobs, and over one-third had changed profession [Sandmark 2011].

A psycho-educational approach to vocational decision-making may be helpful for psychiatric outpatients [Diamond 1998]. Within a group setting, most of the participants were able to identify realistic vocational goals for themselves and, thus, experienced a sense of empowerment, exploring options without feeling the pressure of immediately returning to employment.

Other strategies include "support employment" in which a person is directly placed in the workplace with a support organization to provide supervision and mentoring [Becker *et al.*, 1994]. In order for patients with mental health disorders to return to work, it is considered that they should be able to perform most activities of daily living and have a satisfactory level of social functioning, concentration, persistence and pace. Adequate sleep and control of anger are particularly important.

Full remission is not a requirement for RTW and follow-up with treatment should continue thereafter [Pro 2005]. It is emphasized that with authorization from the patient, discussions between the physician and supervisor or human resources manager can "dramatically improve stress tolerance" [Pro 2005]. In Panel 4.1 summarizes of some possible modifications to meet the needs of persons with mental health disorders, as proposed by [Fabian *et al.*, 1992] and by [Tse 2002].

Possible Work Modifications for Persons with Mental Health Disorders

- Supervisor training: e.g. Work-site meetings with job coach & employee
- Schedules: e.g.flex-time with input from the employee, ↓ hours
- Procedures: e.g. saving job during period of hospitalization
- Performance expectations: e.g. allow more time to learn a job, ↑ tolerance regarding errors
- Job tasks: e.g. allow task alternation
- Supervisor and coworker orientation: e.g. education about mental health disorders especially to identify warning signs, enlist support

Panel 4.1 Suggested categories of workplace modification for persons with mental health disorders [Fabian *et al.*, 1993] [Tse 2002].

4.1.2 *Explicitly stress-related mental health disorders*

In the last two decades, stress-related mental health disorders including burnout have increased as a cited cause of sickness absence, particularly in Scandinavia [Andersen *et al.*, 2012] [Engström & Janson 2007] [Belkić 2011].

4.1.2.1 *Acute stress reactions*

These are described as extreme reactions to "stressful events" often with "preoccupying concerns about the event" (p. 155) [Teasdale & Deahl 2007] (see

Appendix A, Section 1). The manifestations are diverse and may include anxiety, depression and somatic complaints such as palpitations, headache and dizziness *inter alia*. Besides standard medical treatment, a short reprieve from the stressful working conditions may be recommended.

Insofar as a work stressor is the clear trigger of the psychiatric symptoms, work restriction may be temporarily recommended until a solution at the workplace is implemented [Pro 2005]. Whether such situations represent an actual risk to the patient or whether they are issues of choice i.e. tolerance of unpleasant work situations must be carefully weighed by the clinician. Early intervention of these acute stress reactions, by e.g. exposure-based therapy appears to help prevent the development of PTSD [Bryant *et al.*, 2008].

4.1.2.2 *Post-traumatic stress disorder*

Post-traumatic stress disorder is noted to be increasingly common in relation to the workplace, particularly among those who have been assaulted, faced bank robberies or were involved in or witnessed major accidents at work [Pro 2005]. In our clinical experience, these incidences almost inevitably lead to various degrees of PTSD, and require prompt and aggressive treatment. If, e.g., intrusive thoughts impair concentration, work tasks may need to be modified [Pro 2005].

Early intervention after traumatic events has been investigated with regard to reducing subsequent long-term psychiatric morbidity. Among the methods used has been Critical Incident Stress Debriefing (CISD). However, the effectiveness of CISD has not been established in randomized controlled investigations. Possible harm from CISD has even been suggested [Teasdale & Deahl 2007]. There appears to be consensus that education about normal post-traumatic symptoms is appropriate, as well as the need to avoid unhealthy responses such as alcohol or substance abuse. In addition, practical support and help to return to a normal work routine are needed, together with basic health screening. The often-lengthy litigation proceedings associated with the traumatic event can be deleterious to recovery. Exposure to the actual scene of the trauma may exacerbate symptoms and impair work capacity.

Occupational exposure to noise and specific sounds should also be taken into consideration with regard to PTSD, as well as other neuropsychiatric disorders. Excessive noise can disrupt task performance, undermine attention and cause irritability. Warning sounds such as in airplane or train cabins can provoke startle responses [Willcox & Hardy 2007]. "Gradual job reentry" and desensitization by a therapist working with the patient and the communicating employer may be necessary [Pro 2005].

4.1.2.3 Burnout and related disorders

As discussed in Chapter 2, the entity of burnout has been conceptually very closely linked to work conditions. Within the framework of work fitness and occupational rehabilitation, burnout can be viewed as "the end-point in the breakdown of the adaptational process that results from a long-term mismatch between the demands placed upon an individual and the emotional resources that can be brought to bear to cope with these" (p. 160)[Teasdale & Deahl 2007].

Burnout is noted to be among the most common mental health-related causes of impaired work efficiency. Younger workers with less experience are noted to be a risk group for burnout. External locus of control is cited as a frequent concomitant. Disturbed sleep has also been found to predict symptoms, as well as prolonged sick-leave among employees with burnout [Sonnenschein *et al.*, 2008]. A quasi-experimental study of clerical workers from Israel indicates that vacations provide some relief from burnout. However, after a few days back on the job, burnout returned, reaching the pre-vacation levels after three weeks at work [Westman & Eden 1997].

A workplace-oriented intervention study was implemented in southern Sweden among seventy-four patients on long-term sick-leave for burnout [Karlson *et al.*, 2010]. The core intervention was a "convergence dialogue meeting" between the supervisor and the patient, with the main focus on finding short- and long-term solutions. During the 1.5 year follow-up period, the RTW rate increased linearly, with 89% having some RTW by the end of the follow-up period. Among the control group of patients also on long-term sick-leave for burnout, there was no increased RTW after 6 months, and the overall RTW rate was 73%. The authors conclude that the work-place intervention was associated with improved longer-term RTW for this group of patients.

Among physicians, professional help through counselling in conjunction with job interventions such as reduction in work hours are reported to help ameliorate burnout, according to a study from Norway

[Isaksson *et al.*, 2008]. In a comment to the recent study from the U.S. indicating that burnout appears to be significantly more common among physicians than other working adults [Shanafelt 2012], it was suggested that recognizing the heavy cognitive load faced by physicians would help design strategies to ameliorate burnout [Centor *et al.*, 2012].

Chronic fatigue syndrome (CFS) is characterized by diminished energy levels, fatigue and frequently also musculoskeletal complaints, lasting at least 6 months. Graded exercise and cognitive behavioral therapy have been demonstrated to be effective [Teasdale & Deahl 2007]. With regard to employment, low motivation is a frequent concomitant. It is emphasized that requests for disability retirement should be resisted, especially since most persons with CFS will recover. According to the criteria of the Americans with Disabilities Act of 1990, there is no significant risk of imminent, substantial harm associated with work in relation to chronic fatigue syndrome and other common functional disorders. According to some authors [Talmage 2005], work modifications are not likely to improve work capacity, and therefore the efficacy of such is called into question.

4.1.3 *Anxiety disorders*

As noted in Chapter 2, anxiety disorders are among the most prevalent psychiatric disorders seen in the community, and are strongly associated with occupational disability [Braunwald *et al.*, 2002] [Clark *et al.*, 2009] [Horwath & Weissman 2000]. It has been argued that the resultant distress and disability are comparable to that seen in schizophrenia and in chronic medical conditions such as diabetes.

Anxiety disorders are reportedly all too often medicalized. Recovery requires identification of the trigger factors and promoting the patient's active involvement. Counselling and short-term cognitive behavioral therapy can help in "challenging unfounded worries" and problem solving. Relaxation techniques may also be effective [Teasdale & Deahl 2007]. Vocationally-focused cognitive behavioral therapy was implemented among a small group of persons with anxiety disorders in Hamilton, Ontario, Canada [Kidd *et al.*, 2008]. After the intervention, those who were employed reported enhanced sense of mastery in completing their work assignments, but were more dissatisfied with promotion prospects and job security. In a 6-month prospective study of 204 Australian employees with at least one health condition, sickness absence and limitation of work activity were found to be associated with over a two-fold increase in anxiety or depression [Sanderson *et al.*, 2008]. It can thus be inferred that sick leave may well exacerbate the anxiety condition, as is precisely our clinical experience.

4.1.4 *Depression*

Depression is among the leading causes of disability in developed countries [Levav 2009]. Major depression engenders a loss of function that is often far greater than that caused by physical illness. Depression is highly prevalent in the workplace and has a major deleterious impact upon performance, productivity, absenteeism, and disability [Bender & Farvolden 2008] [Gilbody *et al.*, 2012]. In the U.S. alone, it has been estimated that time lost from work due to depressive disorders amounts to $21.4 billion [Pro 2005]. Among Danish employees applying for sick-leave benefits for common mental health problems, those who fulfilled the DSM-IV criteria for depression were likely to have a longer sickness absence [Nielsen *et al.*, 2012]. On the other hand, underperformance at work may be the consequence of depression, also termed "presenteeism." In fact, this is the most frequent manifestation of depression [Pro 2005].

While medication and cognitive behavioral therapy are the usual mainstays, these should not be the exclusive focus. Supportive counseling to help handle major psychosocial stressors may be required. Motivation and confidence need to be bolstered in order to promote RTW [Teasdale & Deahl 2007]. Insofar as there is a serious suicide risk and work is considered to be a psychosocial stressor, it is recommended that work be restricted [Pro 2005].

There is a lack of effective interventions delivered in the workplace setting for patients with depression [Bender & Farvolden 2008]. For example, a recent randomized controlled trial from Amsterdam among 117 employees on sick leave for major depression examined the effect of adjuvant occupational therapy. Whereas the rate of recovery from depression was increased and returning to work in good health were increased by the intervention, overall work participation was not significantly affected [Hees, de Vries *et al.*, 2012]. This same group of investigators [Hees, Koeter *et al.*, 2012] also analyzed the predictors of RTW among these patients over 18 months of follow-up, and found that in addition to diagnostic factors, work motivation and conscientiousness also showed significant multivariate association with RTW. In another

Dutch study of employees sick-listed for major depression, RTW duration was not significantly affected by a collaborative care program applied by the occupational physicians [Vlasveld *et al.*, 2012].

4.1.5 *Bipolar disorders*

Very high rates of unemployment are seen among persons with bipolar disorders [Morselli *et al.*, 2004]. In assessing the employability of these patients, considerations include "frequency of relapse, functional capacity during periods of well-being and adherence to any long-term treatment plan, particularly their compliance with mood stabilizing medication" (p. 158) [Teasdale & Deahl 2007]. It should be also noted that hypomania, with attenuated manic symptoms is greatly under-diagnosed, particularly outside the psychiatric setting [Braunwald *et al.*, 2002].

Disturbed sleep and sleep deprivation are triggers for episodes of mania. Thus, shift work or work involving long distance air travel may not be suitable for individuals with bipolar disorders [Teasdale & Deahl 2007]. Based upon a literature review and clinical research experience, Tse [2002] proposed guidelines for an integrated approach to employment of persons with bipolar disorders. This approach incorporates clinical, vocational training and employment services. Rapid job placement is recommended rather than prolonged pre-vocational assessment and training, in light of frequently high educational level and vocational experiences prior to the onset of illness. Interventions proposed in these guidelines involve working with an individual client, garnering support from workmates, managers, as well as the personal social network, advising the employers on provision of support systems within the actual workplace and liaising with government agencies to reinforce the client's aspiration to work.

Key issues impacting upon employment and occupational rehabilitation of persons with bipolar disorders include: "i) the recurrent nature of their illness; ii) their limited ability to cope with stress and iii) the loss of confidence that results from illness episodes" [Tse & Yeats 2002].

Bipolar disorders have been found to be associated with 2.5 times more lost work days per ill worker compared with major depression. Greater severity and length of depressive episodes were reportedly the major effect upon lost work time [Kessler *et al.*, 2006]. It has therefore been suggested that more attention should be given to bipolar disorders with regard to work fitness and rehabilitation programs.

There is some evidence that social support may be associated with improved clinical outcome among individuals with bipolar disorder. However, due to the complex dynamics of this disorder, it may be that more support is forthcoming to those with initial hypomania or euphoric mania compared to those with both polarities [Goodwin & Jamison 2007].

4.1.6 *Psychotic disorders*

It is estimated that approximately one-third of patients with psychosis will fully recover, particularly if the onset of psychosis is rapid and prior history is normal. Paranoid or delusional disorders are considered to be justifiable causes for disqualification from jobs that are "safety-sensitive" such as police work, commercial driving or work with classified information. The "duty to warn" in these situations, preempts patient consent of release of medical information [Pro 2005].

Anecdotal reports are given of successful maintenance of employment in sectors affecting public safety, despite several severe episodes of psychosis. In these cases, low dose medication, full disclosure to the employer and active support were vital [Teasdale & Deahl 2007]. Overall, for persons recovering from psychosis, finding workplaces where they feel encouraged and comfortable appears to be an important factor in vocational success [Woodside *et al.*, 2006].

4.1.7 *Alcohol and drug misuse*

Sick leave or transfer to a non-safety critical job may be necessary in this context. After treatment of the disorder, the RTW process may include a signed contract with explicit description of the expected behavior. Supervisors and coworkers often identify signs of relapse.

Using this strategy, the London subway system has approximately a 75% success rate at 1-year follow up for workers with serious alcohol or drug-related disorders requiring residential treatment. An 85% success rate (return to flying) is cited for pilots in the U.K. whose fitness certification was withdrawn for alcohol or drug-related reasons, and who underwent treatment and rehabilitation [Carlton *et al.*, 2007].

4.2 Neurological Disorders

Guidelines are not readily available regarding the relationship between work performance and neurological illness. Modified work is recommended, assuming that the patient is mentally competent, with an emphasis upon work autonomy in order to adapt to the constraints of the neurological disorder [Klimek 2005].

4.2.1 *Migraine headaches*

We noted in Chapter 2, that sickness absence is a frequent consequence of headaches in general, and migraine headaches, in particular [Wilcox 2007]. Migraine headaches are also associated with underperformance while at work [Stewart *et al.*, 1995]. Severity appears to be an important determinant of performance decrement [Pransky *et al.*, 2005]. Headaches are often associated with co-morbidity, particularly depression, which is also of relevance to the workplace. Persons with relatively frequent migraines (bimonthly or more) are most likely to be absent from work, as well as underperforming while at work [Stewart *et al.*, 1995].

Workplace factors that can trigger headaches include chemicals, unstable temperature, lighting, irregular sleep and/or meal patterns, *inter alia* [Willcox & Hardy 2007]. The limited data in this regard suggests that psychosocial job stressors may also be triggers of headache [Cheng *et al.*, 2001] [French *et al.*, 2000] [Milutinović *et al.*, 2012].

An important measure at the workplace is to provide a quiet, dark room for rest if the migraine headache attack occurs at work. Safety-critical jobs such as ATC and airline piloting may be precluded by migraine headaches [Willcox & Hardy 2007]. In preparing for RTW, a challenge of graded activity and exercise together with a headache diary or headache scale are recommended [Klimek 2011].

4.2.2 *Epilepsy*

Employment limitations are noted to be a major concern for patients with epilepsy. Even among those without recent seizures, unemployment rates are reportedly high, and often attributed directly epilepsy [Fisher *et al.*, 2000] [Holland *et al.*, 2009] [Strine *et al.*, 2005]. However, among a small cohort of adults in Sweden with newly diagnosed unprovoked epileptic seizures, no adverse consequences upon employment *per se* were noted compared to healthy referents after 10 years of follow-up, although income was lower among the patients with epilepsy [Lindsten *et al.*, 2002]. In contrast, a Japanese study reports that 40 of 278 patients stated that they resigned from their jobs due to epileptic seizures [Wada *et al.*, 2001].

Several of the psychosocial problems cited above in relation to mental health disorders are also noted for epilepsy, namely stigma and fear of other people's reactions, as well as shame and embarrassment [Fisher 2000]. In the U.K. for example, 53% of employed persons with epilepsy chose not to reveal their illness [Dalrymple & Appleby 2000]. Employers are noted to often be reluctant to have employees with epilepsy return to work, for fear of disruption or injury at the workplace [Klimek 2011].

Psychological distress is reportedly more common among U.S. adults with epileptic seizures compared to persons without seizures [Strine *et al.*, 2005]. In our clinical experience, insofar as the patient with epilepsy adheres to the appropriate therapeutic regimen and is free from comorbidities, work capacity can be maintained. In fact, often times, patients with epilepsy show a high affinity towards their work, which provides them with emotional satisfaction and pride.

Seizures frequently occur at the sleep-waking interface. This is particularly observed in idiopathic generalized epilepsy [Brown & Prevett 2007]. There is some evidence that persons with epilepsy may choose to avoid shift work [Dasgupta *et al.*, 1982]. Those who work night shifts may thus be a highly selected group, and for that reason, a significant association between seizure frequency and night shift work has not been documented. However, since sleep deprivation is a frequent concomitant of night shift work, and is also a recognized trigger of seizures, it has been recommended that night shift work be avoided by patients with idiopathic generalized seizures [Brown & Prevett 2007].

There are anecdotal reports of a relation between exposure to stressors and seizure frequency. This is attributed to changes in arousal level that can trigger neuronal discharge. On the other hand, lack of activity can also lead to increased seizure frequency. It is noted that exposure to stressors should be taken into consideration with regard to the work and responsibility of persons with epilepsy [Brown & Prevett 2007].

Photosensitivity may also be increased with sleep deprivation. While photosensitive-epilepsy is rare in adults, when present it can be triggered by exposure to flickering light and glare. Visual display equipment is usually considered to be safe for persons with photosensitive epilepsy. Special circumstances such as exposure to slow flicker from helicopter blades prompted routine EEG recording as part of the medical screening of helicopter pilots.

Some general "common sense" restrictions regarding the work of persons with epilepsy have been outlined. These include avoidance of: climbing and work at heights without protection; driving or operating machinery with motors; work need unguarded machinery, fire or water; working for extended periods of time in an isolated setting. Power tools that are hand-held may be a hazard as well. Overall, sectors in which a single seizure could have serious or even fatal consequences include transport and the building trades or other jobs entailing work on heights. More specific licensing regulations have been formulated, e.g. in the U.K, regarding driver's licenses and epilepsy.

Due to competitive disadvantage, many persons with a past or present history of epilepsy do not disclose this information when applying for work or during work-related medical examinations. The need "to drop old prejudices in favor of current knowledge about epilepsy" is underscored (p. 187)[Brown & Prevett 2007].

4.2.3 *Disorders of sleep and awareness*

Perhaps the most important consideration is the generic finding that sleep disturbances (insomnia symptoms as specified by the DSM-IV) are significantly associated with increased risk of disabling mental health disorders, as well as disability from physical illnesses, including musculoskeletal disorders. This statement is based upon a longitudinal study of over 50 000 public sector employees from Finland, who were free of work disability at the beginning of the study and with adjustment for numerous sociodemographic, behavioral and clinical factors [Salo *et al.*, 2010].

As to more specific disorders of sleep and awareness, obstructive sleep apnea is a major concern. Besides the neurocognitive and cardiovascular consequences, obstructive sleep apnea can interfere with normal work [Caples *et al.*, 2005]. Persons suffering from this disorder usually have difficulty with rotating shift work. Safety considerations are obviously crucial for motor vehicle operations with respect to obstructive sleep apnea and those with suggestive symptoms and obesity should be worked-up with overnight oximetry. The rare syndromes of classical narcolepsy and cataplexy are also potential hazards at work. Attention to adequate nocturnal sleep and planned daytime naps together with medication are warranted [Willcox & Hardy 2007]. The considerations of effect of work hours upon cognitive function, as discussed in Chapter 2, obviously take on a much greater salience among persons with disorders of sleep and awareness.

4.2.4 *Disorders related to neurotoxicity exposure*

It is not considered advisable for a person with pre-existing neuropathy to have any exposure to neurotoxic substances, regardless of the safety precautions. When a toxic exposure is expected to have contributed to or exacerbated a neurological condition, a detailed occupational and environmental history is essential, with attention to the specific tasks, use of protective equipment as well as the chemicals involved.

Preventive actions are recommended such as implementation of proper ventilation systems, ergonomic and tool safety measures and isolation to protect workers against dangerous exposures. Educational programs are also advisable, especially with regard to proper use of protective equipment. It is also vital to ensure that this equipment is suitable and properly functioning [Willcox & Hardy 2007].

4.2.5 *Cerebrovascular disorders*

Clearly, the location and size of an acute stroke will critically determine the recovery process including RTW. Risk of recurrence and sudden incapacitation is considered generally relatively low, although precautions about work in isolation as well as regarding operation of a motor vehicle, etc. are warranted. The specifics of these restrictions depend upon the clinical features to which we allude above [Willcox & Hardy 2007].

In a small qualitative study from Sweden among patients who had suffered a cerebrovascular accident, RTW was found to be facilitated by "understanding and positive attitude of co-workers." "Will" and "self-efficacy" were also found to promote RTW [Medin *et al.*, 2006]. In our clinical experience, insofar as the appropriate modified work conditions can be instituted after a cerebrovascular accident, the majority of patients successfully return to work; indeed, RTW provides them with emotional satisfaction and stability.

4.2.6 *Brain tumors*

Considerations regarding RTW are based upon function, similarly to the approach for stroke. However, the histological characteristics affecting prognosis must be borne in mind. There is a risk of symptomatic seizures particularly post-craniotomy or if the cerebral cortex has been affected by e.g. gliomas or meningiomas [Willcox & Hardy 2007].

There have been a few published studies concerning RTW among patients with treated brain tumors. In one small series, the majority of patients with malignant glioma either took early retirement or had markedly diminished work activity [Davies *et al.*, 2003]. However, in certain individual cases occupational activity proceeded successfully. For example, a self-employed engineer who managed all aspects of his work was able to continue exactly as before the diagnosis, and an illustrator was able to use computer skills to overcome sensory loss in one hand [Davies *et al.*, 2003]. Among 155 patients with treated intracranial meningioma at follow-up telephone interview, at least 75% reported being able to work, concentrate, sleep adequately, as well as make decisions, remember new things, put their thoughts into action, find the right words, write, read and drive as before [Kalkanis *et al.*, 2000].

> Work fitness and occupational rehabilitation in relation to other malignancies are considered in the next section.

4.3 Experience Regarding Work Fitness and Rehabilitation from Other Areas of Medicine

We now examine some other areas of medicine in which insights can be gleaned regarding work fitness and rehabilitation. Attention should be paid to co-morbidity, bearing in mind that mental health disturbances are frequent concomitants of somatic disease, and the close interface with work activity. Regarding chronic somatic disease, a systematic review of cohort studies reveals common prognostic factors for work disability. These include somatic complaints, limitations in daily activity due to the disease, heavy manual work and female gender [Detaille *et al.*, 2009].

4.3.1 *Oncology*

With progress in diagnostics and therapy, increasing numbers of patients return to their jobs after, or even during cancer treatment. Return to work is recognized as an important component of quality of life for patients with cancer, helping them maintain not only economic, but also *emotional* stability. In a study from the U.S. of 1162 survivors of cancer, 81% stated that their job helped them maintain emotional stability during treatment. However, workers with cancer are reportedly fired or laid off at five times the rate than other workers in the U.S., notwithstanding that fact that 40% of those with cancer missed fewer than 5 days during an average month due to treatment. Altogether, 19% felt they couldn't handle the job, although 33% of supervisors thought so and 14% had their work responsibilities decreased due to diagnosis of cancer [Journal National Cancer Institute 1998].

• Fatigue: This is the most common sequela of cancer therapy [Smith & Toonen 2007] and is identified as a barrier to return to work for patients with breast cancer [Tamminga *et al.*, 2011]. Similarly to the observations concerning chronic fatigue syndrome presented earlier in this chapter, graded exercise programs have been helpful for patients with cancer suffering from fatigue. Depression is also highly prevalent among patients with cancer, and has a deleterious effect upon survival [Watson *et al.*, 1999].

• Rehabilitation programs and work: A series of studies from Oslo, Norway was devoted to rehabilitation to working life among patients with breast, prostate and testicular cancer without early relapse after primary treatment. It was confirmed that holding a job was a key prerequisite for maintaining healthy living conditions [Gudbergsson 2007] [Gudbergsson *et al.*, 2006]. In Stockholm, Sweden a team rehabilitation program was developed for women with lymphedema after breast cancer surgery. The team consisted of a physiotherapist, social worker, oncologist, occupational therapist and nurse. A large number of the participants increased the percentage of working time after participating in the program. Several participants considered that this special rehabilitation program played a critical role in their ability to return to work [Johnsson 2003].

• Recommendations against shift work for previous or current breast cancer: As noted in Chapter 2, on the basis of the current evidence, including the experimental evidence that tumor growth is accelerated by suppression of melatonin secretion, it is now recommended that women with previous or current breast cancer be advised against working night shifts [Bonde *et al.*, 2012].

• Systematic review in progress: We are currently performing a systematic review in which we have identified over 50 articles published within the last decade in which empirical data are presented concerning RTW among patients with various types and stages of cancers. The studies have been of various designs: cross-sectional, case-control and longitudinal. However, we have found no intervention studies in which work-related factors were modified as part of controlled clinical trials, which should be the ultimate goal. Moreover, there has not been any *systematic* assessment of work stressors in any of these papers. Nevertheless, some qualitative insights often based upon individual patients could be gleaned. These include the importance of work schedules, support from supervisor and general social support, considerations of physical and chemical exposures, difficulties about privacy (self-disclosure) and role ambiguity for health professionals with cancer, as well as concerns about employment discrimination and perceptions about diminished work capacities from employers and sometimes from colleagues. The importance of these factors *vis-à-vis* cancer risk as well as prognosis [Knutsson *et al.*, 2012] [Lutgendorf *et al.*, 2005] [Schernhammer *et al.*, 2001] [Schernhammer *et al.*, 2003] was underscored in Chapter 2.

• Role of the physician: A recent publication from Belgium regarding RTW for patients with breast cancer indicates that treating physicians do not consider themselves competent to provide advice concerning work-related issues. On the other hand, in some countries, occupational physicians have been precluded from involvement in the RTW process due to legislative constraints [Tiedtke *et al.*, 2011]. Concordantly, qualitative studies from the U.S. and from the Netherlands among patients with breast cancer revealed that little guidance was provided by the physicians regarding the patients' work [Main *et al.*, 2005] and that such guidance is needed [Tamminga *et al.*, 2011].

4.3.2 *Ischemic heart disease and hypertension*

• Psychological factors are closely intertwined with issues concerning work fitness/return to work for persons with cardiovascular disease. First of all, it should be emphasized that negative emotions can act as a mediator in the causal pathway between occupational stressors and ischemic heart disease (IHD) [Kubzansky & Kawachi 2000]. It has been stated that cardiovascular symptoms may be "out of all proportion to the objective evidence of disease" and that this may be due to the "profound psychological disturbance that can follow the development of cardiovascular disease" (p. 381) [Price & Petch 2007]. On the other hand, our clinical experience is that denial of cardiovascular symptoms is also a frequent occurrence, particularly in evaluations of work fitness where fear of losing one's job comes into play [Schnall & Belkić 2000]. Anxiety among patients as well as their families after the occurrence of cardiac events can also impact profoundly upon return to work [Price & Petch 2007]. In light of the focus of the present book, the coexistence of cardiovascular disease and mental health disorders should thus be especially borne in mind. This has been particularly emphasized by Melamed and colleagues who examined in depth the relation between burnout and cardiovascular disease [Melamed *et al.*, 2006].

• Hypertension and IHD must be viewed in a special light for jobs that can impact upon public safety. Unmanaged hypertension can be associated with symptoms such as headaches, dizziness and malaise that interfere with job performance. Importantly, many of these jobs also entail cardionoxious exposures that can exacerbate hypertension as well as other cardiovascular parameters. Risk of cardiac syncope is obviously one of the most critical concerns, requiring appropriate cardiologic workup [De Gaudemaris 2000].

• Most of the clinical guidelines relevant to the interface between the workplace and the patient's cardiovascular system continue to be focused upon levels of physical exertion [Belkić, Landsbergis *et al.*, 2004]. Thus, when assessing limitations of work capacity, these are typically based upon non-invasive evaluation through echocardiography and exercise testing [Hyman 2005] [Price & Petch 2007]. Cardiac rehabilitation is recognized as an important intervention, which improves physical capacity and survival in patient with IHD. However, this does not necessarily lead to return to work [Hyman 2005]. Crucially, as can be noted from Chapter 2, many of the occupations and exposures associated with high risk for IHD or hypertension are unrelated to levels of physical exertion. The challenge remains, as articulated well over two decades ago, to offer the cardiac patient a style of life and of work, which will protect both his or her health and the right to be productive [Maisano 1988]. This concern becomes especially salient with regard to psychosocial workplace exposures, such as job strain, in view of the evidence that chronic exposure to job strain is associated with a significant independent risk of recurrent cardiac events after the 1st myocardial infarction [Aboa-Éboulé *et al.*, 2007] [Lásló *et al.*, 2010] [Theorell *et al.*, 1991].

• Given the importance of these psychosocial and other workplace factors in the etiology and progression of IHD and hypertension, we have developed proposals for an integrated and *graded* approach to occupational cardiologic work-up, based upon the degree of CVD severity [Belkić, Schnall & Uglješić 2000]. This can include laboratory cardiovascular testing of workplace stressors and the use of ambulatory blood pressure and electrocardiographic monitoring during work [Belkić 2003]. Concordantly, Hyman [2005] states: "a trial of return to work with blood pressure monitoring at work is almost always indicated" (p. 254). As per the original formulation by Maisano [Maisano 1988], there is a pressing need to realize the potential of occupational cardiology as a discipline, which would move beyond strictly observational epidemiological studies to evidence-based prevention-oriented clinical practice [Belkić, Schnall *et al.*, 2002]. There have not yet been any larger-scale intervention studies examining the effect of ameliorating exposure to job strain or other cardionoxious factors among those with hypertension, or who are otherwise at high risk for developing IHD, or for patients who have already suffered a cardiac event. Nevertheless, our clinical experience indicates that implementing changes in the work environment, especially with regard to work schedules, together with interventions aimed at the promoting healthy coping strategies and at the standard cardiac risk factors have been effective in protecting working patients from further clinical deterioration, together with maintaining work capacity, including for jobs impacting upon public safety [Belkić, Savić *et al.*, 1995]. We have found that interventions aimed exclusively at the standard cardiac risk factors without concomitant changes in the work environment for workers in highly stressful occupations such as professional driving, meet with limited success [Emdad *et al.*, 1998a] [Uglješić, Belkić, Simeunović-Micković, Vukajlović 1992].

• Modifications of work schedules (timing and length) are among the most immediately feasible ways to ameliorate the effects of job strain and other cardio-deleterious exposures [Belkić, Schnall & Uglješić 2000]. We have suggested that these and other strategies should be explored in randomized clinical trials, which would not only provide a needed link in etiological research, but would also be helpful for developing evidence-based guidelines for prevention-oriented care of working patients at high risk for or with manifest IHD [Belkić, Landsbergis, *et al.*, 2004]. These recommendations are corroborated by Price & Petch [2007], who state: "the conclusion that psychosocial factors are important in the development of [IHD] is now inescapable, such that efforts should be made in the workplace to reduce these factors. The relative contribution as compared with traditional risk factors and how best to ameliorate their impact are questions that merit urgent clarification" (p. 393).

4.3.3 *Rheumatologic / musculoskeletal disorders*

• Depression and anxiety are recognized as frequent concomitants of chronic rheumatologic disorders, including rheumatoid arthritis and systemic sclerosis [Smallwood-Sherrer 2005] [Ostojić *et al.*, 2010]. High pain and depression scores are typically not reflected in the degree of disease severity [Smallwood-Sherrer 2005]. Loss of work in itself has been associated with high levels of depression and pain among patients with rheumatoid arthritis [Fifield *et al.*, 1991].

• Systemic sclerosis has a major impact upon work productivity. A recent study from Los Angeles of 162 patients with scleroderma revealed that 40% reported disability due to the disease [Singh *et al.*, 2012].

• For patients with rheumatoid arthritis, avoidance of heavy manual labor and repetitive motion of the involved joints is recommended [Cox & Nugent 2007]. Handling aids, ergonomic adjustments and relocation and training for physically less strenuous work are cited as possible strategies to help patients with rheumatoid arthritis continue to work [Ryder & Bird 2007]. With regard to osteoarthritis, maintaining flexibility and motion of the involved joints is emphasized, although heavy labor is not advisable. Aids such as dictaphones or other types of voice-activated systems are often helpful when the hand joints are affected. Carpal tunnel syndrome should be managed by avoiding: poor wrist and forearm posture, lengthy flexion and repetitive movements of the wrist, exposure to handheld vibrating tools, as well as direct pressure over the carpal tunnel itself. Minimizing repetitive use of tools, especially those entailing vibration is particularly important for disorders of the shoulder. In general, avoiding or diminishing the precipitating activity, modifications in posture, technique and equipment, as well as appropriate pacing and rest breaks are important considerations for promoting return to work for persons with musculoskeletal disorders [Ryder & Bird 2007].

• Lack of control over work activities and pace is found to be associated with lowered chances of remaining on the job for patients with chronic rheumatologic disorders [Smallwood-Sherrer 2005]. Control within the workplace is reportedly linked to successful return to work among patients with rheumatoid arthritis. A 2-year prospective Swedish study of 110 patients with early rheumatoid arthritis examined an active team support program, including rehabilitation meetings with the employer, together with disease-modifying medications. This program was found to effectively prevent or delay work disability [Nordmark *et al.*, 2006]. Low support from coworkers and employers who are reluctant to retain workers with chronic rheumatologic disorders further compromise the chances of staying on the job. Education can be helpful in this regard [Smallwood-Sherrer 2005].

• Musculoskeletal disorders frequently result in absence from work. In Sweden, e.g., these are the major cause of sickness absence [Holmgren & Dahlin Ivanoff 2004]. Some evidence-based return-to-work guidelines for various musculoskeletal disorders have been formulated by the Royal College of General Practitioners in the U.K. For example, for a new episode of low-back pain without any indication of serious spinal pathology, RTW is advised at an early stage, even if this results in some residual discomfort. It is considered preferable to temporarily transfer the employee to lighter duties or modified work rather than interrupting employment [Palmer & Greenbough 2007]. However, a retrospective cohort study of persons with lower back pain indicates that restricted duties did not diminish the incidence or length of sickness absence [Hiebert *et al.*, 2003]. On the other hand, introduction of preventive measures such as mechanical lifts in hospitals has been shown to diminish sickness absence due to low back pain among nurses [Evanoff *et al.*, 2003]. Other recommended measures for return-to-work including training to improve awareness and implementation of better work practices, providing an "induction" period during which a worker can proceed at a slower pace with unfamiliar tasks; job rotation and rest breaks to avoid sustained repetitive motion; task optimization to reduce heavy lifting and awkward positions, high stools to avoid prolonged standing and the use of lifting aids [Cox & Nugent 2007] [Palmer & Greenbough 2007].

• The physician can play an important role in the RTW process for patients with musculoskeletal disorders. In a study from California, physician recommendation that the patient is ready to return to work after low back injury has been associated with a significantly higher percentage of RTW during the subacute or chronic phase, after adjusting for injury severity as well as for workload factors [Dasinger *et al.*, 2001].

• Early rehabilitation is important for musculoskeletal disorders, since this increases the likelihood of RTW [Lydell *et al.*, 2009]. Six-year follow-up has been performed on a multi-professional 8-week rehabilitation program from Sweden among 122 participants with musculoskeletal disorders [Norrefalk *et al.*, 2007]. Fifty-two percent had returned to work compared to 13% of the referents. Relative to the period prior to rehabilitation, there was a significantly higher level of activity, as well as reduction in pain and analgesic consumption among the participants.

• The effect of modified work upon RTW, among persons with musculoskeletal disorders has received some attention [Loisel *et al.*, 2005] [van Dujin *et al.*, 2005]. The conclusions are somewhat contradictory. Loisel and colleagues [2005] consider that the current evidence indicates that advice to return to modified work and graded activity programs are effective in preventing work disability related to musculoskeletal disorders. However, modified work entailing substantial reduction in work tasks or working hours as the only advice given by occupational health physicians did not influence total duration of sick leave due to musculoskeletal complaints [van Dujin *et al.*, 2005]. The overall conclusion is that more precise and practical recommendations are needed, with "future studies {involving} all relevant stakeholders…{aimed} at developing new strategies that are effective, efficient and have a potential for successful implementation" (p. 507)[Loisel *et al.*, 2005].

4.3.4 *Diabetes, peptic ulcer disease and other gastrointestinal disorders*

• Previously, persons with diabetes reportedly faced problems in relation to employment [Waclawski 1989]. More recently, it has been found that having diabetes does not diminish one's chances of entering the labor market, nor do younger persons with Type 1 diabetes have increased levels of unemployment. In the U.K., the requirements of the Disability Discrimination Act have been "wholly beneficial" in diminishing outright bans against persons with diabetes (p. 351) [Waclawski & Gill 2007]. Nevertheless, certain justifiable restrictions are still in place concerning risk of hypoglycemia and jobs affecting public safety such as airline piloting, truck driving, fire fighting, work in foundries or work on scaffoldings. Even these restrictions have "room for latitude" (p. 351), based upon diabetic control and the cooperation of the patient.

• With regard to shift work, as noted, control of blood glucose was significantly better among 120 day workers in Bangkok compared to 120 shift workers matched for age, duration of DM and use of hypoglycemic agents. The two groups did not differ significantly in BMI; however, there were significantly more shift workers with abnormal GHQ scores [Chalernvanichakorn *et al.*, 2008]. Still, in clinical practice, shift work is not considered to be completely contraindicated for persons with diabetes. Rapidly rotating shifts appear to be particularly undesirable for persons with insulin-treated diabetes [Waclawski & Gill 2007].

• As the therapy for peptic ulcer disease has become more effective, less attention has been given to contributory psychosocial factors. Nevertheless, work stressors are recognized as potential triggers of symptoms related to peptic ulcer disease, PUD. It is therefore suggested that when these factors are identified as the source of these symptoms, they "should be addressed through management intervention in preference to controlling symptoms with long-term medication" (p. 316) [Astbury & Southgate 2007]. As discussed in Chapter 2, there is a strong association between peptic ulcer disease and shift work [Knutsson 2003]. However, many persons with PUD are able to work the night shift without notable exacerbation of their condition. Therefore, *a priori* exclusion from shift work is not necessarily warranted solely on the basis of a diagnosis of PUD [Astbury & Southgate 2007].

• Inflammatory bowel disease can create problems that lead to sickness absence. Patients with severe disease are less likely to be able to work [Astbury & Southgate 2007]. Practical issues such as the access to restroom facilities and flexibility regarding when breaks are taken can play in important role in maintaining work capacity. Production line work and jobs involving public safety may be therefore precluded for persons with symptomatic inflammatory bowel disease. Although typically milder, irritable bowel syndrome can create similar problems.

4.3.5 *Respiratory disorders*

A relatively well-developed, integrated approach to work fitness and occupational rehabilitation exists with regard to respiratory disorders. This is incorporated into the clinical practice of pulmonary medicine and more broadly into general internal medicine, as evidenced by a full chapter on "Environmental Lung Disease" included in the more recent editions of Harrison's Principles of Internal Medicine [Balmes & Spiezer 2011]. Within these more recent editions of Harrison's Principles of Internal Medicine, including the 18th Edition, 2012 it is only for lung disease that a full chapter focusing on the relation to the environment, with a focus on occupational disease, is provided.

Of fundamental importance is the recognition that job-related and other environmental hazards contribute to many pulmonary disease processes, and that "unless the underlying connection with hazardous exposures is identified and mitigated, treatment of the manifestations rather than the cause at best only ameliorates the condition. At worst, the neglect of hazardous exposures may lead to both failure of treatment and failure to recognize a public health problem with wide significance" (p. 19) [Hu & Speizer 1998].

A large number of pulmonary disorders are defined and managed according to these principles. These include occupational asthma, hypersensitivity pneumonitis, pneumoconiosis and reactive airways dysfunction syndrome [Hyman 2005]. Pulmonary medicine sub-specialists are mandated to carefully inquire about workplace exposures [Spiezer 1998]. The need for a high index of suspicion regarding occupational asthma is emphasized, with recommendations for measuring forced expiratory volume in 1 second (FEV1) before and after a work shift, as well as for laboratory pulmonary function studies to identify responses to potentially broncho-constricting agents to which the patient is exposed [Palmer & Pearson 2007]. Protection from exposure is viewed as the fundamental intervention, both on the individual level as well as wider measures to protect the workforce. A classical example is byssinosis, due to exposure to cotton dust, as briefly summarized in Panel 4.2.

Pulmonary Medicine in Clinical Practice: A Key Example

• Symptom: "Monday chest tightness"

Prompts query about:

• Exposure to cotton dust—Byssinosis

• Up to 80% of exposed workers can have a fall in FEV_1 as a sign of bronchial airway constriction

• Therapeutic Measures: "*Clearly, reduction of dust exposure is of primary importance.*"

Panel 4.2 An approach to work fitness and the work environment from pulmonary medicine (Quotation from p. 1433 [Speizer 1998]).

The distinction also needs to be made between actual sensitization asthma whereby exposure to minute amounts of the substance elicits severe bronchospasm versus substances that act more non-specifically as irritants. In the latter case, return to work within the same industry is potentially more feasible [Palmer & Pearson 2007].

The International Labor Organization (ILO) has an established classification system for evaluating chest x-rays to detect and monitor pulmonary responses to mineral dusts. Although these roentgenographic findings do not always correspond to the extent of functional impairment, this system is very useful for screening large numbers of workers [Speizer 1998].

It is also within the realm of pulmonary medicine that the relationship between exposure to respiratory carcinogens and occurrence of specific cancers has been especially well-recognized. It has often been the "astute clinician" who noted an increased incidence of the malignancy within a given occupational setting [Speizer 1998]. A classic example is that of Dr. Irving Selikoff and colleagues in the relation between asbestos exposure and mesothelioma, as well as pulmonary interstitial fibrosis (asbestosis).

These efforts have lead to legislative actions to protect workers as well as the wider public from exposure to asbestos and many other substances.

As a result of U.S. federal legislation, the levels of dust in coal mines have been substantially reduced. Moreover, the Black Lung Trust Fund taxes coal companies on a per-ton-of-coal basis and uses these funds to pay the medical and indemnity benefits for persons who have developed pneumoconiosis [Leigh & Schnall 2000]. Despite these advanced measures and integrative approach, far more advanced than for most areas of medicine, as briefly reviewed in this chapter, it is still considered that the contribution of occupation/environmental factors to respiratory disease is "generally underestimated" (p. 20) [Hu & Speizer 1998].

4.4 Special Issues for Work Fitness and Occupational Rehabilitation

We conclude this chapter with attention to two special issues regarding work fitness and occupational rehabilitation. The first is public safety, to which we alluded frequently. Next, we revisit the discussion of women and work within the rehabilitation framework, and segue into a broader and more grounded clinical approach to work and mental health, as informed by cognitive ergonomics and brain research, via the Occupational Stressor Index [Belkić 2003] to which the next chapter is devoted.

4.4.1 *Further considerations about public safety*

We have noted throughout this chapter that whenever public safety may be affected, particular caution is needed in approaching questions of work fitness and occupational rehabilitation. In general, such work tasks fall into the category of "safety critical," meaning that impairment can place others at risk [Carter, Major *et al.*, 2007]. This is especially the case with regard to neuropsychiatric and cardiovascular disorders, as well as hypoglycemia associated with diabetes mellitus, where sudden loss of consciousness or impaired judgement or cognitive function could occur. Normal corrected vision, hearing and vestibular function are also of obvious concern in this framework.

In the U.S. federal law may prohibit workers in safety-sensitive occupations, such as professional drivers or nuclear power plant operators, from taking medications that could impair safe performance of their work [Aronoff *et al.*, 2005]. In particular, psychoactive medications may affect psychomotor and driving ability, and therefore may require work restrictions. Tricyclic antidepressants should be avoided. Only under the stringent review of a neuropsychiatrist qualified in this area should neuroleptics be permitted for a professional driver. Sedating anxiolytics are considered incompatible with professional driving, and should only be used if the half life is < 5 hours for less than 2 weeks, under medical supervision and with the lowest possible dose. Stimulants such as those prescribed for attention deficit disorder also preclude professional driving, unless the patient is exempted after expert review.

Many of these occupations have highly developed and tested medical licensing standards. Among the most extensive and rigorous protocols for selection and licensing are for airline pilots, with internationally accepted standards of work fitness, particularly with respect to cardiovascular disease, hypertension, psychiatric and metabolic disorders as well as substance abuse [Dark 1987] [Johnston 2007] [Joy 1992]. Stringent licensing standards are also in place for air traffic controllers and sea pilots [Johnston 2007] [Carter 2007]. Commercial or professional ground transport licensing protocols are in place as well. Within the European Union, there are more stringent fitness requirements for driving vehicles over 3.5 tons or with more than eight passenger seats. The rationale is that accidents involving such vehicles result in greater damage as well as potential harm to a larger number of passengers. In various settings, similar restrictions are in place for taxi drivers and for drivers of high-speed vehicles [Carter, Major *et al.*, 2007a].

The U.S. Department of Transportation have developed specific criteria for permitting commercial drivers with hypertension to continue work. A one-year medical certification is permitted for drivers with blood pressure between 140 – 159 / 90 – 99 mm Hg. With levels of 160 – 179 / 100 – 109 mm Hg, a three-month medical certification is permitted. In both of these conditions, the certifying physician is mandated to refer the professional driver for treatment, such that blood pressure levels are lowered prior to expiration of the certification. These criteria may be amended insofar as concomitant diabetes or renal disease is present [Hyman 2005]. At the same time, it should be noted that many anti-hypertensive medications can cause dizziness, hypotension and fatigue mandating particular caution at the initiation of therapy. Clonidine, prazosin and some other anti-hypertensive medications can have major central nervous system effects that impact upon driving safety. Dehydration and electrolyte disturbances can also impair driving ability [Aronoff *et al.*, 2005].

Our particular concern has been that many of these occupations also entail exposure to job stressors that contribute to the development of the very disorders that would preclude work fitness, as reviewed in Chapter 2. The clinician is then faced with an exceedingly difficult dilemma when called upon to assess the work fitness. In attempting to make an informed judgment, the salient question must also be raised: "is the work environment fit, or conducive to health?" [Belkić, Landsbergis *et al.*, 2004].

4.4.1.1 *Suggestions for a safer return to work for professional drivers*

Modified work becomes imperative, with a view towards returning to or continuing with safer, healthier working conditions. Clearly, depriving persons of their occupational activity, often during the most productive years, can have devastating consequences for themselves and their families. Some proposals for return to work for professional drivers after e.g. clinical stabilization following an acute cardiac event have been suggested [Belkić *et al.*, 1998]. Many of these are in line with general suggestions for improving the working conditions of urban transit operators [Kompier & DiMartino1995] [Kompier *et al.*, 2000]. These include providing regular work assignments with two days off between blocks of work days, rest breaks after every two hours of work, *inter alia.* It has also been emphasized the "judicious choice of line assignments might also be a means of attenuating stress levels for the professional driver returning to work" [Belkić *et al.*, 1998] (p. 50). In particular, we recommended that a previous accident or near accident on a given route is ample cause for avoiding that route. The social support network can be of crucial importance in this process.

A small-scaled intervention study among city bus drivers in Stockholm revealed that improving bus routes and technological conditions were associated with a clinically important fall in blood pressure [Rydstedt *et al.*, 1998]. Tellingly, the study was denoted as "the human side of the road." In San Francisco, motivated by the high prevalence of hypertension among the urban transit operators related to number of years on the job [Ragland *et al.*, 1987], a special line was created to ameliorate the contributory stressors. Unfortunately, under-funding of public transportation impeded these efforts [Fisher & Belkić 2000].

An expanded occupational public-health role of the clinician could be crucial in this realm. One of the most urgent needs is for clinicians, together with occupational ergonomists and other specialists, to have greater influence to recommend and implement protective guidelines about work conditions for these jobs [Fisher & Belkić 2000]. A composite view to health promotion, improvements in the work environment and rehabilitation has been described in this light [Kristensen 2000]. As it now stands, the clinician is continually faced with the dilemma of making a judgment about the individual's work fitness, knowing full well that the job itself is contributing to the patient's work incapacity. The proactive approach which will be developed in this book offers the possibility of ameliorating this dilemma.

4.4.2 *Women, work fitness and return to work*

In the previous chapter, we began by a brief review of gender in relation to work stressors and health. These considerations have not yet made their way into the current standard of care regarding work fitness and occupational rehabilitation. Mainly, attention within this framework has been given to obstetric and gynecological issues, especially protection during pregnancy. Concerns include exposure to ionizing radiation, chemical and physical hazards, including risk of accident and violence at the workplace. With regard to workload and other psychological work stressors *vis-à-vis* the pregnant employee, it is noted that "where work is perceived to be more stressful than home life, giving time off may be pragmatic. However, for working women with small children at home, coming to work may be less demanding than 'rest' at home" (p. 451) [Coomber & Harris 2007]. Post-natal return to work issues are multi-faceted and complex, but some practical considerations include the feasibility of breastfeeding, the mandated availability (in the U.K.) of needed facilities, as well as potential hazardous substances. The need to screen for post-partum depression is emphasized, given that its prevalence is estimated at well over 10%.

The increasing numbers of women at work and the fact that there are slightly higher sickness absence rates among women, render the issues of work fitness and occupational rehabilitation particularly salient for women. In Sweden, persons exposed to work-related strain frequently become long-term sick listed, and this is especially the case for women [Holmgren & Dahlin Ivanoff 2004].

- **Remark in transition**

A critical factor for persons with mental and/or somatic health disorders can be the possibility of returning to modified, ***healthier*** work conditions. Conversely, it has been noted that presenteeism can be more dangerous for a person with ill-health with respect to exposure to adverse occupational factors, compared to healthy persons [Järvholm 2012].

A more advanced, integrative approach based upon an in-depth, comprehensive analysis of work stressors is clearly needed. Our experience within the clinical setting of burnout, depression, cancer, rheumatologic disorders and cardiovascular disease is that a strategy based upon the Occupational Stressor Index [Belkic 2003] can be effective in helping identify and ameliorate occupational stressors during RTW. This will be reviewed in the next Chapter.

Chapter 5

The Occupational Stressor Index (OSI): A Comprehensive Model derived from Cognitive Ergonomics for Clinical Practice

Looking at the previous three chapters together, we must admit that a certain incongruity emerges.

- If the work environment is so clearly associated with mental and somatic health and if we understand quite a bit about the mechanisms mediating exposure to occupational stressors and health outcomes, why is the current standard for medical evaluation of work fitness and return to work still relatively undeveloped in this regard?
- In particular, in light of our sophisticated knowledge about central mechanisms, why are we not better able to protect the mental health of working populations?
- Most specifically, would it not be possible to more effectively ameliorate those work stressors that trigger or exacerbate mental health disorders?

In the rest of this book, we will strive to address these challenges.

Here in Chapter 5, we present the Occupational Stressor Index (OSI) [Belkić 1989] [Belkić 2003], which is a clinically-applicable questionnaire-based tool for comprehensively evaluating the work environment.

The OSI incorporates key components of the sociologically-based work-stressor models: Job Strain [Karasek 1979] and Effort-Reward Imbalance [Siegrist 1996]. In contrast, however, the underpinnings of the OSI are cognitive ergonomics and brain research. Thereby the OSI focuses upon allocation of mental resources, analyzing how human beings process information, make decisions and carry out actions. Thus, many of the neurophysiologic insights from Chapter 3 are reflected in the OSI. From these insights, implementable workplace modifications become readily apparent.

In this Chapter we are presenting the key methodology that will be applied in the series of clinical cases that comprise Part II of this book.

5.1 Basis and Organization of the OSI

The OSI[1] provides an index of the total stressor load of the work environment, as well as an in-depth analysis of the nature of that burden. Within the OSI, the work environment is viewed as a whole, including task-level issues, work schedule, and physical, chemical and broader organizational factors that can all contribute to total burden. OSI. The OSI is quite akin to theory-guided observational approaches such as the RHIA/VERA method[2], which examines the mental structure of work tasks [Greiner & Krause 2000] [Volpert 1982]. However, since the Occupational Stressor Index is questionnaire-based, it does not require on-the-job analysis. Insofar as these are available, direct work-site measurements and other objective data about the workplace can be effectively incorporated into the OSI, and will improve its precision [Belkić 1989].

5.1.1 *The axes of the OSI: formation of a two-dimensional matrix*

There are two axes of the OSI: the vertical axis comprised of levels of information transmission and the horizontal axis composed of seven stressor aspects. These axes are merged to form a two-dimensional matrix. We will now review these two axes, and then show the complete OSI model in Figure 5.1.

5.1.1.1 Levels of information transmission: the vertical axis

The levels of information transmission [Welford 1960], that constitute the vertical axis of the OSI, were first presented in Chapter 3. Therein it was noted that these reflect how incoming signals are received, processed and acted upon (Panel 3.1).

---

[1] The OSI as of now is termed the "occupational stressor index", which is most consistent with the focus upon work place exposures, i.e. stressors, according to the definitions provided in Chapter 1.

[2] German abbreviation for "regulation barriers at work / methods to investigate regulation requirements at work".

The basic cognitive ergonomic processes are reflected in the three levels of information transmission. These can be mapped over time using neurophysiologic methods. These levels of information transmission provide a very useful format for categorizing a broad range of occupational endeavor, and have been used e.g., in work simulation analysis [Luczak 1971].

Recall that the first two levels (sensory input and decision making) are often "invisible," and are likely to be missed unless the queries are purposefully directed to capture them. Thus, for example, when people report working fast, they mainly look at the task performance level.

In the OSI we have added a fourth "General" level for elements that are related to the overall work environment and not localized to a specific level of information transmission. As will be clearly seen, this general level often is critical for identifying modifiable stressors.

5.1.1.2 Stressor aspects: the horizontal axis

The horizontal axis of the OSI contains the stressor aspects. These seven stressor aspects in the OSI are shown in Panel 5.1.

Stressor Aspects of the OSI Model

- Underload
- High demand
- Strictness
- Extrinsic time pressure
- Aversive/noxious exposures
- Symbolic aversiveness/threat-avoidant vigilance
- Conflict/uncertainty

Panel 5.1 Stressor aspects of the OSI model.

> Each of these stressor aspects contains individual elements organized according to the four levels of the OSI, as will be seen in the forthcoming.

- Underload

The first stressor aspect of the OSI is underload, the elements of which are shown in Panel 5.2. The three input level elements of underload are: homogeneous signals, low frequency of incoming signals and working alone without the need to communicate with others.

As noted in Chapter 3, not only exceedingly rapid, but also very slow rates of incoming signals can impair correct and timely performance. This is especially the case if the low flow of information is prolonged in duration. This observation coincides with the well-known "U" shaped-curve. Therein, it is shown that optimal performance is associated with moderate arousal levels, whereas a performance decrement, together with heightened catecholamine excretion, occur not only with overload but also with understimulation [Frankenhaeuser & Gardell 1976] [Hebb 1960].

The Underload Aspect of the OSI

- Input level
  - --Homogeneous signals
  - --Low frequency of incoming signals
  - --Working alone: without need for communication
- Central decision-making level
  - --Decisions automatic from input
- Task performance level
  - --Homogeneous tasks
  - --Simple tasks
  - --Nothing to do (including waiting time)
- General level
  - --Fixed pay
  - --Inadequate pay
  - --No chances for upgrade
  - --Lack of recognition of good work

Panel 5.2 Elements of the underload stressor aspect of the OSI.

Underload or monotony is characteristic of many types of automatic production work or long-distance driving, in which a high level of vigilance must be maintained to detect infrequently or irregularly occurring signals. Recall that task alternation and other countermeasures are needed to protect the health and safety of workers in such occupations [Braby *et al.*, 1993] [Levi 1981].

The general level elements of underload are quite similar to the reward component of Effort Reward Imbalance [Siegrist 1996]. These underload elements can coexist with demanding tasks, leading to the unhealthy combination of high effort and low reward.

Other combinations of high demands and underload can also be harmful [Levi 1981] [Braby *et al.*, 1993], including abrupt changes in work tempo from very slow to exceedingly rapid. Moreover, time spent at work waiting to perform one's tasks (an element of task performance underload in the OSI) is destimulating and frustrating. With improved organization, this stressor can often be ameliorated with enhanced productivity as well as job satisfaction.

- High demand

In Chapter 3, an in-depth review of psychological work demands was presented based upon cognitive ergonomics and neurophysiologic studies. Thereby, we demonstrated that it is possible to go much further than asking whether one "works hard" and "works fast," to analyze tasks in terms of time and allocation of mental resources. Recall once again that this is particularly vital for the first two levels (sensory input and decision-making) that are often "invisible." As seen in Panel 5.3, on the input level besides the number of signals to be processed, we consider their modality, complexity, dynamics, and sources. For example, the visual modality is known to place the greatest demands upon attentional resources, as do heterogeneous signals, especially if they come from various sources.

Proceeding to the level of central decision-making, we consider how many elements are involved (complicated) and their interrelation (complex), whether these affect the work of others, and how quickly the decision needs to be made. Next, we consider the nature, heterogeneity and time exigencies involved in task performance. Several of the modifiable stressors implicated in adverse mental health outcomes are found at the general level of the high demand aspect. These include long work hours, night shift work, lack of rest breaks or paid vacations, *inter alia*, as reviewed in Chapter 2.

The contribution of these stressors to fatigue was implicated in the event-related potential paradigms discussed in Chapter 3.

The High Demand Aspect of the OSI

- Input level
  - –Several sources of information
  - –Heterogeneous signals
  - –Heavy burden on the visual system
  - –High frequency of incoming signals
  - –Three sensory modalities
  - –Communication essential
- Central decision-making level
  - –Complex decisions
  - –Complicated decisions
  - –Decisions affect work of others
  - –Rapid decision-making
- Task performance level
  - –Heterogeneous tasks
  - –Simultaneous task performance
  - –Complex tasks
  - –Rapid task performance
- General level
  - –Piece rate work
  - –Long work hours
  - –Holds 2+ jobs
  - –Lack of rest breaks
  - –Night shift/irregular work hours
  - –Lack of paid vacations

Panel 5.3 Elements of the high demand stressor aspect of the OSI.

- Strictness

The strictness aspect of the OSI (Panel 5.4) is akin to lack of decision-making latitude, as per the Job Strain Model [Karasek 1979]. Once again, the levels of information transmission more precisely define the nature of the stressor and how it impacts upon the human nervous system. It is insufficiently appreciated, e.g., that strict requirements to detect incoming signals impose a heavy burden upon the CNS. Substantial mental resources are consumed whenever incoming signals cannot be ignored, as is the case, e.g. when sitting being the wheel of a motor vehicle.

When there is little or no room for deviation from a precise standard in decision-making or task performance, creativity and imagination are stifled. This is especially stressful when imposed arbitrarily, without a well-defined rationale for such strictness.

Physical constraints such as work in a fixed body position within a confined, crowded workspace are clearly unphysiological and can generate claustrophobia as well as potentially impacting upon self-esteem and dignity, as discussed in Chapter 3 [Brooker & Eakin 2001]. Possibilities for counter-measures are often quite easily implemented, and because physical change is readily apparent, this can have an immediate positive effect upon the individual employee as well as the work team.

The Strictness Aspect of the OSI

- Input level
--Strict requirements for signal detection

- Central decision-making level
--Strict problem-solving strategy
--Strictly defined correct decision

- Task performance level
--Work must meet a strictly defined standard

- General level
--Fixed body position
--Confined, windowless workspace
--Lack of autonomous workspace
--Limited in taking time off from work
Low influence over
--Schedule
--Tasks
--Policy
--With whom one works

Panel 5.4 Elements of the strictness stressor aspect of the OSI.

Particularly for those who are afflicted by mental health disorders, the possibility to take time off from work when needed is imperative [Tse 2002]. For many jobs, however, especially in the face of cutbacks in work staff, lack of backup personnel has severely limited this possibility. Influence over scheduling, work tasks, with whom one works as well as larger policy issues, can be improved within the context of e.g. "communicative action" [Habermas 1981], a practical method for democratic decision-making to provide employees with an opportunity for influence over their work situation [Gustavsen 1990].

- Extrinsic Time Pressure

In Chapter 3 we paid substantial attention to the impact of external time pressure upon mental workload. Based upon neurophysiologic evidence [Hohnsbein *et al.*, 1995], the potential of imposed time pressure to compromise safe performance was clearly seen. The mechanisms were outlined in Figure 3.5.

These experimental observations corroborate the documented increase in accident rate associated with external time pressure [Gardell *et al.*, 1983] [Green *et al.*, 1991] [Greiner *et al.*, 1998]. Because of its critical importance, within the OSI we treat extrinsic time pressure as a distinct stressor aspect. We thereby coalesce some features of both the high demand and decision-latitude dimensions of the Job Strain Model [Karasek 1979].

Panel 5.5 displays the five elements of extrinsic time pressure. On the input level, there is lack of control over speed of incoming signals in e.g. traffic or in other settings in which one does not have control over the number or nature of interactions with other people or with devices. In emergency situations of various types, as well as driving, decisions cannot be postponed.

Lack of control of rate of task performance is typical of paced work, as is still the case e.g. in many factories. An important consideration is whether the work is performed directly on an assembly line as opposed to those tasks that can be carried out off the line (on a separate desk or work station). In the latter case, the worker will usually have more moment-to-moment control over speed of performance.

Deadlines and speed-up can be viewed as exacerbating the overall time pressure, with possible deleterious consequences for health of the individual worker as well as for his or her performance, and potentially for public safety, as well.

The Extrinsic Time Pressure Aspect of the OSI

- Input level
  --No control over speed of incoming signals
- Central decision-making level
  --Decisions cannot be postponed
- Task performance level
  --No control over rate of task performance
- General level
  --Deadline pressure
  --Speed-up

Panel 5.5 Elements of the extrinsic time pressure stressor aspect of the OSI.

- Noxious exposures

Noxious physical exposures also contribute to the stressfulness of the work environment. Neurophysiologic data indicate that these exposures can consume substantial attentional resources. In Chapter 3, it was noted, e.g., that exposure to hypoxia, turbulence or noise during task performance was associated with a prolongation of P300 latency [Gunter *et al.*, 1987] [Kramer *et al.*, 1987] [Polich & Kok 1995].

Exposure to headlight glare has been shown to elicit EEG desynchronization indicative of central arousal, particularly among professional drivers [Belkić, Ercegovac *et al.*, 1992]. Besides being unpleasant and often distracting, numerous adverse somatic effects are well-recognized in association with exposure to various physical and chemical agents.

In constructing the OSI, we made particular note of the deleterious impact of these noxious physical and chemical factors upon the cardiovascular system [Belkić 1989] [Belkić, Savić *et al.*, 1995]. More recent reviews of this topic can be found in [Fine 2000a] and [Muzi *et al.*, 2004].

Panel 5.6 shows the noxious exposures included in the OSI, according to levels of information transmission. On the input level these include the visual and auditory stressors: glare and noise, respectively. Vibration and lifting are exposures directly associated with task performance. The overall work environment becomes physically uncomfortable insofar as the ambient temperature is not adequately regulated, or in the presence of noxious gases, fumes or dusts. Data about these physical factors may be available in the occupational records of a given workplace. In many countries, these are subject to control from the regulatory agencies, such as the National Institute for Occupational Safety and Health (NIOSH) and the Occupational Health and Safety Administration (OSHA) in the U.S. [Fine 2000b], or *Arbetsmiljöverket* in Sweden.

The Noxious Exposure Aspect of the OSI

- Input level
  --Glare
  --Noise
- Task performance level
  --Isometric Lifting
  --Vibration
- General level
  --Heat
  --Cold
  --Noxious gases, fumes, dusts

Panel 5.6 Elements of the noxious exposure stressor aspect of the OSI (also termed aversiveness, referring to these physical exposures).

- Threat avoidant vigilance

In Chapter 3, we reviewed the neurophysiologic concomitants of "threat-avoidant vigilance," TAV, noting that when the potential consequences of one's actions can include disaster, work becomes a "threat-avoidant" activity whose primary goal is self-protection. This is inevitably associated with negative emotions [Lazarus 1967] and often with adverse mental health outcomes. Recall that TAV places the heaviest burden upon conscious attentional resources. This is because, for survival reasons, our nervous systems are constructed to selectively allocate mental resources to threatening stimuli, even if the threat is only symbolic. We reviewed illustrations of this hidden burden upon attentional resources in studies of human electrocortical brain activity during simulated traffic situations [Belkić, Savić *et al.*, 1992] [Martin *et al.*, 1992].

The "symbolic-aversiveness" (or TAV) aspect is incorporated into OSI, but is not part of sociological work-stress models. Insufficient appreciation of TAV in occupational psychosocial research has lead to underestimations of the stressor burden of many occupations at increased risk for mental and somatic health disorders [Belkić 2003] [Belkić & Savić 2008].

The elements comprising the TAV dimension of the OSI are presented in Panel 5.7. Besides having to maintain high levels of attention, viewing visually disturbing scenes or listening to emotionally disturbing accounts comprise input level TAV.

The Threat Avoidant Vigilance Aspect of the OSI

• Input level
--High level of attention (Serious consequences of momentary lapse)
--Visually-disturbing scenes
--Listens to emotionally-disturbing accounts

• Central decision-making level
--Serious consequences of a wrong decision

• Task performance level
--Hazardous task performance

• General level
--Work Accident
--Witnessed work accident
--Suicide occurrence
--Work-related litigation/Testifying in court
--Lack of functioning emergency system

Panel 5.7 Elements of the threat avoidant vigilant stressor aspect of the OSI (also termed symbolic aversiveness or disaster potential).

Potentially serious consequences from a wrong decision represent TAV on the central level. Task performance level TAV is related to associated hazards. The five elements that contribute to general TAV are mainly cumulative over working life, such as having experienced or witnessed work accidents, the occurrence of suicide at work or involvement in litigation. Without a functioning emergency system, the general sense of safety at work is compromised.

- Conflict

From the vantage point of cognitive ergonomics, conflict and uncertainty add a qualitatively new stressor dimension. As stated by Neerincx and Griffoen [1996] "task load is not a simple summation of the load of the individual processes. Interference between concurrent information processes increases task load" (p. 545). In contrast to a normal, smooth work routine, in which there is reinforcement of the correctness of work decisions and actions, conflict or uncertainty arises when untimely or inaccurate correlations disrupt work and its rhythm. Pavlov [1951] has termed this the difficult meeting of excitation and inhibition in the brain.

The Conflict Aspect of the OSI

- Input level
--Signal/noise conflict
--Signal/signal conflict

- Central decision-making level
--Missing information needed for decision
--Contradictory information
--Unexpected events change work plan

- Task performance level
--Conflicting Demands
Task Performance hampered by:
--Extrinsic Problems
--Interruptions from people

- General level
--Emotionally charged work atmosphere
--Lack of help with work-related difficulties
--Opposition to career advancement
--Violations of behavioral norms/abuses of power
--Lack of mechanisms for redress of grievances
--Threat of job loss
--Job lacks coherence

Panel 5.8 Elements of the conflict stressor aspect of the OSI (also termed uncertainty).

Panel 5.8 shows the elements of conflict/uncertainty. On the input level these are 1) interference in identifying an incoming signal because of "noise"(signal/noise conflict) and 2) uncertainty in distinguishing the signal of interest from signals that should be ignored (signal/signal conflict).

On the central decision-making level the three elements are: missing information, contradictory information and unexpected events that cause a change in work plan. Task level conflict arises from conflicting demands in time and space, and from problems and interruptions that hamper task performance.

We have included 7 elements that create general conflict. All of these are far too familiar in working life. Many of these have been directly implicated in mental health disturbances, as reviewed in Chapter 2. These include interpersonal conflicts and lack of support with difficulties at work, career blocking, other violations of the norms of behavior or abuse of power, as well as lack of possibilities to redress grievances, threat of job loss and performing work which is bereft of meaning and coherence.

5.1.2 *The OSI model in its entirety*

Having completed a brief review of the levels and aspects of the OSI, we now combine these two axes to form the 2-dimensional matrix. This is the complete OSI model, as shown in Figure 5.1.

5.1.2.1 *General principles for scoring/coding the OSI*

Each element of the OSI is scored on a scale from 0 to 2, with zero being "not present" and 2 as "strongly present." To give an example of the scoring, we take the element of inadequate pay. (This is on general level of the underload aspect), and the question reads as follows:

C2 My salary:
a. Covers substantially more than my needs and those of my family.
b. Covers a bit more than my basic needs and those of my family.
c. Just barely covers my basic needs and those of my family.
d. Totally inadequate to meet my basic needs and those of my family.

The coding is as follows:
0 C2 = a Covers substantially more than basic needs
0.5 C2 = b Covers a bit more than basic needs
1 C2 = c Just barely covers expenses
2 C2 = d Totally inadequate.

Aspects Information Transmission Level	Underload	High Demand	Strictness	Extrinsic Time Pressure	Aversiveness/ Noxious Exposures	Avoidance/ Symbolic Aversiveness	Conflict/ Uncertainty
Input	• Homogeneous signals • Low frequency of incoming signals • Works alone--without need for communication	• Several info. sources • Heterogeneous information • Heavy burden on visual system • High frequency of incoming signals • 3 sensory modalities • Communication essential	• Strict requirements for signal detection	• No control over speed of incoming signals	• Glare • Noise	• High level of attention (Serious consequences of momentary lapse) • Visually-disturbing scenes • Listens to emotionally-disturbing accounts	• Signal/noise conflict • Signal/signal conflict
Central Decision-Making	• Decisions automatic from input	• Complex decisions • Complicated decisions • Decisions affect work of others • Rapid decision-making	• Strict problem-solving strategy • Strictly defined correct decision	• Decisions cannot be postponed		• Serious consequences of a wrong decision	• Missing information needed for decision • Contradictory information • Unexpected events change work plan
Output/ Task performance	• Homogenous tasks • Simple Tasks • Nothing to do	• Heterogeneous tasks • Simultaneous task performance • Complex tasks • Rapid task performance	• Work must meet a strictly defined standard	• No control over rate of task performance	• Isometric lifting • Vibration	• Hazardous task performance	• Conflicting demands *Task performance hampered by*: • Extrinsic problems • Interruptions from people
General	• Fixed pay • Inadequate pay • No chances for upgrade • Lack of recognition of work	• Piece rate work • Long work hours • Holds 2+ jobs • Lack of rest breaks • Night shift/irregular work hours • Lack of paid vacations	• Fixed body position • Confined, window-less, workspace • Lack of autonomous workspace • Limited in taking time off from work *Low influence over*: • Schedule • Tasks • Policy • With whom one works	• Deadline pressure • Speed-up	• Heat • Cold • Noxious gases, fumes, dusts	• Work Accident • Witnessed work accident • Suicide occurrence • Work-related litigation/Testifying in court • Lack of functioning emergency system	• Emotionally-charged work atmosphere • Lack of help with work-related difficulties • Opposition to career advancement • Violations of behavior norms/abuses of power • No grievance redress • Threat of job loss • Job lacks coherence

Figure 5.1 The Occupational Stressor Index (version 2013), slightly revised from [Belkić 2003].

5.1.2.2 *Calculation of the additive burden of occupational stressors*

- OSI stressor aspects:

The elements within a given aspect are first summed to give the total aspect score. As will be discussed later in this chapter, these total aspect scores are highly informative in indicating the nature of the stressor burden and its association with adverse health outcomes.

- The total OSI stressor score and its clinical usefulness:

The total OSI score is the sum of all 7 stressor aspects, i.e. the grand total of the entire OSI matrix. In the clinical context, this score is the most useful indicator of the overall burden of work stressors. It is particularly helpful when formulating and implementing worksite modifications. The OSI can provide an in-depth profile of the fixed, as well as potentially modifiable workplace stressors, identifying the level at which the burden primarily occurs, and the major contributing aspects. This information helps pinpoint where modifications in the work environment would be most beneficial. These intervention strategies can be developed in a flexible way, based upon feasibility, with the key being to lower the burden. Lowering the total stressor burden has positive effects on worker health, well-being and productivity. This applies even to a relatively low total OSI score. However, insofar as the total OSI exceeds certain levels, interventions are urgently needed. In our experience, total OSI scores > 90 require urgent intervention. Insofar as the total OSI score exceeds 100, the work environment is acutely dangerous.

5.2 The Occupation-Specific OSI Instruments

Thus far we have presented the OSI model in its general or generic form. The Generic OSI Questionnaire [Belkić 2003][Belkić & Savić 2008] is applicable to workers of any occupational profile, and it functions well in that capacity, as will be discussed later on in this chapter. A further improvement is provided by the occupation-specific instruments, the need for which has been strongly emphasized [Landsbergis *et al.*, 2000].

5.2.1 *Generic versus occupation-specific instruments*

The OSI provides a bridge between two divergent approaches in occupational psychosocial research. One of these encompasses the theory-based, generic approaches. These are frequently far removed from actual work experiences, and therefore may not be helpful for assessing *within-occupation variance,* which is precisely how intervention strategies are developed, in practice. The other approach is occupation-specific. Here, detailed information is provided but often with a narrow focus. Based upon one occupation, the more generalizable conclusions requiring between-group analyses are difficult to generate.

The OSI offers a viable solution, through occupation-specific instruments that are mutually compatible within the OSI theoretical framework. This promotes between-occupation comparisons. At the same time, the occupation-specific OSI questionnaires are more operationalized and streamlined than a single generic instrument. In the occupation-specific questionnaires, queries about the fixed aspects of a given line of work can be omitted, so that the focus is upon the variable features. The occupation-specific OSI's are especially helpful for targeting modifiable stressors in a given profession.

5.2.2 *The process of developing occupation-specific OSI's*

As will be seen in this sub-section, developing occupation-specific OSI's is a multi-step process, which is labor intensive and time consuming. Nonetheless, it should also be said that the effort is indeed rewarding, and this is particularly the case in the clinical setting.

5.2.2.1 *Initial steps: qualitative analysis together with the generic OSI*

- Review of the single-occupation literature:

Reviewing the literature is a vital step from which one can garner invaluable insights into the key stressors concerning the occupation in focus. One can learn how these may vary from worksite to worksite as well gleaning information about the unchanging or relatively fixed characteristics of the profession.

- Pilot study using the generic OSI:

A pilot study is then performed with a small group of persons employed within the occupation. These persons complete the generic version of the OSI, and should be willing to put in the needed time to comment and explain their answers in relation to their actual work environment.

This process is facilitated by the open-ended questions as illustrated in Panel 5.9.

Open-Ended Queries in the OSI Questionnaire

- What is the best part(s) about your job?
- What is the most difficult aspect of your job?
- What do you think could be done to make that difficulty less of a burden?
- What could be done to improve working life at your current job?
  --Immediately
  --Long-term
  --Which of these changes do you consider most important?
- If attempts were made to improve the conditions for your job, what would you suggest to preserve the good aspects of your work as it now stands?
- Other comments

Panel 5.9 The open-ended queries that are part of the OSI questionnaire.

- Taking a participatory action research approach:

Whenever persons from the occupation are motivated to develop a specific OSI, this process can be viewed within the participatory action research perspective [Israel *et al.*, 1996]. In fact, this is the optimal setting, with the deepest insights generated into the actual working conditions and strongest motivation to improve these. The OSI for physicians, for example, was developed in this way, and was termed "*for physicians by physicians*," as will be discussed later on.

5.2.2.2 *The three major modifications by which the occupation-specific OSI's differ from the generic OSI instrument*

- Identification of fixed elements of the specific occupation:

First, the unchanging characteristics of a given occupation can be assigned a fixed score. In the physician-specific OSI, there are 12 fixed-score elements, indicating that these are unchanging characteristics of physicians' work. For example, since potential human injury or fatality from an error is an essential feature of physicians' work (TAV on the central decision-making level) this element is always scored maximally (2 points). Other fixed score items include the need to make complex and complicated decisions (high demand on the decision-making level) and receiving contradictory or unclear information. This step shortens/streamlines the specific-OSI, omitting superfluous or obvious questions.[3]

• Operationalization of variable elements–occupation-specific questions: The variable features of a given occupation can be operationalized according to the specificities of that profession. For professional drivers, e.g. several of the variable elements of the OSI are directed towards the traffic environment (such as road and vehicle conditions, type of routes, passengers, accidents, work schedules, timetable stringency, rest breaks).

The queries are presented in a neutral manner so that reporting bias is minimized. One example here is how the questions are presented for elements of high demand versus underload at the input level. Here, the scoring of the frequency of incoming signals is according to where the driving predominantly takes place—within a city signifies rapid incoming signal speed (high demand), whereas driving mainly on long, intercity routes represents a low frequency of incoming signals (underload). Heterogeneous signals (high demand) are encountered when a person drives on various routes, while when driving takes place on the same route day after day, the signals are relatively homogeneous (underload).

• Identification of elements with a narrowed score range:
The range of possible scores can also be narrowed within an occupation-specific OSI. In the OSI for physicians there are 27 elements with narrowed-score ranges.

An example is hazardous task performance indicating threat avoidance on the task-performance level. The maximum score of 2

[3] This step appears to be helpful for obtaining complete data, as has been achieved among physicians and professional drivers. Thus, in these specific OSI's by e.g. not asking whether an error could have fatal consequences, we avoid a question which would indicate "cluelessness" about the person's actual work. The specific OSI instead focuses on the stressors that may truly vary within the specific occupation, and this heightens the interest and involvement in completing the questionnaire. See subsection 5.4.2 on face validity of the OSI.

points is given if there are threats of violence from psychotic patients, risk of infection from close contact with blood/other bodily fluids, or work entailing exposure to ionizing radiation. This element is assigned a minimum score of 1 since even without these clearly dangerous situations, there are always some potentially hazardous tasks related to the work of physicians.

5.2.2.3 *Making use of objective information about the workplace*

Objective information about the workplace can be used as cross-validation of the self-reported questionnaire items of the OSI. Insofar as a specific OSI will be used for a larger number of employees at a given workplace, further refinement of the specific-OSI is sometimes possible.

- On-site observation:

On-site observation is obviously time-consuming, but provides very helpful insights that can further streamline the OSI for a given worksite. Furthermore, because of its "hands-on" nature, on-site observation is often the best way to pinpoint needed interventions that would be most feasible in practice. Theory-guided observational approaches such as the RHIA/VERA instrument [Greiner & Krause 2000] [Volpert 1982] can also be useful for identifying objective measures of, for example, workload, hindrances, and the like, that best coincide with the elements of an occupation-specific OSI. It should also be emphasized that visiting a worksite is an invaluable experience for a clinician whose patient clientele is heavily represented by a given occupation or worksite.

- Defined features of a given worksite (further streamlining):

It is often found that there are certain features that are defined or constant for a given worksite. For example, it may be that teachers working at a given institution all have paid vacation at specified intervals when the school is closed. Nevertheless, it is vital to ensure that e.g. preparatory time for courses or grading exams performed at home during the official vacation period is taken into account. It should also be queried as to whether such vacation time is actually free from work obligations at another job.

- Variable elements that can be gleaned from occupational records:

Occupational records can often provide information about physical and chemical exposures, work schedules including night duty, vacation time, *inter alia*. These data can be used as cross-validation of the self-report items from the OSI. In certain instances, finer gradations can be instituted for elements of the OSI. For example, for urban mass transit operators there could be finer gradations to the scoring of high frequency of incoming signals based upon actual traffic density measures. By a similar logic, data about the average number of passengers on a given route could improve quantification of the burden of communicating with the public.

5.2.3 *Available occupation-specific OSI's and those in development*

We have fully tested specific OSI instruments for physicians, teachers, nurses, professional drivers and for those who work daily with computers. The specific OSI's for scientists and for control panel workers have undergone initial pilot testing. The OSI's for factory workers, airline pilots, artists and fire fighters are in development. Translation and validation of OSI instruments have been completed or are currently on-going into Spanish, Chinese, Mongolian, Italian, French, Serbian, Slovenian, Swedish, Rumanian, Bulgarian and Japanese. The OSI is included in the data base of the National Institute of Occupational Health and Safety (NIOSH), USA. http://www2a.cdc.god/niosh-workorg/detail.asp?id=85 and the Job Stress Network www.workhealth.org.

> Permission to use any of the OSI instruments should be obtained from the authors. Our policy is to provide permission free-of-charge for all clinical and research endeavors aimed at improving the job conditions and health of working people. We are happy to answer questions concerning its application, and to discuss how the OSI might be best implemented in a given setting. A sample of a completed OSI questionnaire and score sheet for a clinical case study from Part II is provided in Appendix B.

5.3 Reliability of the OSI

The reliability of the generic and specific OSI's has been assessed in a multi-faceted manner. The OSI is observer coded, and on many occasions, more than one observer has independently scored the questionnaires. Inter-observer variation has usually been quite minimal, and arises mainly for certain input and central elements of the high demand aspect. Our procedure has been to discuss any point of divergence and come to consensus. A third observer sometimes served as arbiter, although this has rarely been needed. Two independent observers coded the OSI's in several studies of professional drivers [Belkić *et al.*, 1996] [Emdad 1997] [Emdad *et al.*, 1997], physicians [Savić 2002] [Nedić 2006a] [Belkić & Nedić 2007] [Belkić 2009] [Nedić *et al.*, 2010], teachers [Belkić 2003], as well as heterogeneous groups of employed persons (generic OSI) [Belkić 1995b].

The internal consistency of the various OSI aspects and the total OSI has been examined in a number of studies, and the values are shown in Table 5.1. For the physician-specific OSI only the variable elements are included. The Cronbach α is also listed for the variable features of the OSI for professional drivers [Belkić *et al.*, 1996].

Table 5.1 Internal consistency of the OSI instruments (Cronbach α values). From references: [Belkić 1995b] [Belkić *et al.*, 1996] [Belkić 2003] [Nedić 2006][Belkić & Nedić 2007].

	Generic OSI	OSI for physicians		OSI for professional drivers
Underload	0.62	Could not be calculated		
High demand	0.80	0.84		
Strictness	0.41	0.67		
Extrinsic time pressure	0.54	0.41	Input-Central-Output= 0.58	
Noxious exposures	0.67	0.57		
Threat avoidance	0.67	0.62		
Conflict/ uncertainty	0.80	0.57		
Total OSI	0.81	0.89	The 7 aspects= 0.74	0.84

The overall internal consistency of the OSI is within the optimal range for each of the examined instruments. In addition, for the OSI for physicians, the Cronbach α of the seven aspects is very good. The high demand aspect for these OSI instruments also has an excellent internal consistency. This point is particularly important because, as mentioned, it is with this aspect that the most inter-observer variability is seen.

Most of the other aspects have shown acceptable internal consistency. The exceptions include the strictness aspect for the generic OSI, and extrinsic time pressure aspect, particularly for the physician-specific OSI. Factor analysis of the extrinsic time pressure aspect revealed two factors that explained 63% of the variance: one was comprised mainly of the input, central decision-making and output level elements: lack of control of incoming signals, making non-postponable decisions and low control over rate of task performance—these are elements related to patient load and work in the emergency setting. As seen in Table 5.1, these elements show an acceptable level of internal consistency. The second factor was comprised of the 2 elements on the general level: deadline pressure and speed up. For the underload aspect of the physician-specific OSI questionnaire, there were only 3 variable elements, two of which were not normally distributed, so that the Cronbach α was not calculated.

Test-retest reliability of the OSI's has been examined in pilot studies for the specific OSI's. Repeated application of the OSI has also been performed in the clinical setting. The elements that remained unchanged, as well as the changes in working conditions over time were correctly reflected in the OSI, as was confirmed by follow-up queries to the study participants [Belkić 1989][Savić 2002][Belkić 2003]. Moreover, the OSI has been used as the basis for intervention studies [Uglješić, Belkić, Simeunović-Micković & Vukajlović 1992] [Belkić *et al.*, 1996] [Emdad, *et al* 1998a], in which the working conditions at follow-up were reliably reflected.

5.4 Validity of the OSI

5.4.1 *Construct validity of the OSI: theoretical/biological coherence*

The construct validity of the OSI is clear from both a theoretical vantage point and from its biological plausibility. In fact, these two, usually divergent perspectives are well integrated within the OSI.

This is achieved, in part, by the two-dimensional matrix structure of the OSI, by which the stressor aspects are elucidated according to the level of information transmission. As discussed in detail in Chapter 3, these levels were formulated as a theoretical framework within cognitive ergonomics by Welford [1960], and fully reflect the mental chronometric processes that are well established from neurophysiology. By so doing, the OSI captures the relatively silent burden of many stressful occupations. The OSI incorporates key facets of well-established, sociologically based stressor models [Karasek 1979] [Siegrist 1996].

The OSI is coherent with the theory of cognitive energy mobilization [Gaillard 1993] which confirms the indelible coupling between psychological demands and the possibilities for control, such that with sufficient decision-latitude, or control, a worker can modulate even a fairly onerous, *though not overwhelming*, psychological workload to meet his or her moment-to-moment needs and capacities.

The OSI includes vitally important stressor aspects such as threat avoidant vigilance and conflict/uncertainty that are missing from the sociological models. Thereby, a more complete assessment of the burden of work is provided. The additive burden reflected by the total OSI score is in line with the construct of "resources" or total burden upon the human operator, with a view as to how this burden impacts not only upon performance, but also in relation to fatigue and mental as well as somatic health consequences [Hockey 1997] [Belkić, Schnall, Savić & Landsbergis 2000].

5.4.2 *Face validity of the OSI*

The generic OSI has good face validity. Working people consider the questions relevant to their daily life on-the-job and they understand quite well even the somewhat more abstract questions. The generic OSI questionnaire can be used for between-occupation comparisons, especially when evaluating a heterogeneous working population with a wide range of profiles, including blue collar, white collar and service workers, with various educational levels. The face validity of the generic OSI has been confirmed among heterogeneous populations of both women and men [Belkić 1989] [Belkić 1995b] [Belkić 2003].

A striking feature of the specific OSI instruments is their strong face validity. This is where the invested effort to develop these specific questionnaires is truly reflected. Patients and participants in research investigations consistently express their appreciation that the specific OSI's focus upon the relevant conditions of their work and that superfluous or trivial queries are avoided. Of particular note, the physicians who completed the specific OSI confirmed that this instrument captures the key stressors that they experience at work. As a likely consequence, participation rates of studies using the OSI for physicians has been remarkably high, consistently over 85% with no missing data [Savić 2002][Nedić 2006a][Belkić & Nedić 2007][Nedić, *et al.*, 2010].

The face validity of the specific OSI instruments is also clearly seen in their capability to reflect the actual working conditions of subgroups within a given profession, e.g. surgeons and anesthesiologists versus clinicians in the non-surgical specialties [Savić 2002][Nedić 2006a][Belkić & Nedić 2007][Belkic & Nedić 2012], urban mass transit operators versus long-route truck drivers [Belkić 1989][Belkić, Savić *et al.*, 1995][Belkić, *et al.*, 1996][Emdad 1997], teachers of various profiles [Belkić 2003], *inter alia.*

5.4.3 *Criterion validity of the OSI: empirical results*

In a number of empirical studies, the total OSI, its aspects and many of the elements are significantly associated with risk behaviors and health outcomes. Moreover, the total OSI scores and OSI profiles help identify and characterize the work conditions of occupational groups at elevated risk for stress-related disorders.

5.4.3.1 *Results among physicians*

The OSI for physicians has been applied in a case-control study design among 208 physicians employed at clinical institutions in Novi Sad [Nedić 2006a]. The cases were physicians with one or more of the so-called acquired (potentially stress-related) cardiovascular disorders (ACVD) (myocardial infarction, angina pectoris, arterial hypertension or certain arrhythmias) [Eliot 1979]. The referents were physicians without diagnosed ACVD.

The total OSI was significantly higher among the cases than controls. Two aspects: high demands and threat avoidance were dominant in showing higher exposure among the cases. The most consistent and significant stressors that distinguished physicians with ACVD from referents were long work hours, speed-up and threat of job loss.

We concluded that physicians are a heavily burdened occupational group and that several occupational stressors assessed by the physician OSI are significantly associated with case status [Nedić *et al.*, 2008b].

In gender-stratified analysis, the relationship between working conditions assessed by the OSI and ACVD was most apparent among the women physicians [Nedić *et al.*, 2008a].

• Associations between work stressors and unhealthy behaviors:
The relationship between work stressors assessed by the OSI and lifestyle-related risk factors for cancer and heart disease (LRCRF): smoking, obesity, lack of recreational physical activity and alcohol consumption, has also been examined. This was done first among 112 female physicians working at the Novi Sad clinical center [Belkić & Nedić 2007]. The total OSI and several OSI aspects, particularly threat-avoidance alone or in combination, showed significant multivariate associations with the LRCRF, as did individual OSI elements. The latter included long work hours, restricted problem-solving strategies, insufficient help with clinical difficulties and supervisory responsibility (overweight and/or lack of physical activity) and problems hampering patient-care (smoking). We concluded that diminishing the work stressor burden, as assessed by the OSI, should be incorporated into intervention strategies aimed at these risk factors.

These analyses have been expanded to include both male and female physicians at the Novi Sad clinical center [Belkić & Nedić 2012]. Altogether 191 physicians without manifest coronary heart disease were included in that study. Only 23 physicians (12.0%) had a low lifestyle-related cancer/cardiovascular risk. The surgeons and anesthesiologists faced a heavier total work stressor burden than physicians in other profiles (total OSI = 87.7 ± 8.8 versus 74.1 ± 10.5, p=0.000). Among the 56 surgeons/anesthesiologists, lower nightshift work scores were associated with low lifestyle-related cancer/cardiovascular risk (F=4.19, p=0.046). A lower total OSI score was associated with low risk among the other 135 physicians (F=4.06, p=0.046). The findings were most pronounced among the female physicians.

• Associations between work stressors and clinical hypertension:
In a comparison of 35 female physicians with, and 74 without clinically-diagnosed hypertension, adjusting for covariates including body mass index, BMI, having an OSI high demand score above the mean yielded an OR = 3.14 (95% CI=1.05–9.43) for hypertension. However, overweight physicians *without* diagnosed hypertension were more often current and heavier smokers. The total OSI score was significantly lower among the physicians with the favorable risk profile defined in that study as not a current smoker and without diagnosed hypertension. The strongest multivariate model for favorable risk profile (FRP) included having a

hobby and lower BMI, with total threat avoidant vigilance score below the mean showing a highly significant adjusted association (OR = 0.30, CI = 0.12 – 0.78, p=0.01)). Disturbances from other people and listening to emotionally disturbing occurrences also showed significant inverse multi-variate associations with FRP [Nedić *et al.*, 2010]. In Figure 5.2 we display the total OSI scores that differed significantly according to risk profile among the 112 female physicians examined in Refs. [Belkić & Nedić 2007][Nedić *et al.*, 2008a][Nedić *et al.*, 2010]. The mean total OSI scores was 77.3 ± 11.8 among the 112 female physicians, ranging from 46.8 to 103.3.

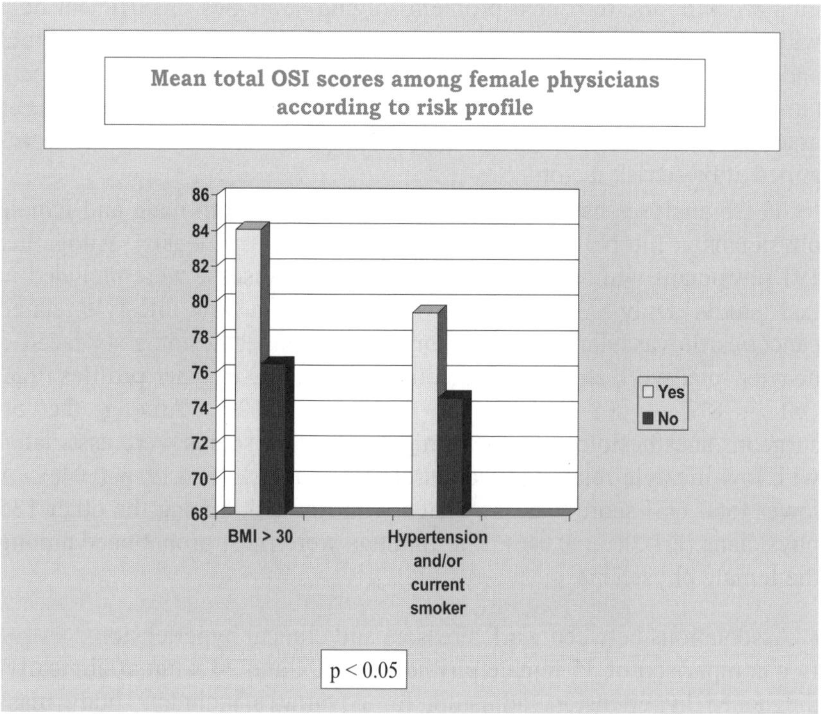

Figure 5.2 Mean total OSI scores that differed significantly according to risk profile among the 112 female physicians from Refs. [Belkić & Nedić 2007][Nedić *et al.*, 2010].

5.4.3.2 *Results among professional drivers*

- Associations between work stressors and unhealthy behaviors:

In our first studies using the OSI, 258 male professional drivers up to age 40 working in Belgrade completed the specific OSI for that occupation

[Belkić 1989][Belkić, Pavlović *et al.*, 1992] [Belkić, Savić, Micković & Uglješić 1992]. The participants also completed a questionnaire comprised of scales concerning somatization, sleep disturbance, coronary-prone behavior and maladjustment to their job. These four scales based upon validated instruments [Cornell Index 1985] [Roffwarg 1979] [Zyzanski & Jenkins 1970] were summed into an adverse behavioral index, which was associated with the total OSI scores ($p<0.001$). In turn, the adverse behavioral index was associated with smoking intensity ($p < 0.05$). These results suggested that the overall burden of work stressors, as assessed by the total OSI, may impact upon smoking, and that this relation could be mediated by the above-described adverse behavioral index. More recent studies among 69 male professional drivers in Stockholm revealed a direct multivariate association between the total OSI score and smoking intensity ($p = 0.02$), with adjustment for number of smoking years [Emdad *et al.*, 1998].

- Associations between work stressors and hypertension or CHD:

As reviewed in Chapter 2, professional drivers are at very high risk for hypertension, CHD and cerebrovascular disease. The relation of this risk to their occupational activity is well appreciated [Belkić, Savić *et al.*, 1994] [Ragland *et al.*, 1997] [Tüschen *et al.*, 2006]. Generic work stressor models have not succeeded in explaining this relation. Using generic instruments, professional drivers are not consistently classified as a high strain occupation [Belkić, Savić *et al.*, 1994] [Karasek & Theorell 1990]. In contrast to non-significant results obtained for the demand and control dimensions using a questionnaire based on the Job Strain Model, the OSI total high demand scores were nearly three times greater for professional drivers (16.1 ± 2.1) compared to referents of similar socio-economic status (6.4 ± 3.8) ($p < 0.001$) [Emdad *et al.*, 1997]. Professional drivers in Belgrade and Stockholm had ~ twice the mean total OSI scores (67.2 ± 4.3) and (63.6 ± 4.0) compared to heterogeneous groups of workers of similar socioeconomic levels (33.0 ± 7.9) and (34.8 ± 6.1) ($p < 0.001$) [Belkić 1989] [Belkić, Savić *et al.*, 1995] [Emdad *et al.*, 1997]. Pressure to stay on schedule and long work hours were identified via OSI as key modifiable stressors within this occupational group, associated respectively with professional drivers having hypertension and ischemic heart disease [Emdad *et al.*, 1997].

5.4.3.3 *Published studies among heterogeneous occupational groups*

As discussed, the Generic OSI Questionnaire can be used for between-occupation comparisons, especially when evaluating a heterogeneous working population with a wide range of profiles. We have collected and analyzed data using this questionnaire among 345 workers of various occupations and of both genders, in several countries [Belkić 1989] [Belkić, Savić *et al.*, 1995] [Belkić 1995b] [Belkić 2003]. More recently, the results of Djindjić and colleagues [2012] have been published in which the OSI was applied in a heterogeneous group of nearly 1 000 employees from Serbia.

- Associations between work stressors and unhealthy behaviors:

As noted, in our first studies, 227 male blue-collar workers up to age 40 of various profiles completed the Generic OSI Questionnaire. Similarly to the professional drivers, we found that the total OSI scores were significantly associated with the adverse behavioral index [Belkić 1989] [Belkić, Pavlović *et al.*, 1992] [Belkić, Savić *et al.*, 1995]. In turn, among these blue-collar workers, the adverse behavioral index showed a significant association with number of days of sick leave in the past year ($p < 0.001$). These findings suggested that the overall burden of work stressors, as assessed by the total OSI, impact upon sick leave, and that this relation could be mediated by the adverse behavioral index. It should also be noted that the mean number of sick days was significantly greater among the blue-collar workers compared to the professional drivers.

Our stratified analyses among the professional drivers and among the blue-collar referents reveal different patterns for these two groups. On the one hand, the total burden of work stressors appears to affect sickness absence among the referents. Since the drivers had more limited possibilities to take sick leave due to very strict scheduling, the burden of work stressors appears to impact through unhealthy behaviors leading to greater smoking intensity. These insights can be helpful for informing intervention strategies.

- Associations between work stressors and components of the cardiovascular metabolic syndrome:

In the recently-published study from Serbia [Djindjić *et al.*, 2012], significant cross sectional associations were found in both male and female employees between the total OSI scores and components of the cardiovascular metabolic syndrome, namely, arterial hypertension, type 2 diabetes mellitus and dyslipidemia. The reported odds ratios were adjusted for age. Among men only, the OSI high demand and extrinsic time pressure scores were significantly linked to hypertension, whereas only among the women, each of the OSI aspects was significantly related to type 2 diabetes. Among the women only, the strictness and conflict dimensions were significantly linked to dyslipidemia. In both men and women, the OSI total underload score was significantly associated with dyslipidemia and hypertension.

5.4.4 *Clinical validity of the OSI*

From its inception, the OSI has been envisioned as a clinical tool. The OSI model and its operationalization through the generic and specific instruments were developed primarily by physician specialists [Belkić 1989] [Belkić 2003] [Belkić, Savić *et al.*, 1995] [Savić 2002]. In clinical applications, the OSI has been repeatedly found to be useful as a diagnostic tool and for formulating and implementing realistic work place modifications needed for patients with stress-related disorders.

Within this framework, the first questions to be posed are:

- Is this a stressful workplace?
- Is this workplace contributing to the patient's disorder?
- Can workplace modifications help improve the patient's clinical status?

We will begin this line of inquiry by a brief comparison with the Job Strain Model. Earlier we noted that professional drivers did not significantly differ from referents with regard to the demand and control dimensions using a questionnaire based on the Job Strain Model [Emdad, Belkić et al 1997].

We also noted that they are not consistently classified as a high strain occupation [Belkić, Savić *et al.*, 1994] [Karasek & Theorell 1990]. In fact, professional driving is classified as a "passive job," namely low demands and low decision-making latitude, according to U.S. imputational data [Karasek & Theorell 1990].

Also, according to these imputational data, natural scientists are classified as "relaxed jobs" (low demand and high decision-making latitude), while physicians and teachers are classified as an "active jobs" (high demands and high decision-making latitude), which are predicted to promote healthy coping strategies through active learning [Karasek & Theorell 1990], as discussed in Chapter 2.

We summarize the job strain classifications of these four occupations in Figure 5.3.

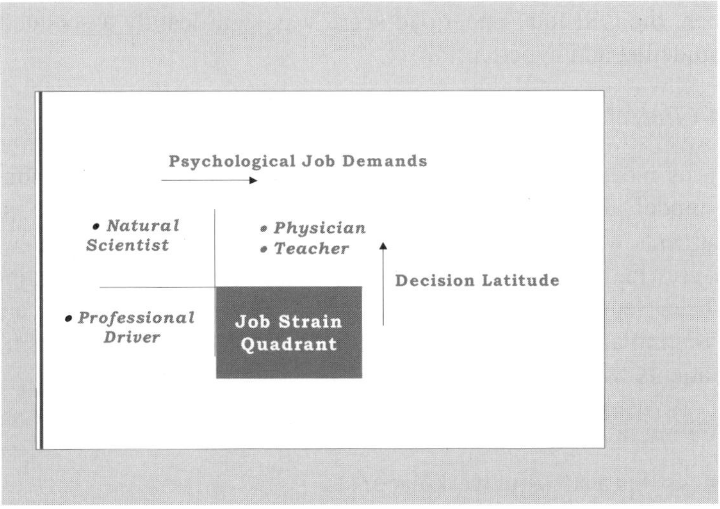

Figure 5.3 Classification of Psychological Job Demands vs. Decision Latitude quadrants of selected occupations according to Ref. [Karasek & Theorell 1990].

In contrast to classifications according to the Job Strain Model, using the OSI, professional drivers and natural scientists both are found to face high demands, but they do so in very different ways. It should also be emphasized that the reputed decision-making latitude of teachers and physicians is becoming ever more compromised [Belkic, Schnall *et al.*, 2000].

Crucially, the overall burden of occupational stressors, as assessed by the total OSI is often very high among scientists, teachers, physicians, and professional drivers. In answer then to the questions posed at the beginning of this subsection: Indeed, there are highly stressful work situations among these occupations, namely with total OSI scores > 90 and even over 100.

Some prototypical total OSI scores for patients with mental health disorders from these occupations are given in Figure 5.4. In our clinical experience, these stressors often contribute to the patient's disorder, particularly in the realm of mental health.

And, finally, with regard to the third question: Yes, workplace modifications can often help improve the patient's clinical status.

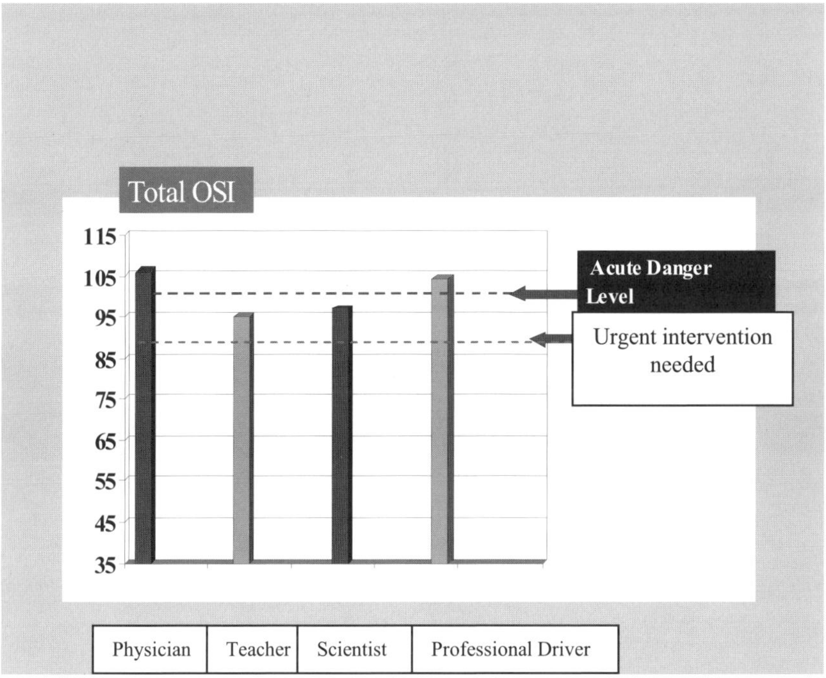

Figure 5.4 Prototypical total OSI scores for clinical cases involving mental health disorders among physicians, teachers, scientists and professional drivers.

Part II of this book will be devoted to these clinical issues through a series of cases studies among physicians and other occupational groups, based upon the OSI.

Part II

The Clinical Case Studies

Chapter 6

Introduction to Part II: The Clinical Case Studies

6.1 A Brief Recapitulation

In Part I we focused upon theoretical models, together with the epidemiologic and physiologic evidence concerning the work environment and mental health, as well as selected comorbidity. Thereby, first, conceptual plausibility was provided for the premise that job stressors impact upon mental well-being. The empirical data, including a substantial number of longitudinal studies, supporting this relation were shown to be strong and consistent. We then explored the potential mechanisms, mediated by the central nervous system, as to how exposure to various occupational stressors can affect cognitive and emotional function. Taken together, it can be said that there is convergent validation via the essential elements of causal inference [Rothman & Greenland 1998] to conclude that work stressors indeed contribute to mental ill-health.

In Part I we also reviewed the established clinical practice in the field of work fitness and occupational rehabilitation. We noted that the current standard for medical evaluation of work fitness and return to work for persons with mental health disorders is still relatively undeveloped, and we queried as to why this is so. The Occupational Stressor Index was presented as a comprehensive methodology grounded in the cognitive neurosciences, and which can be applied in the clinical setting. We suggested that the OSI could be used to formulate and implement more effective return to work strategies for these patients.

6.2 Aims, Scope and Organization of Part II

As we now transition to Part II, the tack is substantially different. *Herein, the individual, the person himself or herself becomes the center of our attention.* The abiding question is how to translate what has been presented in Part I into a new, evidence-based approach towards the work environment, an approach which can truly help patients faced with neuropsychiatric disorders.

In Part II, we present a series of case studies, informed by our clinical experience. The OSI, the Occupational Stressor Index, is used in each of these case studies to assess the work environment, as well as to formulate and implement the interventions. We highlight successful interventions, namely, those that have had a clear positive impact for the individual. Since our emphasis is upon the interface between the individual and the work environment, there will be only brief mention of psycho-pharmacology and other standard aspects of clinical therapy.

Disclaimer:
These standard therapeutic procedures as well as the described workplace modifications are presented for scientific and educational purposes, and should not be considered explicit advice for any actual individual patient. All identifying data in these cases, including initials used in each case, have been changed to protect patient anonymity. Thus, none of the case studies can be traced to any specific person.

6.2.1 *The structure of the clinical case studies*

The clinical case studies begin with an introductory page comprised of a very brief summary of the current situation together with the total OSI score. For most of these cases, a set of initial queries is posed, upon which we recommend that the reader reflect while reviewing the case:

- Is this a dangerously stressful work situation?
- Is the patient's work situation contributing to his/her disorder? *If so, how*?
- Could workplace modifications help improve the patient's clinical status? *If so, how*?

This is followed by a classical case presentation, history plus objective findings. The latter include a standard neuropsychiatric evaluation, neuropsychological testing including relevant questionnaire findings, and, for most of the case studies, neurophysiologic and/or psychophysiologic evaluation.

In the next segment, the patient's work situation is evaluated based upon the OSI. This evaluation is presented in a succinct, narrative form and proceeds by aspect, starting with underload (left-most column of the OSI model) and proceeding through to the conflict/uncertainty aspect (right-most column of the OSI model). After the corresponding aspects have been presented, conclusions are made about whether or not effort-reward imbalance and job-strain are present, as well as concerning the threat-avoidant vigilance and conflict/uncertainty burden. Within this segment, the baseline OSI is summarized in a single-page figure, in which the modifiable and fixed stressor elements are summarized according to the OSI model.

The subsequent segment(s) of each clinical case study outline(s) the therapeutic intervention process, focused upon the workplace. The measures implemented to lower the occupational stressor burden in line with the needs of the patient are summarized in one or more OSI figures.

In several of the cases, the workplace interventions are formulated jointly by the patient and the clinician. The latter is a neuropsychiatrist with expertise in stress medicine and occupational medicine, and is termed an "occupational neuropsychiatrist" an appellation which we will discuss in more detail in Part III of the book.

Chapter 7

An Exhausted Psychiatrist Thinking about Suicide: Our First Clinical Case Study

Dr. R, a psychiatrist in her early 50's working in a leading training hospital, presents with extreme exhaustion.

She can hardly get herself out of bed.

She feels empty and admits that suicide has crossed her mind.

An initial query about her work elicits a grimace.

Her status remains unimproved after standard pharmacologic and cognitive-behavioral therapy.

Total OSI = 106

Questions for reflection while reviewing this case:

- Is this a dangerously stressful work situation?
- Is the patient's work situation contributing to her disorder? *If so, how?*
- Could workplace modifications help improve the patient's clinical status? *If so, how?*

7.1 The Case: Dr. R is Extremely Fatigued and Admits to Thoughts of Suicide

For the past few years, Dr. R has felt increasingly fatigued particularly during and after work, but also at home while performing her usual household chores. It is difficult for her to fall asleep. She wakes up several times per night, after which she has trouble going back to sleep. In the mornings she awakens feeling drained. Upon repeated questioning, she admits to suicidal thoughts, but denies having any definite plan or previous attempts

Effort has been needed for her to communicate with patients and colleagues at work, as well as with family. She spends progressively less time with friends and attends fewer cultural events. These activities, which had previously been a source of pleasure, now require much greater effort and have ceased to provide satisfaction. On the contrary, they are exhausting for her.

→These difficulties intensified three weeks ago after night call in the psychiatric emergency room, during which several patients were admitted in acute exacerbation. One of these patients had a known history of suicide attempts. Despite Dr. R's conclusion, which she clearly communicated to her colleagues, that inpatient care was imperative, the patient was discharged the next morning by the ward team. The patient committed suicide right after leaving the hospital. Dr. R. was immediately told about the patient and that there would be a meeting to review the case. When Dr. R arrived home later that day, her strength was totally depleted. For two days thereafter she could not get out of bed, lost her appetite and could barely get 2 to 3 hours sleep per night.

This is Dr. R's second episode of severe exhaustion. The first occurred at the end of her psychiatry residency, while preparing for board certification. She had occasional thoughts of suicide at that time, but did not seek treatment and the symptoms subsided spontaneously. Past medical history is otherwise unremarkable.

Dr. R. lives with her husband, an engineer and their 15 year-old daughter. She has never smoked cigarettes and does not drink alcohol. She performs most of the household chores, entailing substantial physical exertion, but engages in no recreational physical activity. Her parents are retired physicians, in good health, and live in another town. She is an only child. Most members of her genetic family are healthy, to her knowledge.

- What is missing from this history?

7.1.1 *Objective findings*

Dr. R. appears exhausted, somewhat apathetic, and slightly older than her stated age. She is asthenic, blood pressure: 110/70 mmHg, pulse: 85/min, unremarkable physical examination. Laboratory values including sedimentation rate, complete blood count, electrolytes, liver function and T3, T4, TSH within normal limits.

- Initial psychiatric evaluation:

Depressive affect, anhedonia, impaired concentration, pessimistic view to the future, sleep disturbance, suicidal ideation. No neurological abnormalities. Diagnosis: Depression up to moderate intensity (F32.1) [World Health Organization, 1993] (Appendix A, Section 1).

- Neuropsychological testing:

Right-handed, normal memory span, reaction time and attention.

7.1.2 *Initial assessment, management and clinical course*

- Depression with suicidal ideation:

Dr. R considers (and her physician agrees) that currently she cannot return to work, so she goes on sick leave. She is placed on anti-depressives and has a few sessions of cognitive behavioral therapy. Thereafter, her days seem empty and she becomes even more dysphoric. Her self-esteem deteriorates, as she feels that she does not perform anything useful and that her best days are past. Peri-menopausal symptoms become apparent from which she becomes even more exhausted and she sees herself as "old". Recreational physical activity was recommended but not implemented; she is so de-energized and also experiences vasomotor instability, so that she just cannot get herself going.

- Do you agree with this initial diagnosis? Why or why not?
- Why was this management strategy unsuccessful?
- What may be an iatrogenic aspect of this approach?
- Another diagnosis to be considered? What else is needed to evaluate this?

7.1.3 *Additional psychometric and neurophysiologic evaluation*

- Questionnaire findings:

→ Oldenburg Burnout Inventory "Mini-Olbi":
Exhaustion score = 17, Disengagement score = 13
She "totally agrees" that there are days when she already "feels tired before going to work", and after work she "feels worn out and weary" "needs more time to relax than in the past, in order to feel fit again". This is consistent with resource depletion [Demerouti *et al.*, 2001].
Findings consistent with burnout syndrome–exhaustion component predominant.
→General Health Questionnaire (GHQ12) = 7
Indicative of high psychological distress, of particular note, is that "much more than usual" she has lost much sleep over work, has felt constantly under strain, has been feeling unhappy and depressed, and felt that she could not overcome her difficulties. She has "much *less* often that usual" been able to enjoy her normal day-to-day activities.

- Neurophysiologic evaluation:

→Quantitative electroencephalographic findings:
Overall low peak alpha frequency (9.5 Hz) in eyes open and eyes closed conditions, most markedly reduced in the frontal regions, no frontal asymmetry. Reduced beta power (3.2 μVolts).
→Auditory Event Related Potential Odd Ball Paradigm:
Low amplitude (55 μVolts) and normal latency.
Findings consistent with burnout syndrome [van Luijtelaar *et al.*, 2010].

- What are the new insights provided by this additional evaluation?
- Is this information sufficient for you to proceed with a new plan for this patient? Why or why not?

7.2 Dr. R's Case Re-visited: Insights from the OSI

The clinical history/presentation of Dr. R's case in Section 7.1 provides important insights, but is incomplete. We learned therein about the acute trigger: a difficult night call with a patient fatality due to suicide. We also learned that Dr. R's clinical judgment was not properly heeded. However, most psychiatrists have had such experiences during and after night call, on one and usually many more occasions. To understand the reasons for Dr. R's current status, we return to the question: Is this a dangerously stressful work situation? Indeed, the overall burden of work stressors as indicated by the total OSI score of 106 is well above the acute danger level. In other words, the total burden of work stressors surpasses the absolute tolerance limit.

When this extreme work stressor burden is viewed together with Dr. R's clinical picture, the diagnosis of "work-related burnout" (Appendix A, Section 3) is inescapable. The scores on the exhaustion and disengagement scales of the Mini-Olbi and the neurophysiological findings further corroborate this diagnosis. Adequate management of Dr. R's case requires identification of the occupational triggers. Those that are fixed need to be distinguished from modifiable stressors. It is from the latter that an integrative assessment and management plan focusing on the work environment can be developed. In Figure 7.1, each OSI stressor for Dr. R. is identified and categorized as either fixed or as modifiable. The completed OSI questionnaire and score sheet for this case are provided in Appendix B.

- Underload:

As seen in the left-most column of Fig. 7.1, all 7.5 points for underload are related to five factors that could potentially be ameliorated. Low, fixed pay would require substantial organization intervention. On the other hand, waiting time occurs mainly during night call, due to frequent delays before an announced patient arrives. During that time, typically well after midnight, Dr. R is awakened, and in a state of aroused readiness. Low chances for upgrade are due to career blocking, because, in fact, there are opportunities for promotion. Another destimulating stressor is lack of recognition of good work. On the contrary, attention is mainly focused upon poor patient outcomes and errors. The underload burden of Dr. R is over twice higher than the mean for university hospital physicians [Nedić 2006a][Belkic & Nedić 2007].

- High demand:

Over half of the high demand burden is fixed. Several of the modifiable factors are associated with work in the emergency room and intensive care unit (high flow of information, need for rapid decision-making and task performance, corresponding to input, central and output levels, respectively). Teaching, scientific research and administrative duties without separate time allocated for these activities, further contribute to the high demands.

The other modifiable high demand stressors are on the general level: long work hours (including work at home), lack of rest breaks, weekly night call without guaranteed relief and frequently immediately following dayshift work.

> The high demand burden is heavy but typical for university hospital physicians. Together with the high underload score:
>
> EFFORT-REWARD IMBALANCE is present
>
> [Siegrist 1996] [Nedić, *et al.*, 2001].

- Strictness:

Most of the strictness burden is modifiable. On the input, central and performance levels, this is related to rules and regulations and having several persons oversee her work.

The general strictness factors reflect low influence over her schedule, tasks, policy, the colleagues and staff with whom she directly works as well as limited chances to take time off when needed. Her office is windowless and shared with a colleague, so that she must look for rooms in which to see patients.

- Extrinsic time pressure:

This is nearly the maximum possible (9.5 of 10). Well less than half of this burden is fixed.

The modifiable factors are related to lack of control over number of patients and how they are scheduled, as well as work in the emergency room and intensive care unit, together with deadlines. The latter are mainly related to administrative, teaching and scientific duties. The total extrinsic time pressure score is more than one standard deviation above the mean for university hospital physicians [Belkić & Nedić 2007].

> We use the total (high demands + extrinsic time pressure) score above the mean plus lack of decision-making latitude (high strictness scores) as an operational definition of JOB STRAIN for physicians:
>
> JOB STRAIN is present.

	Underload	High Demand	Strictness	Time Pressure	Noxins	Threat avoidance	Conflict/ Uncertainty
Input		Information: • Several sources • Heterogeneous • Rapid inflow (ER) • Communication essential	• Strict requirements for detecting information --ER/ICU	• Limited control over speed of incoming information --Can't control patient scheduling, # inpatients	Sporadic: •Noise (ER)	• Grave consequences of momentary lapse -ER/ICU • Visually-disturbing scenes (suicide, trauma) • Listens to emotionally-disturbing occurrences --Most severe patients	Incoming information conflict: • Signal/noise • Signal/signal
Central Decision-Making		Decisions: • Complex • Complicated • Affect others • Rapid --Supervises --ER/ICU	Strict: • Problem-solving strategy • Definition of correct decision -Rules -Many over-seers	• Can't postpone decisions --ER/ICU		• Potentially fatal consequences of wrong decision	Information: •Contradictory •Missing --Can't get history, language barriers • Unforeseeable events require new plan -ER/ICU
Output/ Task Perfor-mance	• Waiting time	Tasks: • Complex • Varied --Clinical, teaching, research, administration •Simultaneous & rapid tasks: ER/ICU	• Strict evaluation of performance -Many over-seers	• Limited control of performance rate --Can't control which clinical tasks assigned, # patients, other duties		• Hazardous tasks (psychotic patients, infection)	• Conflicting tasks (no time aside for teaching or non-clinical tasks) *Hampered by **many**:* • Extrinsic problems • Interruptions from people
General	• Fixed pay • Inadequate pay • Low chance for upgrade (due to active opposition) • Little recognition of good work	• >48 h/work week • No true rest breaks • Night shift 4x / month – works before & after, no guaranteed relief after	• Shares window-less office & looks for room to examine patients • Limited in taking time off from work *Low influence over*: -With whom she works –Schedule -Tasks -Policy	• Deadline pressure • Speed-up	Mild: • Heat • Cold	Past work exposures: • Harmed by psychotic patients • Witnessed serious accidents • Patient suicides • Work-related court testimony • No system for non-medical emergencies	• Emotionally-charged work atmosphere • Little help with clinical difficulties • Opposition to career advancement • Behavior norm violations, power abuses • No grievance redress • Some pointless tasks
Total	Modifiable: 7.5 Underload = 7.5	Fixed: 15.5 Modifiable: 13 High Demand = 28.5	Fixed: 4 Modifiable: 14 Strictness = 18	Fixed: 3.75 Modifiable: 5.75 Time pressure = 9.5	Modifiable: 1 Noxious = 1	Fixed/past :12.5 Modifiable: 4 Threat avoidance = 16.5	Fixed: 8.5 Modifiable: 16.5 Conflict = 25

Figure 7.1 Summary of the baseline OSI for Dr. R: Total OSI = 106.

- Noxious exposures:

There is somewhat less than optimal heating and air-conditioning, and sporadic noise in the emergency room. Overall, however, exposure to noxious physical factors is fairly minimal for Dr. R.

- Threat Avoidant Vigilance:

The TAV score is exceedingly high, over 3 standard deviations above the mean for female university hospital physicians [Nedić 2006a][Belkić & Nedić 2007]. Most (but not all) of this TAV burden is an intrinsic part of Dr. R's work as a psychiatrist, coupled with past work experience: having been harmed by a psychotic patient, having seen colleagues and staff assaulted by patients, having seen several patient suicides (notably, the most recent which could have been prevented, had colleagues heeded her advice) and having testified in court regarding patients and a colleague.

- Conflict and uncertainty:

The conflict/uncertainty score is also exceedingly high, over 4 standard deviations above the mean for female university hospital physicians. Most of the conflict/uncertainty burden is due to potentially modifiable factors. In particular, there are numerous barriers that frequently hamper providing adequate patient care, numerous interruptions often at critical moments and a tense atmosphere, especially with display of knowledge (colleagues keep this for themselves and don't help one another), active opposition to career advancement (colleagues step over each other in this competitive atmosphere). Besides career blocking, demeaning comments are frequent from some colleagues and supervisors, with clinical assessment and recommendations often ignored.

The TAV and CONFLICT aspects are a major source of Dr. R's work stressor burden. In our experience working with colleagues suffering from burnout, these two aspects are: THE MOST CRITICAL CONTRIBUTORS TO PSYCHOLOGICAL DISTRESS.

7.3 How to Proceed? Return to Healthier Work with Bolstered Coping Strategies

Dr. R has become burned-out, in large measure, due to her work. Yet, return to work is pivotal for her recovery. We present a realistic plan for modifying the conditions under which she works, tailored to her clinical status, capacities and affinities. This is an iterative process; we start with the steps that can be immediately implemented, in order for Dr. R to get back to work with reasonable safety.

7.3.1 *Immediate steps*

These measures are outlined in Figure 7.2, according to the OSI model. Dr. R's acute deterioration was associated with handling patients at extremely high risk for suicide during night shift work in the psychiatric emergency room. At least temporarily, she should not take night call and avoid ER duty with exposure to the most severely ill patients.

She should work a regular day shift, starting half-time. In order to function effectively, she needs her own office and it must be assured that she is not interrupted when seeing patients. At least ten minutes of rest break must be scheduled between patients. During break time, Dr. R. needs to be completely free from disturbance. Implementing these measures for Dr. R is reasonably straightforward. The rationale that only under such conditions can her work capacity be preserved is accepted by the hospital administration.

As seen in Figure 7.2, the stressor burden has been lowered considerably, altogether by over 17 points, so that the total OSI score is now below the acute danger level. This is due not only to the direct interventions outlined above (marked with frames on Fig. 7.2) but also due to the impact of these measures on other stressors (marked with arrows on Fig. 7.2). This is seen most clearly for work in the emergency room, which influenced 13 other factors.

Overall, it was the high demand score which was reduced to the greatest extent by these interventions. With a reduction of nearly 8 points, the total high demand score is now below the mean for university hospital physicians. Thus, exposure to both JOB STRAIN and EFFORT REWARD IMBALANCE has been effectively lowered. Most importantly, with these measures, Dr. R goes back to work, which positively affects her self-confidence. Since she is now working reduced hours, she has the time (and it is firmly recommended) that she regularly engages in recreational physical activity. She also has time scheduled to meet with the occupational neuropsychiatrist twice per week to pursue the next phases of the process of creating a healthier work environment.

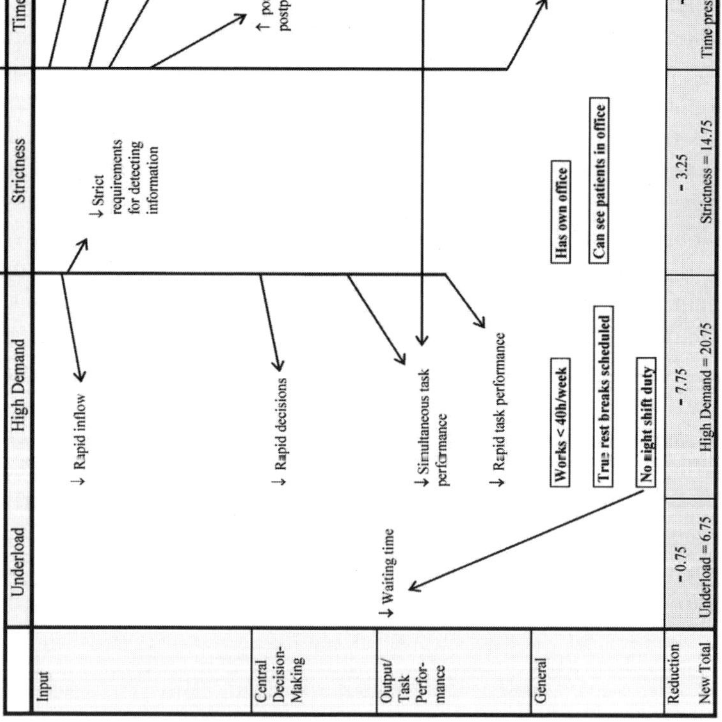

Figure 7.2 Immediate steps for Dr. R's initial return to work: Total OSI (106 – 17.125) = 88.875.

7.3.2 *Step II–Cognitive/behavioral therapy focusing on psychosocial work stressors*

The immediate measures outlined above created the preconditions for addressing the more complex, psychosocial work stressors. Here, Dr. R gains deeper insight into the work she performs and its toll upon cognitive and emotional resources.

She more objectively assesses the milieu in which she works, identifying strategies to handle the difficulties that exist. As her coping mechanisms are bolstered, she better distinguishes those stressors upon which she can have a direct influence from those that are not within her immediate domain. (The latter will be addressed in Step III).

Beginning with the underload aspect, lack of recognition of good work and low chance for position upgrade (due to active opposition) are brought into focus. Here, Dr. R is encouraged to think about the innumerable patients she has helped. She is also encouraged to savor and appreciate her pedagogical and scientific achievements and their positive impact. With this, Dr. R is given the assignment to upgrade her Curriculum Vitae, including an extensive narrative and to describe her accomplishments in an oral presentation. This helps lay the basis for a formal application to upgrade her academic and clinical position. Dr. R is also asked to describe the good work and contributions of colleagues and staff and to elaborate how these are complementary to her own.

Next, Dr. R analyses her actual workload and tasks. Besides clinical work, she was teaching physicians on specialization training and medical studies in an informal setting, as well as lecturing, performing clinical research and administrative duties. Work time was not allocated for these other tasks, but rather "sandwiched in" between clinical activities. Consequently, she often stayed late at the hospital or came in early in the morning to complete this work. She also did a good deal of preparation at home, in the evenings and weekends. She was frequently called at home by the hospital staff, as well as by patients and sometimes even their families.

In parallel with the workload analysis, Dr. R prepares a diary during a workday. She notes that "bottlenecks" occur when difficult patients come early in the day to outpatient clinic. Scheduling these patients at the end of the workday circumvents this problem.

Figure 7.3 summarizes the processes involved in Step II.

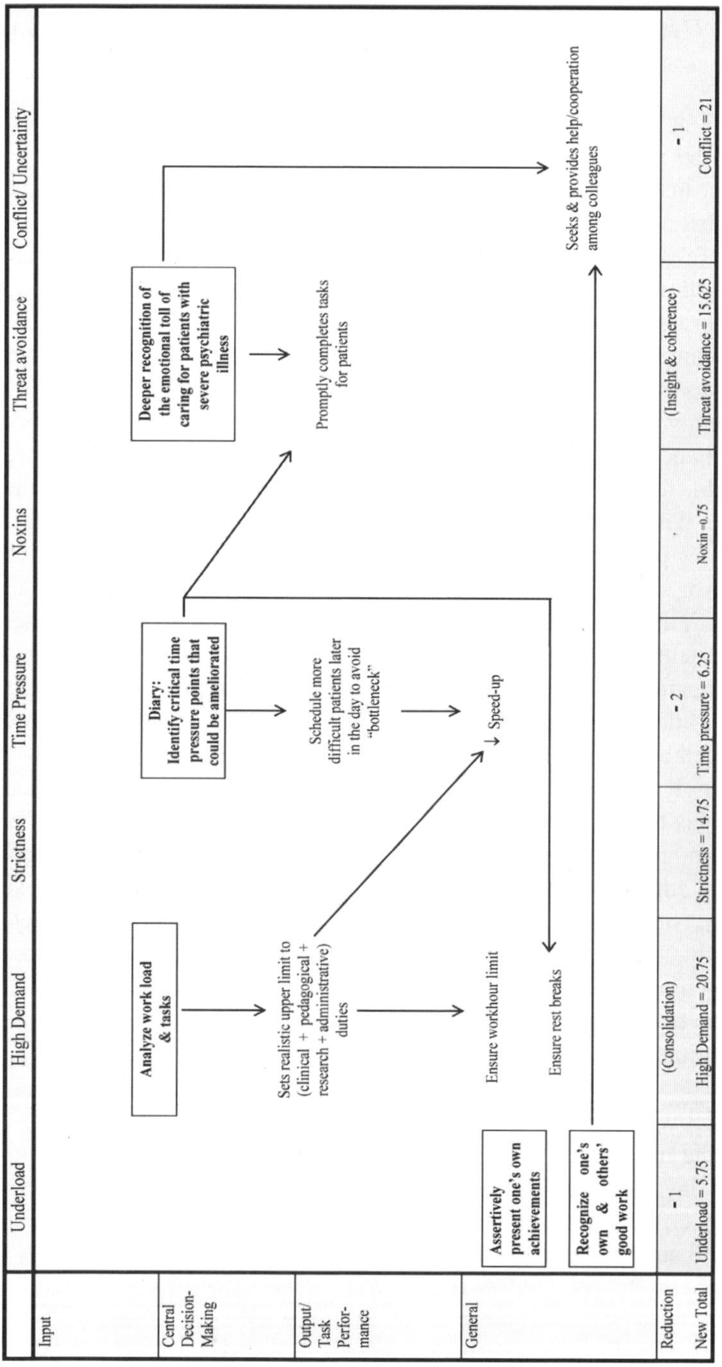

Figure 7.3 Cognitive/behavioral therapy with a focus on psychosocial stressors: Total OSI (88.875 – 4) = 84.875.

Dr. R more deeply considers the emotional toll of caring for patients with severe psychiatric illness. She revisits the events that triggered her own illness. She realizes that she did everything she possibly could to help the patient who later committed suicide, and that the outcome was due to the colleagues' failure to heed her advice. She recognizes the need to accept this reality. By scheduling the most difficult patients at the end of the workday, Dr R can immediately complete the medical report and all other work needed for these patients. Thereafter, she has the time to discuss difficult cases with colleagues.

Dr. R selects those colleagues with whom she can comfortably exchange experiences and share her feelings. Although the atmosphere at work is competitive and tense, there are a few such colleagues. Dr. R's self-confidence is enhanced and a positive process is initiated whereby colleagues begin to help one another. Not only does she thereby receive the support which she needs, Dr. R also provides that support, in return.

7.3.3 *Step III – Outreach: Initial efforts towards improving work organization*

Dr. R is now back to work and the overall burden of occupational stressors, as reflected in the total OSI of 84.875 although still high, is within one standard deviation above the mean for university hospital physicians [Nedić 2006a]. However, a number of the stressors (night call, ER duty, etc.) contributing to high demands she had faced prior to her present illness have been offloaded onto other colleagues.

The conditions under which Dr. R was working prior to her present illness are not at all atypical. The total OSI scores of other colleagues in her unit range form 95 to 108. Of particular note is that the TAV and conflict/uncertainty scores remain exceedingly high for Dr. R, as well as for her colleagues.

The next step is to enumerate all the possible organizational measures that could be taken to lower the stressor burden for Dr. R. and for her colleagues. This comprehensive overview is presented in Figure 7.4.

From this overview, Dr. R makes some decisions about the initial steps that she considers most vital. She begins by returning once again to the event that immediately triggered her illness. She realizes that there is a major breakdown in communication between senior colleagues like her, and the junior colleagues such as those who did not heed her advice.

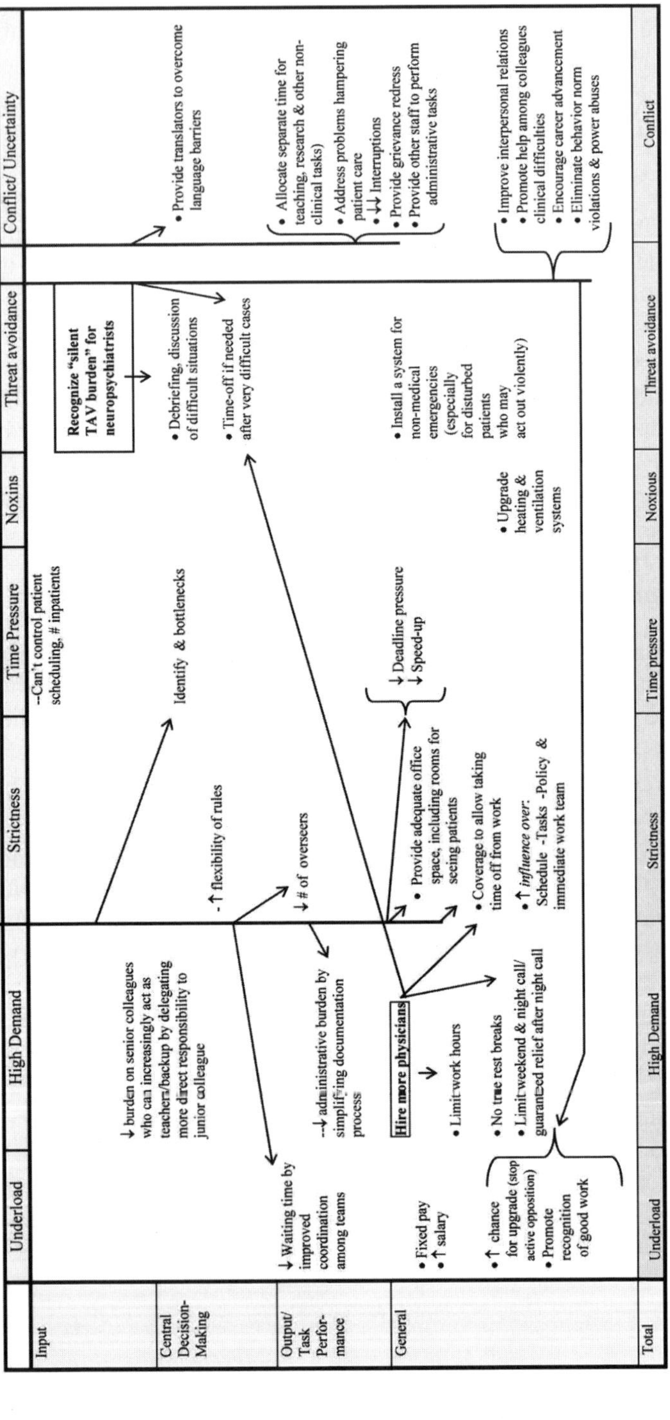

Figure 7.4 A comprehensive view of occupational stressors faced by Dr. R, that could be ameliorated by organizational measures.

She notes that rounds and other meetings frequently evoke tirades between these two groups. The younger colleagues want to "prove" their competence and knowledge by acting independently, while the senior colleagues feel slighted in that their experience is belittled. As a response to these feelings, some of the senior physicians make demeaning comments about their younger colleagues.

An underlying tension is related to the competition for career advancement. This tension is exacerbated when some of the younger physicians acquire higher academic positions through their research and view clinical work with a certain disdain. This attitude is actively supported by a segment of the hospital department leadership since these younger colleagues who are more involved in research often secure prestigious research grants. At the same time, several of the senior physicians including Dr. R and some of the younger colleagues as well face career blocking initiated by a sector of the department leadership.

Dr. R now feels ready openly discuss this situation with those colleagues who provide mutual support for the difficult clinical cases. Overall, they agree with her assessment and express their appreciation that Dr. R has articulated the situation so accurately.

The process of implementing organizational change is difficult and slow. The colleagues know that there will be many roadblocks and conflict ahead. They decide that the best next steps would be:

- To meet with those in the department leadership who are most likely to give an ear to their observations about the present situation.

- To help each other prepare their CV's and other formal documents to apply for position upgrade.

7.4 Comments and Further Thoughts

We leave the rest of the development regarding Dr. R open. Many outcomes are possible, based upon very many factors. We encourage the reader to ponder further in relation to his/her own experience and realistic possibilities for improvement.

While her own efforts are obviously essential, a favorable outcome for Dr. R will also be influenced by the efforts of her colleagues, those of the occupational neuropsychiatrist as well as the goodwill and integrity of those in positions of leadership and organizational responsibility.

Within the framework of the developing field of "occupational neuropsychiatry," it must be explicitly emphasized that *empathy* is the vital ingredient, the "glue" as it were, for promoting coherence and healthy return to work for Dr. R, and for so many whose situation is much like hers.

Further Reading

Section 2.2.4.1, Section 3.4.3.2, and Section 4.1.2.3 are recommended as cross-references within part I of this book. References of particular relevance for this case study include: [Fridner *et al.*, 2009] [Kumar, *et al.*, 2005], [Maslach et al. 2001] [Maslach & Leiter, 2008][Nedić 2006b][Rosenberg & Godhramri 2001] [Savić 2002] [Shirom 2011].

> With these insights gleaned about the work environment and mental health within our own profession, we now proceed to the next cases, which concern other occupations and the impact of working conditions upon patients within the domain of neuropsychiatry.

Chapter 8

Middle School Teacher with Panic Attacks and Migraine Headaches: Second Case Study

M.A., in her late 30's, teaches mathematics and natural science in a middle-school.

She faces her workdays with trepidation—fearful that she cannot fulfill her obligations.

The ensuing panic attacks are associated with ever more frequent migraine headaches.

Total OSI = 96

Questions for reflection while reviewing this case:

- Is this a dangerously stressful work situation?
- Is the patient's work situation contributing to her disorder? *If so, how?*
- Could workplace modifications help improve the patient's clinical status? *If so, how?*

8.1 The Case: M.A.'s Panic Attacks and Severe Migraines

For the last 3 to 4 years, M.A. has felt increasing psychological tension and worry that she will be unable to fulfil her daily obligations. Recently, she has begun to fear losing control, both at work and at home with her children. This fear is episodic and associated with palpitations, sweating, lack of air and pressure in the chest. She often wakes up during the night and is thereafter unable to go back to sleep. With increasing frequency, she finds herself overwhelmed by negative thoughts that bring on subsequent migraine headaches. These, in turn, indeed prevent M.A. from fulfilling her obligations, since she then must lie down in a dark, quiet room. The headaches have a rather insidious onset. They are pulsating and accompanied by photophobia, phonophobia, nausea and often also vomiting. No aura is described. She usually takes sumatriptan after the headache has lasted for at least 1-2 hours.

Migraine headaches were first diagnosed at age 13, at which time they occurred about 1-2 per month, usually premenstrually. After age 25, the headaches became more frequent, approximately 3-4 times per month, and over the last year 2-3 times per week.

M.A. is very engaged with her regular work as a teacher. She also gives private lesions several days per week. She performs all the housework tasks alone and is very involved with her own two children, sons age 8 and 11.

She has been pregnant three times with two normal childbirths and one spontaneous abortion. Menses are regular and heavy. Past medical history and review of systems are otherwise unremarkable. Her mother has suffered from migraine headaches since adolescence and at age 60 had a transitory cerebrovascular crisis. Her sister has occasional migraine headaches. M.A. lives with her husband who is a project manager for a multi-national natural gas systems company and their sons. She has smoked about 20 cigarettes per day for the past 15 years, and drinks 4 to 5 cups of coffee per day. She does not drink alcohol. With regard to eating habits, she rarely eats breakfast on workdays and is quite irregular in eating other meals. Lunch often consists of yogurt and a sandwich.

8.1.1 *Objective findings*

M.A. appears anxious, thin, has pressured speech and appears older than her stated age. She is slightly tachypnic, blood pressure: 130/80 mmHg, pulse: 95/min. There are scattered wheezes on forced expiration. The remainder of the physical examination is unremarkable. Except for serum ferritin at the lower limit of normal, all other hematologic as well as biochemical and endocrinological laboratory values including T3, T4, TSH are within normal limits.

- Neuropsychiatric findings:

Neurological: Symmetric hyperactive deep tendon reflexes, otherwise normal neurological examination.

Psychiatric: Sudden, recurrent paroxysmal anxiety attacks lasting for several minutes and occurring up to 3 to 5 times per day. These attacks have an unexpected onset with chest discomfort, palpitations, feelings of choking and light-headedness. The attacks are associated with feelings of loss of control and fear of dying. Some underlying obsessive ideation and sleep disturbances are present.

Diagnoses:
Migraine headaches without auras (G43.0),
Panic attacks--episodic paroxysmal anxiety (F41.0)
Tobacco dependence (F17.2)
[World Health Organization, 1993] (Appendix A, Sections 1 and 2)

- Neuropsychological testing:

Left-handed, normal memory span, reaction time and attention.

- Questionnaire findings:

→Spielberger State Anxiety Score = 55 (extremely high) [Spielberger *et al.*,1983].

→Panic Disorder Severity Index Composite Score = 1.5
corresponding to moderately ill [Keogh *et al.*, 2012].

→General Health Questionnaire (GHQ12) = 6
indicative of high psychological distress.
Much more than usual she has: “lost much sleep over worry,” felt that she “could not overcome [her] difficulties” and “felt constantly under strain.”

- Psychophysiologic and neurophysiologic evaluation:

→Electroencephalographic and polygraphic findings: Maximally desynchronized EEG indicates psychological tension. Respirations 13/min, ECG 102/min, sinus tachycardia. Heart rate variability: ↓ 0.15 – 0.4 Hz component, ↑ 0.04 – 0.15 Hz component, indicating elevated sympathetic tone and withdrawal of vagal input.

→Visual Event Related Potential Odd Ball Paradigm:
High amplitude, short latency of N2 and P3 components, rapid reaction time, intense involvement in task performance. Consistent with arousal and heightened vigilance.

8.2 M.A.'s Work Situation: Insights from the OSI

M.A. has worked as a middle-school teacher for ten years, five years at her present job in a low-income school. In Figure 8.1, each OSI stressor for M.A. is identified and categorized as either fixed or as modifiable.

- Underload:

There are no inherent underload factors in a teacher's work environment. In the case of M.A., however, as seen in the left-most column of Fig. 8.1, 8.5 points for underload are related to five modifiable factors. M.A. performs some monotonous administrative tasks, has inadequate, fixed pay with no chances for upgrade. There is little recognition of good work.

- High demand:

Over three quarters of the high demand burden is fixed for M.A.'s teaching profile and work setting. Most of the modifiable factors are on the general level. M.A. spends 30 hours per week actively teaching in the classroom and changes weekly between mornings and afternoons. She spends another 10 hours per week grading homework and exams, and another 10 hours per week preparing course plans, plus other duties (performing administrative tasks, communicating with parents and meetings with colleagues and staff). Work time is not allocated for these other duties besides classroom teaching, so that *de facto* she works through breaks, intersperses these tasks with teaching and brings home work daily. She does not have true rest breaks because there are always work-related interruptions. The usual class size is between 26 and 30 pupils, and she has 6 different classes. Besides this regular work, she does private tutoring, and remedial teaching over the summer.

The combination of high demands plus underload suggests that: EFFORT-REWARD IMBALANCE is present.

	Underload	High Demand	Strictness	Time Pressure	Noxins	Threat avoidance	Conflict/ Uncertainty
Input		Information: • Several sources • Heterogeneous • Communication essential	• Strict requirements for detecting information: --special needs pupils --accident risk -behavioral threats	• Limited control over speed of incoming information --Can't control # pupils, # classes	Sporadic: • Noise	• Vigilance required ∝ accident risk & unpredictable pupil behaviors • Listens to emotionally-disturbing occurrences	Incoming information conflict: • Signal/noise (actual noise)
Central Decision-Making		Decisions: • Complex • Complicated • Affect others • Rapid: special needs, violence risk	-Rules require strict: • Problem-solving strategy • Definition of correct decision	• Sometimes cannot postpone decisions: --accident risk -behavioral threats		• Potentially serious consequences of wrong decision regarding pupil behaviors, laboratory	Information: •Contradictory • Unforeseeable events require new plan: frequent curriculum Δ
Output/ Task Perfor-mance	• Some monotonous administrative tasks	Tasks: • Complex • Varied • Rapid: laboratory-technical --Teaching + administration	-Many over-seers: • Strict evaluation of task performance	• Limited control of performance rate # pupils, # classes	• Lifting	Hazards: • Small but present risk of violence from pupils • Poor electrical installation	• Conflicting tasks (no time aside for tasks besides classroom teaching) *Effective teaching hampered by **many***: • Extrinsic problems • Interruptions from people
General	• Fixed pay • Inadequate pay • Low chance for upgrade • Little recognition of good work	• >48 h/work week • No true rest breaks • Irregular work schedule • 2nd job	• Changes classrooms • Very limited in taking time off from work *Low influence over*: -Support staff with whom she works –Schedule -Tasks -Policy	• Deadline pressure • Speed-up	Mild: • Heat • Cold • Dust, chemicals (lab. work)	Past work exposures: • Heard about serious accident • No system for emergencies	• Little help with difficulties • Behavior norm violations, power abuses • Ineffective grievance redress • Some pointless tasks • Threat of job loss
Total	Modifiable: 8.5 Underload = 8.5	Fixed: 22 Modifiable: 6.5 High Demand = 28.5	Fixed: 3 Modifiable: 15 Strictness = 18	Fixed: 3 Modifiable: 6 Time pressure = 9.0	Modifiable: 4.5 Noxious = 4.5	Fixed: 6.5 Modifiable: 3 Threat avoidance = 9.5	Fixed: 3 Modifiable: 15 Conflict = 18

Figure 8.1 Summary of the baseline OSI for M.A. Total OSI = 96.

• Strictness:
M.A. teaches a substantial number of pupils with behavioral and social problems. This, plus laboratory work create strict requirements for information detection. The remainder of the strictness burden is modifiable. Her influence over all important aspects of work is minimal or none, and she is overseen by administrators who have never worked as teachers and who often criticize her work and judgment, as well as that of her colleagues. The curriculum is administratively pre-determined. It is very difficult for her to take any time off at all during the regular school year. She must change classrooms several times per day, carrying along with her all needed materials. Altogether, these factors create a high strictness burden.

• Extrinsic time pressure:
A major proportion of the heavy external time pressure load is modifiable. Contributory factors include the large number of classes taught, large class size over which she has no control, together with frequent administrative deadlines. Due to these factors and the above-described heavy demands, M.A. must often work at an accelerated pace.

> The total (high demands + extrinsic time pressure) score together with low decision-making latitude (high strictness scores) indicate that: JOB STRAIN is present.

• Noxious exposures:
The classrooms are run down with a number of structural problems. Heating is sub-optimal and there is no air conditioning. The rooms are drafty and they are dusty since janitorial services have been cut back. M.A. must occasionally lift heavy laboratory equipment. Overall, the noxious exposure load is not inconsequential.

• Threat Avoidant Vigilance:
Substantial TAV burden is present, mainly related to the nature of M.A.'s work. Vigilance is needed because of unpredictable behaviors of some pupils and because of accident risk associated with the laboratory work. She has not, however, had or seen a work-related accident. If a system were in place to handle emergencies and if the electrical installation were repaired, the TAV burden could be somewhat ameliorated.

- Conflict and uncertainty:

Almost all of the heavy conflict/uncertainty load would be lightened. Frequent administratively-mandated curriculum changes require new plans and approaches. The work-related instructions are often confusing and contradictory. Effective teaching is hampered by large class size, lack of appropriate textbooks, administrative constraints, poor infrastructure and lack of teaching assistants to provide the individualized attention needed by many of the pupils. Some of the administrators make demeaning comments about the teachers. There is a grievance system in place; however, it is not effective or confidential. Due to budget cuts for education, there is a threat of job loss.

The TAV and CONFLICT burden is high and likely to be a major CONTRIBUTOR to M.A.'s PSYCHOLOGICAL DISTRESS.

8.3 M.A. Meets with the Occupational Neuropsychiatrist

Even though M.A. is still working, she is well aware that her current situation is untenable. Meetings with the occupational neuropsychiatrist proceed as follows:

8.3.1 *Assessment*

The total OSI score is close to the acutely dangerous level. While M.A.'s work situation is not the sole source of her current clinical condition, it is a major contributor. The two neuropsychiatric disorders are anxiety with panic attacks and migraine headaches without aura. Smoking, unhealthy eating habits and sub-clinical iron deficiency also warrant attention.

8.3.2 *Therapeutic measures: Cognitive-behavioral therapy, immediate work-related and lifestyle changes and pharmacotherapy*

The therapeutic approach begins with one week away from work, during which M.A. starts on serotonin reuptake inhibitors as well as oral iron supplements, especially prior to menses. She is also is referred to a professional smoking cessation center, to a dietician and to a relaxation training group.

Within the framework of cognitive-behavioral therapy, she concretely addresses the inter-relation among the work environment, unhealthy lifestyle and her clinical status. Work-related interventions that could be most feasibly implemented are identified, through analysis of workload and tasks, together with a review of the results from the baseline OSI. These changes are summarized in Fig. 8.2.

Firstly, since it is under M.A.'s full control, demand levels are lowered by stopping the private tutoring and summer teaching. Regarding the latter, this would allow her a full summer vacation of recreation and rest, which she greatly needs.

Next, the number of classes is reduced from six to five. This is achieved by meeting with the school principal and presenting the workload analysis and time obligations involved.

As a consequence, classroom teaching is reduced from 30 to 25 hours, and six hours are reduced from other duties. Thereby, a modicum of relief is provided from the speed up and deadline pressure. She maps out the new schedule and includes times for obligatory rest breaks.

The other request made to the school principal is to have her own classroom. With the description of the extra burden involved in moving from room to room, and that this would improve her functioning, plus the fact that this request would entail no extra cost, the principal agrees.

The prospect of having her own classroom, as a "home-base," prompts M.A. to begin thinking about some physical improvements that could be made quite simply. For the beginning, she takes a few hours on the weekend to come in and prepare the classroom. She does this with the help of her sons, who bring some of their extra youth-oriented science and math posters.

She prepares a small heater / fan which will somewhat ameliorate temperature extremes. She also brings in an alarm which could be used in case of emergencies. M.A. then makes a plan to organize an action session with her pupils to thoroughly clean and decorate the classroom.

Thereafter, she plans to initiate a strategy used by her own teachers when she was a pupil. Namely, each day, one pupil is assigned the responsibility for classroom neatness. Insofar as the pupil does not fulfil this obligation, he or she would be called upon to solve a really tough math problem. M.A. recalls very distinctly that this strategy indeed provided the needed motivation for the pupils to maintain a tidy classroom.

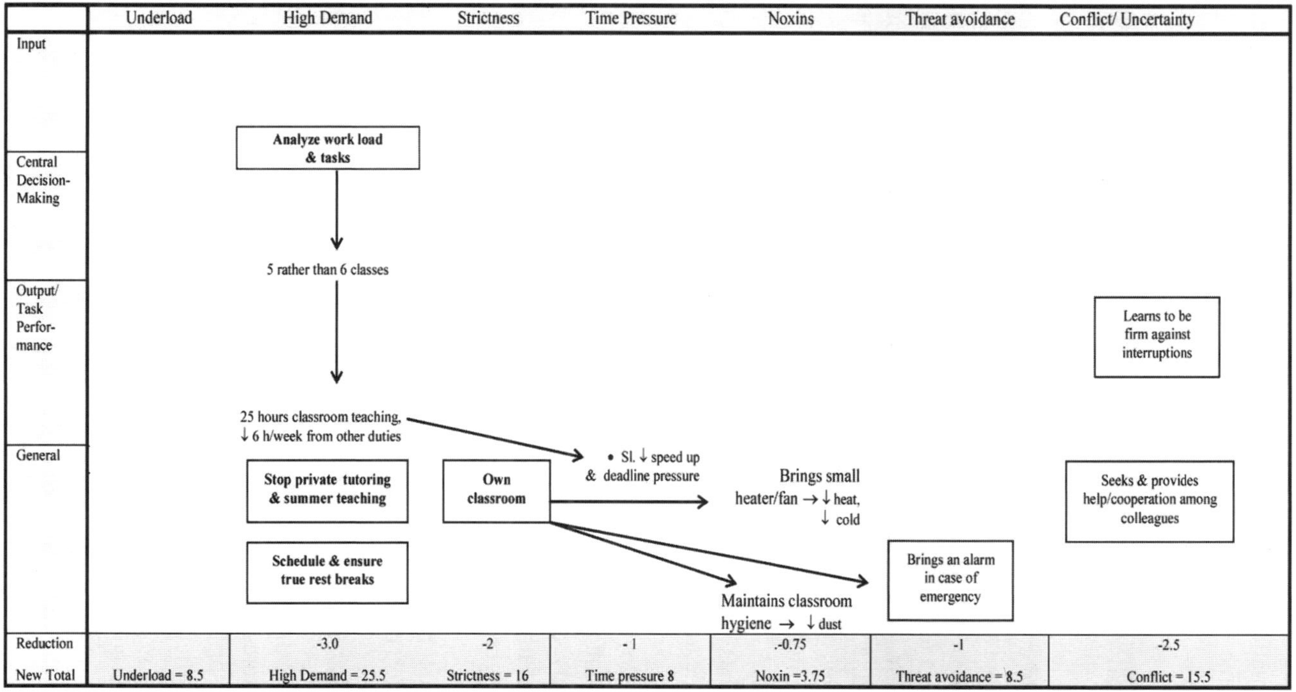

Figure 8.2 Initial modifications in M.A.'s work situation integrated with cognitive-behavioral therapy: Total OSI (96 – 10.25) = 85. 75.

During the cognitive-behavioral therapeutic sessions with the occupational neuropsychiatrist, M.A. revisits her original decision to become a science and mathematics teacher and to work in a low income school. She describes her initial enthusiasm about this "calling," which was much more than "just a job."

She also recalls the inspiring teachers from her own schooling and their innovative strategies for handling pupils with widely different levels of knowledge. In particular, she remembers how her mathematics teacher would engage all the pupils in solving a given problem, and that the one who solved it first was given the privilege of writing a mark of "excellent" on his or her school record. She also recalled the highly effective "buddy" system to encourage the pupils to help one another.

Now, with more time and calm, she begins to think about how to institute these strategies into her own teaching practice. In particular, she reflects on how interruptions and rowdy behavior could be thereby effectively held in check.

M.A. shares these thoughts with several of her colleagues with whom she has a good rapport. She also asks their advice about how to best handle interruptions and disruptions. This give-and-take initiates a process of cooperation and better appreciation among the teachers.

Altogether, with these measures the total OSI is lowered by just over 10 points. M.A. sees clearly that the occupational burden and lifestyle are closely connected. She is given some scientific papers on this topic, especially on the association between total OSI and smoking. She adopts a suggestion from her smoking cessation group. Namely, she puts aside two money jars, one for classroom needs and one for a personal reward. Each time she successfully overcomes an urge to smoke, she puts the money, which would have been spent for cigarettes, into the two jars.

8.3.3 *Outreach: Initial efforts towards improving work organization*

The clinical status of M.A. is substantially improved with the therapeutic measures described in the previous subsection 8.3.2. However, the work stressor burden is still high, as evidenced by the total OSI score over 85. In particular, the conflict and uncertainty burden remains heavy.

Now that the panic attacks and migraine headaches are more or less under control, M.A. begins to probe more deeply into the root causes. She considers lack of job security to be underlying trigger of her fears. Some teachers have already been laid off, creating a "chilling effect."

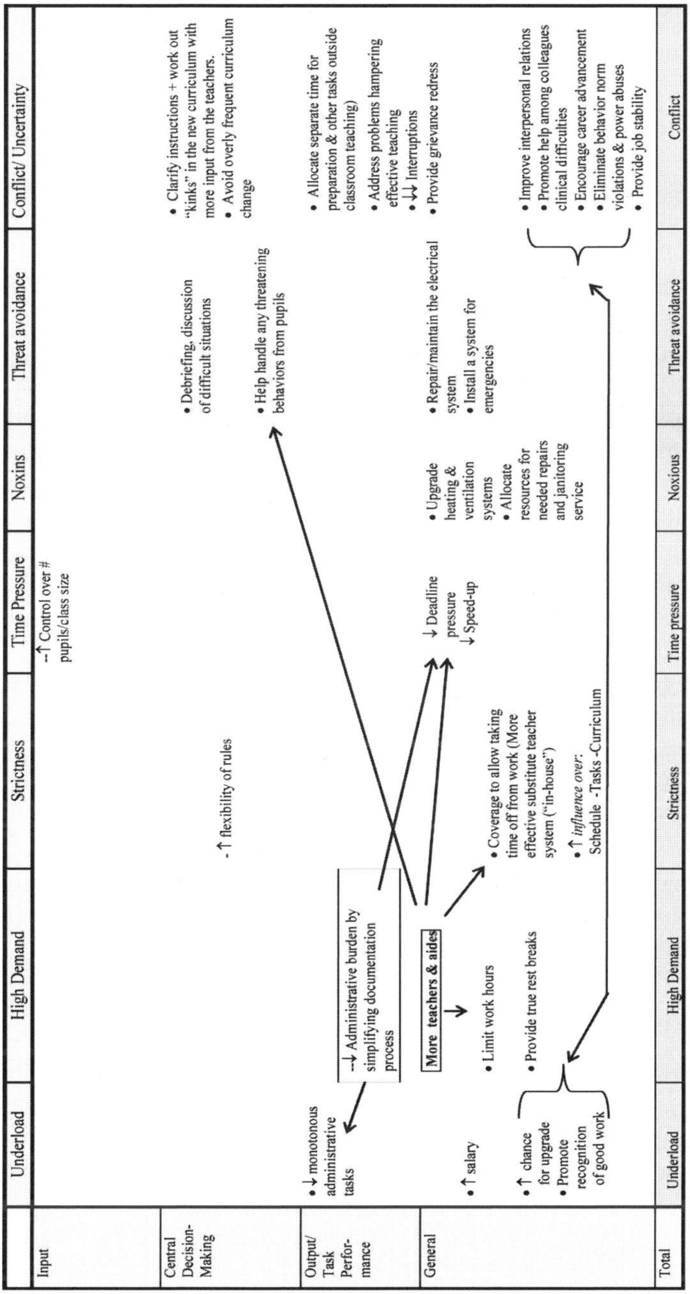

Figure 8.3 A comprehensive view of occupational stressors faced by M.A., that could be ameliorated by organizational measures.

The teachers who remain are then not only saddled with more work, but also there is a general trepidation about "*who will be next*?" More often than not, this fear is unarticulated. Instead, it has contributed to a breakdown of morale and less cooperation and help among colleagues.

It is clear to M.A. that the cutbacks in the school budget need to be addressed in a broader way, with outreach to parents, community groups as well as the teachers' union. With an adequate and more stable school budget, not only would the teachers be secure in their jobs, but it would be possible to reinstate the teaching positions that were cut back and also to hire needed support staff, such as teachers' aides, as well as janitorial services.

At the same time, M.A. sees outreach to the community as a key to improving the overall situation of the school. As community groups become more actively involved, many creative solutions could arise. Senior citizen groups, for example, could mobilize their members to provide one-on-one tutoring for pupils in need. Vital to these efforts is to create a healthy atmosphere, whereby community volunteers are given their deserved respect and validation. The broader context of support for public education, promoting quality education, especially for children who are left far behind is underscored [Ravitch 2010].

Figure 8.3 comprehensively summarizes the possible organizational measures that could be taken to lower the stressor burden for M.A. and other teachers at the school. The process which has begun with M.A. has been an impetus for positive change. M.A. feels gratified about this. She realizes that this process goes well beyond her own work situation. Therefore she allows herself to pull back when needed, to relax, "recharge her battery" and enjoy other aspects of life. Thereby, she strives to more calmly assess the situation and formulate more effective strategies for the challenges ahead.

Further Reading

Sections 2.2.3, 2.2.4.2, 2.3.1, 3.4.1, 3.4.6, 4.1.3 and 4.2.1 are recommended as cross-references within part I of this book. Further references of particular relevance for this case study include:

[Innstrand *et al.*, 2012] [Messing *et al.*, 1997] [Pas *et al.*, 2012] [van der Bergh & Huberman 1999].

Chapter 9

Computer Programmer with Epilepsy and Agoraphobia: Third Case Study

S.P., in his late 20s is a computer programmer & systems manager for a leading communications company.

He has had epilepsy since childhood.

A month ago he had a seizure at work. He took unpaid leave of absence thereafter & has been afraid to go out of his house.

Total OSI = 53.5

Questions for reflection while reviewing this case:

- Is this a dangerously stressful work situation?
- Is the patient's work situation contributing to his disorder? *If so, how?*
- Could workplace modifications help improve the patient's clinical status? *If so, how?*

9.1 The Case: S.P.'s Epilepsy and Agoraphobia

One month ago, S.P. had a generalized tonic-clonic (GTC) seizure while at work and in the presence of his colleague, who called for emergency care. S.P. was taken by ambulance to the local hospital where he was admitted to the neurology ward. EEG findings at that time revealed slowed baseline activity, with irregularly occurring generalized spike and sharp wave activity lasting up to 2 seconds, without clinical correlates. MRI findings (including fMRI) were normal. An increased dose of his anti-epileptic medication (Valproate) was prescribed for outpatient therapy.

The day prior to the occurrence of the seizure was described as fairly typical, aside from being somewhat more strenuous than usual. He had stayed up late (after midnight) since there were visitors at home. S.P. states that he had been taking Valproate as prescribed and denies use of alcohol or illicit drugs.

The first day after having been discharged, on his way to work, S.P. suddenly experienced acute fear of phobic dimensions, that he would have another epileptic seizure at that very moment. He took a taxi and went home. Since then, he has not left his house, and has sought the constant physical presence of his wife. He complains of feeling "continuously uneasy and distracted" and of having difficulty sleeping.

Past medical history and review of systems are remarkable only for epilepsy. Fetal history and delivery were normal and uncomplicated, with no seizures during the peri- or post-natal period. Psychomotor development was normal. S.P. was described as having been in good health until the age of 6 years, after which he had short episodes of being "absent" diagnosed as "*absence*." Since these episodes were relatively infrequent and of short duration, it was predicted that they would disappear spontaneously and no medications were prescribed. At the age of 8, he had the first GTC seizure, followed by the second 6 months later, after which his parents realized that this was indeed epilepsy. They fully accepted the advice of the epileptologist, which included a medication regimen of Valproate and regular follow-up. Thereafter, S.P. was seizure free until age 18. Then, while on vacation with friends, his belongings containing his medications were damaged. As a consequence, he did not take his medications for 5 consecutive days, after which he had a GTC seizure, which occurred without warning. Thereafter, he resumed taking his medications regularly, which were well-tolerated. He felt well and remained seizure-free until the presently described episode. Family history is negative for epilepsy and is otherwise unremarkable.

S.P. completed obligatory schooling on schedule and obtained an undergraduate university degree in mathematics and informatics. He is married and his wife is expecting their first child in five months.

9.1.1 *Objective findings*

S.P. is a well-developed, well-nourished male, who seems somewhat reticent and appears to be approximately his stated age. Blood pressure is 125/70, pulse 82/minute. Physical examination entirely unremarkable. Biochemical, hematologic and endocrinologic laboratory findings all within normal limits.

- Neuropsychiatric findings

Neurological: Normal.

Psychiatric: Phobic anxiety that the epileptic seizures will occur in a public place. Some associated sleep disturbances are present. The anxiety is interfering with the patient's ability to function in daily life.

Diagnoses:
Generalized tonic-clonic epilepsy (G40.3),
Agoraphobia (F40.0).
[World Health Organization, 1993] (Appendix A, Sections 1 and 2).

- Neuropsychological testing:

Right-handed, normal memory span, reaction time and attention.

- Questionnaire findings:

→Epilepsy Self-Efficacy Scale-2000 = 245 (low) [Pramuka *et al.*, 2007].

→Modified Fear Survey Schedule Total Score = 1,
upper quartile for patients with epilepsy. Maximum fear score (4) on seizures, crowds and failure [Hixson *et al.*, 2006].

→General Health Questionnaire (GHQ12) = 4,
indicative of some psychological distress.
Much more than usual he has: "lost much sleep over worry."
Much less than usual has he: "been able to concentrate on whatever [he is] doing."

- Psychophysiologic and neurophysiologic evaluation:

→Electroencephalographic and polygraphic findings:
Normal baseline EEG activity. A few occurrences of regular generalized spike slow wave activity (approximately 3 Hz) lasting 0.25 to 2 seconds without clinical correlates.
Respirations: 9/min, ECG: 80/min, normal sinus rhythm.

→Magnetic resonance findings:
Diffusion tensor imaging, fMRI and magnetic resonance spectroscopic imaging on 3T scanner reveal no epileptogenic focus. Very slight overall reduction in n-acetyl aspartate and choline in the left mesial temporal lobe compared to the right, otherwise entirely unremarkable.

→Visual Event Related Potential Odd Ball Paradigm:
Normal P300 amplitude, slightly prolonged latency, typical of patients with epilepsy and without psychotic symptoms [Halford 2003].

9.2 S.P.'s Work Situation: Insights from the OSI

S.P. has worked as a computer programmer and systems manager for six years, all at his present job with a leading communications company. In Figure 9.1, each OSI stressor for S.P. is identified and categorized as either fixed or as modifiable.

- Underload:

There are no inherent underload factors in S.P.'s work environment. However, as seen in the left-most column of Fig. 9.1, the total of 3 points for underload is related to two potentially modifiable factors. One is occasional waiting time and the other is fixed pay irrespective of the amount worked, since he is a salaried employee. On the other hand, the pay is entirely adequate, there are opportunities for career advancement and good work is recognized and openly appreciated.

- High demand:

Most of the high demand burden is fixed for S.P.'s profile and work setting. The modifiable factors are on the general level, with the exception of some simultaneous task performance (related to the tasks of system manager and computer programmer, plus supervising other employees). The work hours are long, sometimes over 60 hours per week.

	Underload	High Demand	Strictness	Time Pressure	Noxins	Threat avoidance	Conflict/ Uncertainty
Input		Information: • Several sources • Heterogeneous • Very heavily visual • Quite high frequency • Some communication needed	• Information sometimes hard to retrieve		Sporadic: • Glare		
Central Decision-Making		Decisions: • Complex • Complicated • Affect others (supervises)				• Material damage could result from wrong decision	Information: • Missing • Contradictory • Unforeseeable events require new plan
Output/ Task Performance	• Waiting time	Tasks: • Complex • Sometimes simultaneous • Varied	• Work must meet a strictly-defined standard	• Limited control of performance rate			• Conflicting tasks (system manager + programming + supervising) • Interruptions from people
General	• Fixed pay	• >48 h/work week • No true rest breaks • Irregular work schedule • Short vacations	• Sedentary work • Limited in taking time off from work *Low influence over:* –Schedule –Policy	• Deadline Pressure • Some speedup		Past work exposures: • Work accident (seizure) • Work-related litigation (testified in court about a colleague)	• No grievance redress
Total	Modifiable: 3 Underload = 3	Fixed: 17 Modifiable: 5.5 High Demand = 22.5	Fixed:2.75 Modifiable: 4.5 Strictness = 7.25	Fixed: 0.75 Modifiable: 2.0 Time pressure = 2.75	Modifiable: 1 Noxious = 1	Fixed: 5 Threat avoidance = 5	Fixed: 2 Modifiable: 10 Conflict = 12

Figure 9.1 Summary of the baseline OSI for S.P. Total OSI (Fixed = 27.5 + Modifiable = 26) = 53.5.

True rest breaks are lacking partly because S.P. becomes so involved in his work that he sometimes forgets to take them, and also because colleagues and staff inevitably come to him with computer related problems when he does try to take a break. In relation to system management related duties, S.P. has a somewhat irregular work schedule. Paid vacation time is three weeks per year.

> JOB DEMANDS are HIGH, but rewards are ample.
> Effort-Reward Imbalance is not present.

- Strictness:

There are a few inherently strict elements in S.P.'s job: needed information can sometimes be difficult to retrieve so that it must be picked up right away, the work must meet a strictly-defined standard and while working S.P. is sedentary. It is rather difficult for him to take time off from work and he has little influence over scheduling and company policy.

- Extrinsic time pressure:

The global market is the milieu in which the company "thrives or sinks." Deadlines and some speed-up of work tasks consequently ensue. Since the work which S.P. performs affects the work of his team, the rate of task performance is not entirely under his control. Thus, some extrinsic time pressure on the task performance and general levels is present.

> This is an ACTIVE JOB with high demands and some time pressure, but with substantial, albeit not full decision-making latitude. Full-blown job strain is not present.

- Noxious exposures:

Overall, the physical working conditions for S.P. are comfortable, as seen from a review the elements from general strictness as well as noxious exposures.

There is however one important exception for S.P., namely glare. This comes from the fluorescent lights shining onto stationary computer screen and for lack of adequate curtains or Venetian blinds to block the afternoon sun.

- Threat Avoidant Vigilance:

Since material damage could result from a serious error, the underlying TAV burden is not entirely negligible. The TAV burden from past work experience is due to two factors. One is the seizure which occurred at work, as described earlier in this case presentation. It therefore can be broadly considered a work accident. The other source of TAV from past work experience was that S.P. had to testify in court about a colleague who divulged company-developed patented software to a competitor.

- Conflict and uncertainty:

There is some conflict/uncertainty burden, most of which could be lightened. The work-related instructions are often contradictory. S.P.'s duties as a system manager, computer programmer plus supervising other employees frequently create conflicting demands in time and space. There are frequent interruptions from people, mainly related to the computer-related problems. There is no grievance system in place. On the other hand, inter-personal relations are good, the work atmosphere is pleasant, and there is a strong code of appropriate conduct to which those in positions of power and authority abide. S.P. is permanently employed and the job is coherent and meaningful for him.

There is some, though not extreme TAV and conflict burden.

9.3 S.P. Meets with the Occupational Neuropsychiatrist

S.P. has informed only a few of his closest friends regarding his epilepsy, about which is feels shame and stigma. He did not inform his employer when hired. This meeting with the occupational neuropsychiatrist is the first time he has been out of the house since the seizure occurred.

9.3.1 *Assessment*

The most important barrier to S.P.'s return to work is his fear of a repeat seizure. This fear has rendered him housebound, his self-esteem spiralling downward. Avoiding work because of his feelings of shame and stigma deprives him of a major source of confidence and satisfaction. He has been a valued employee and his work environment is overall quite healthy, although some modifications are needed for S.P. to thrive optimally. The latter would be best implemented together with disclosure of epilepsy. Given that inter-personal relations are good, the company leadership behaves responsibly and that S.P. is legally protected against discrimination for having epilepsy, disclosure is a viable option.

9.3.2 *Integrative therapeutic approach: Supportive/cognitive-behavioral therapy, disclosure and targeted workplace modifications*

The therapeutic approach begins with support and reassurance. This is coupled with an open discussion of the relatively high prevalence of epilepsy in the general population and the need to address and overcome stigmatization.

S.P.'s work achievements and capacity are reviewed, emphasizing the fact that these are indeed appreciated by colleagues and leadership within the company. S.P. has chosen a field in which there would be no major contraindication with regard to epilepsy. Neither public safety nor performance would be compromised if a seizure were to occur. In fact, his own safety would be best protected by informing his co-workers and formulating a contingency plan. Since there is an emergency system in place at work, realization of such a plan would be entirely feasible. Starting from this cognitive vantage point, the fear of a recurrent seizure is then further explored and demystified.

Next, modifiable work stressors are reviewed via the OSI, and potential triggers for seizures are identified. The latter include: fatigue from long work hours, deadline pressure and conflicting demands from his duties as a systems manager, supervisor and computer programmer, as well as glare from the computer screen and the afternoon sun.

As summarized in Figure 9.2, a realistic plan is made for implementing workplace modifications that would optimize conditions for S.P. A meeting with S.P., his immediate supervisor and the occupational neuropsychiatrist is scheduled. S.P. has decided to inform the supervisor about his epilepsy and to present the workplace modification plan. He first "rehearses" the meeting and develops contingency plans for various scenarios in active discussions with the occupational neuropsychiatrist. S.P. plans to direct the meeting himself, and explicitly formulates the circumstances under which he will need active involvement of the occupational neuropsychiatrist. Before the meeting and his return to work, S.P. and his wife decide to take a short vacation.

	Underload	High Demand	Strictness	Time Pressure	Noxins	Threat avoidance	Conflict/ Uncertainty
Input							
Central Decision-Making							
Output/ Task Performance		• Separate time for computer programming and system manager responsibilities					• ↓ conflicting tasks (system manager + programming + supervising) • ↓ Interruptions from people
General		• Limit work hours to 40/week • Plan & ensure true rest breaks • Regularize work schedule	• Facilitate taking time off from work when needed				
Total	Underload = 3	− 5 High Demand = 17.5	− 1.5 Strictness = 5.75	Time pressure = 2.75	−1 Noxious = 0	Threat avoidance = 5	− 4 Conflict = 8

Figure 9.2 Summary of measures taken to lower OSI for S.P. Total OSI (53.5 – 11.5) = 42.

9.4 The Outcome

With the support of his wife and the occupational neuropsychiatrist, S.P. returns to his job and he thrives.

Even though the total burden of occupational stressors was not excessive, improvements in his work environment created conditions for him to perform his job more effectively as well as avoiding potential triggers of seizures.

Further Reading

Sections 2.3.2, 3.4.1.1, 3.4.7, 4.1.3 and 4.2.2 are recommended as cross-references within part I of this book. Further references of particular relevance for this case study include:

[Brown & Previtt, 2007] [Fisher *et al.*, 2000] [Halford 2003][Strine *et al.*, 2009].

Chapter 10

Oncology Nurse with Breast Cancer and Disturbed Sleep: Fourth Case Study

C.G., in her late 50's is an oncology nurse.

She was recently diagnosed with Stage I breast cancer.

Since then, she has had difficulty falling asleep,
her sleep is discontinuous and
the dreams that she recalls
are cancer-related and disturbing.

Total OSI = 85

Questions for reflection while reviewing this case:

- Is this a dangerously stressful work situation?
- Is the patient's work situation contributing to her disorder? *If so, how?*
- Could workplace modifications help improve the patient's clinical status? *If so, how?*

10.1 The Case: C.G. has Breast Cancer and Disturbed Sleep

C.G. underwent routine biennial mammography six weeks ago, on which a non-palpable microcalcified lesion in the upper middle segment of the right breast was found. Excisional biopsy revealed invasive ductal carcinoma. The definitive surgical treatment was breast-conserving therapy and all the final margins were negative. Contrast-enhanced MRI showed no other suspicious lesions. No involvement of the ipsilateral axillary lymph nodes was revealed based upon sentinel node biopsy plus lymphoscintigraphy. The tumor was 0.9 cm in diameter and was estrogen receptor positive and *HER-1/neu* receptor negative. Subsequently, C.G. was treated with standard radiation therapy (25 fractions of 2.0 Gy over 5 weeks) and aromatase inhibitors.

Ever since she was told that the lesion was suspicious, C.G. has had difficulties sleeping. She complains of trouble falling asleep and of waking up repeatedly. The dreams she can remember have all been cancer-related, including remembrance of patients with metastatic disease and terminal outcomes.

Despite these sleep problems, C.G. has continued working. She gets through her work shifts "by drinking strong coffee and by a strong will" to complete her duties. She is determined not to let her colleagues down, since she knows that they are counting on her. She has not disclosed the breast cancer diagnosis to anyone at work.

C.G. states that she has "always been healthy" and denies any previous illness including any sleep disturbances. Review of systems is unremarkable.

During the peri-menopausal period several years ago, she took hormone replacement therapy for about two years upon the recommendation of her primary care physician. She is nulliparous, has never been married and lives alone.

C.G. immigrated to her present country of residence in her mid-twenties. Most of C.G.'s family lives in her country of origin and she has limited knowledge about their medical status.

She has never smoked cigarettes or drunk alcohol. She states that she is "careful" about her diet, but "enjoys sweets, maybe a little too much." She engages in recreational physical activity (folkdance) about once or twice per month and has "many good friends" with whom she socializes as often as she can, within the constraints of her work schedule.

C.G. has shared the cancer diagnosis with two of her closest friends, one of whom became very distraught.

C.G. is referred to the occupational neuropsychiatrist because of the sleep disturbances subsequent to the breast cancer diagnosis. The treating physician did not feel competent about advising on mental health questions, particularly as they may relate to her work.

10.1.1 *Objective findings*

C.G. is an alert, communicative, slightly overweight woman who appears somewhat younger than her stated age. Blood pressure is 130/80, pulse 82/minute, BMI = 27.8. Except for the surgical incision of the right breast and mild radiation-induced skin reaction, the physical examination is entirely unremarkable. Biochemical, hematologic and endocrinologic laboratory findings are all within normal limits.

- Neuropsychiatric findings:

Neurological: Slightly increased startle response, otherwise unremarkable.

Psychiatric: Sleep-onset and sleep-offset insomnia, with recurrent intrusive dreams with flashbacks related to breast cancer diagnosis.

Diagnoses:
S/P Surgical excision and radiation therapy of invasive adenocarcinoma of the right breast (Stage I) (C50),
Post-traumatic stress disorder with predominantly intrusive symptoms and sleep disturbances (F43.1)
[World Health Organization, 1993] (Appendix A, Sections 1 and 2).

- Neuropsychological testing:

Right-handed, normal memory span, reaction time and attention.

- Questionnaire findings:

→Penn State Worry Questionnaire: 11-item positively worded score = 44. High score, notably: maximum score (5) on the items: "As soon as I finish one task, I start to worry about everything else I must do" and "When I am under pressure, I worry a lot" [Wu *et al.*, 2012].

→General Health Questionnaire (GHQ12) = 2
(indicative of some psychological distress)

Much more than usual she has: "lost much sleep over worry."

- Psychophysiologic and neurophysiologic evaluation:

→Polysomnographic findings after night shift:
Disturbed sleep pattern with prolonged sleep latency, sleep fragmentation, diminished REM and slow wave sleep [Åkerstedt *et al.*, 2007] [Marzano *et al.*, 2008].

→Visual Event Related Potential Odd Ball Paradigm:
Selective attention (increased P3 amplitude) to cancer-related word probes but not to other threatening or neutral words [Stanford *et al.*, 2001].
Increased P3 amplitude to visual pain prick stimuli, suggesting loss of down-regulation of the pain empathy response. This down-regulation is expected in health professionals [Decety *et al.*, 2010].

10.2 C.G.'s Work Situation: Insights from the OSI

C.G. is a senior oncology nurse who has worked in the same cancer hospital for the past 30 years. Because of her experience and willingness to do so, she covers nearly all the services in the hospital: from the emergency room to the ICU, to the various inpatient services including the palliative ward, as well as outpatient clinics. In Figure 10.1, each OSI stressor faced by C.G. is identified and categorized as either fixed or as modifiable.

- Underload:

There are no inherent underload factors in C.G.'s work environment. However, as seen in the left-most column of Fig. 10.1, the total of 4.5 points for underload is related to three potentially modifiable factors. One is waiting time, albeit fairly rare, and the others are inadequate and fixed pay. On the other hand, there are opportunities for career advancement and albeit not financially rewarded, good work is recognized and appreciated in other ways.

- High demand:

The demand burden for C.G. is exceedingly high, about half of which is fixed. Several of the modifiable factors are associated with work in the emergency room and intensive care unit, including assisting in invasive procedures. C.G. serves as a supervisor and must also complete a substantial amount of administrative work for which no separate time is

	Underload	High Demand	Strictness	Time Pressure	Noxins	Threat avoidance	Conflict/ Uncertainty
Input		Information: • Several sources • Heterogeneous • Communication essential • Rapid inflow (ER + many seek her attention) • 3 sensory modalities • Visual burden (assists invasive procedures)	• Strict requirements for detecting information --ER/ICU /assists in invasive procedures	• Somewhat limited control over speed of incoming information	• Sporadic noise (ER)	• Potential consequences of momentary lapse --ER/ ICU • Visually-disturbing scenes • Listens to emotionally-disturbing occurrences --Most severe patients	Incoming information conflict: • Some signal/noise • Some signal/signal
Central Decision-Making		Decisions: • Complex • Complicated • Rapid • Affect others: Supervises --ER/ICU	Strict: • Definition of correct decision	• Can't postpone decisions --ER/ICU		• Potentially fatal consequences of wrong decision	Information: •Contradictory •Missing --Can't get history, language barriers • Unforeseeable events require new plan --ER/ICU
Output/ Task Perfor-mance	• Waiting time	Tasks: • Complex • Varied Administration •Simultaneous & rapid task:	• Strict evaluation of performance	• Somewhat limited control of performance rate	• Lifting	• Hazardous tasks (infection)	• Conflicting tasks (Carrying out physician orders, other aspects of patient care, needs of families) *Hampered by:* • Some extrinsic problems • Many interruptions from people
General	• Fixed pay • Inadequate pay	• Occasional overtime work when short-staffed (to 48 h/week max.) • Holds 2 jobs • Works 4 consecutive night shifts every 3rd week	•Some fixed posture --Assists invasive procedures • Somewhat limited in taking time off from work • Limited influence over: Policy	Occasional • Speed-up • Deadlines	Occasional • dust, fumes and heat	Past work exposures: • Harmed by needle stick • Witnessed serious (including fatal) accidents • Patient suicides related to cancer diagnosis	• Some pointless tasks (administration)
Total	Modifiable: 4.5 Underload = 4.5	Fixed: 16.5 Modifiable: 15.5 High Demand = 32	Fixed: 3.5 Modifiable: 4 Strictness = 7.5	Fixed: 4 Modifiable: 3 Time pressure = 7	Modifiable: 3 Noxious = 3	Fixed/past:14 Modifiable: 1 Threat avoidance = 15	Fixed: 8.5 Modifiable: 7.5 Conflict = 16

Figure 10.1 Summary of the baseline OSI for C.G. Total OSI (Fixed = 46.5 + Modifiable = 38.5) = 85.

set aside. She also serves as a teacher and role model for her younger colleagues, for nurses in training as well as sharing her experience with physicians at various levels of training. The remainder of the modifiable high demand stressors are on the general level: some overtime work at her primary job, working a second job (due to the inadequacy of pay on her primary job), and four consecutive night shifts every third week. As do her colleagues, C.G. takes regular rest breaks (including for meals) in a specially-designated quiet room.

> JOB DEMANDS are EXCEEDINGLY HIGH, and there are some rewards but these are FINANCIALLY INADEQUATE.
>
> Some EFFORT-REWARD IMBALANCE IS PRESENT.

- Strictness:

The overall strictness score is not excessive, particularly since rules, regulations and overseeing are kept to the necessary minimum. There are a few inherently strict elements in nursing work: obviously, information needs to be properly detected and registered, the correctness of a given decision cannot be entirely flexible and a modicum of strictness in evaluation of task performance is necessary. C.G. has her own small but comfortable office, in which she spends much less than half her work time, since she is mainly involved in patient care of various settings, as described above. Fixed posture is mainly related to assisting in invasive procedures. There are some limitations in taking time off from work, mainly due to C.G.'s commitment to "be there" for the hospital whenever possible. Influence over hospital policy is also limited.

- Extrinsic time pressure:

There is substantial external time pressure. Nevertheless, this is still less than the maximum seen for health professionals.

More than half of this burden is due to the nature of C.G.'s work, including her obligations in the ER and ICU. Deadlines and speed up occur occasionally.

> This is an ACTIVE JOB with high demands and some time pressure, but with substantial, albeit not full decision-making latitude. Full-blown job strain is not present.

- Noxious exposures:

The main sources of physical stressors are from lifting patients, sporadic noise when working in the ER and occasional dust, fumes and heat. Otherwise, the physical working conditions are comfortable.

- Threat Avoidant Vigilance:

The TAV score is exceedingly high. Almost all of this TAV burden is an intrinsic part of C.G.'s work as an oncology nurse, together with past work experience. C.G. has suffered a few needle stick injuries. One of the patients had acute Hepatitis A infection and she was therefore treated prophylactically with immunoglobulin. A number of colleagues and staff have also incurred needle stick injuries. In the early 1980's, one of her close colleagues subsequently succumbed to AIDs. During C.G.'s many years of work in the cancer hospital, she knows of some patient suicides related to receiving a cancer diagnosis. Because she works on all the services of the hospital, C.G. sees many patients with metastatic disease in the terminal phases. Needless to say, emotionally disturbing accounts and visual disturbing scenes are innumerable.

- Conflict and uncertainty:

Due to her many duties, C.G. is frequently faced with conflicts among tasks such as carrying out physician orders, addressing other aspects of patient care, attending to the needs of families and supervising other staff. There are some external problems that hamper providing adequate patient care, especially lack of beds and short staffing and frequent interruptions during work. On the other hand, inter-personal relations are very good, the work atmosphere is supportive and those in positions of power and authority consistently abide by a code of ethics. C.G. is permanently employed and, aside from some administrative tasks, the job is coherent and meaningful for her.

> There is a heavy TAV burden and some conflict.
> A supportive social climate and responsible leadership are important buffers that bolster team work and coherence.

10.3 C.G. Meets with the Occupational Neuropsychiatrist

As noted, C.G. is referred to the occupational neuropsychiatrist by her oncologist who is concerned about the sleep disturbances and intrusive dreams subsequent to the breast cancer diagnosis. The question is what should be modified in C.G.'s work situation, and how should this process be carried out?

10.3.1 *Assessment*

Although C.G. is managing, with maximal effort, to continue work, the sleep disturbances sooner or later are likely to hamper her ability to function safely and effectively. Albeit high, the total OSI is not at the acutely dangerous level. Moreover, C.G.'s work is a major source of her well-being and self-esteem, especially in view of her high level of competence and involvement. As discussed in Chapter 4, return to work is recognized as an important component of quality of life for patients with cancer, helping them maintain not only economic, but often also *emotional stability*, during treatment and its aftermath.

There are, however, elements of C.G.'s current work situation that are likely to be exacerbating her clinical status. By caring for terminally ill patients, she is repeatedly exposed and sensitized to the worst potential consequences of cancer. The cancer-related nightmares reflect this exposure and sensitization. Night shift work disrupts normal circadian rhythm and sleep disturbances are a well-recognized consequence. It has also been demonstrated that nurses who had worked night shifts for 30 or more years are at a significantly elevated risk for breast cancer [Schernhammer *et al.*, 2001]. Combined with other recent evidence [Knutsson *et al.*, 2012], it is now recommended that women with breast cancer be advised against working night shifts [Bonde *et al.*, 2012]. Therefore, these two exposures (night shift work and palliative care for terminally-ill patients) should be eliminated for C.G.

Given that the social climate is healthy, that the hospital leadership behaves responsibly and that C.G. is legally protected against discrimination for having breast cancer, disclosure is an entirely realistic option. In the setting of a cancer hospital, it is expected that she would receive the needed support and understanding.

Within that framework, C.G.'s lifelong professional commitment to fight against the scourge of cancer would acquire a new dimension of poignancy and urgency if she were to be open about her own situation. For the beginning, she should choose those colleagues and staff with whom she has the best rapport and who are most likely to accept this disclosure without excessive emotion.

10.3.2 *Integrative therapeutic approach: Supportive/cognitive-behavioral therapy, disclosure and targeted worksite modifications*

The therapeutic approach begins by providing C.G. with the chance to articulate her cancer-related fears and describe the nightmares. She needs some emotional release in a secure setting. The occupational neuropsychiatrist provides this with empathy and reassurance.

C.G. also describes her sadness at the reaction of her close friend whom she told about her breast cancer diagnosis. She feels guilty that she caused her friend distress. The need to be selective about disclosure is discussed, and also to be prepared for some unexpected reactions, even among health professionals. C.G. thereby articulates the need to give herself and colleagues "more room to be human," including the admission of fear.

C.G.'s competence and dedication are discussed, emphasizing the fact that these are highly appreciated by patients, colleagues, staff, and leadership within the hospital. C.G. articulates the satisfaction she feels from her work.

Next, the OSI is reviewed. In view of the above, and starting from the underload aspect, it becomes clear to C.G. that she deserves better pay. She admits that she never has requested such; rather, she tends to be self-effacing and reluctant to state her own needs. Given the current financial difficulties facing the hospital, she had felt it would be "selfish" to ask. Now, with the encouragement of the occupational neuropsychiatrist, she realizes that this is essential. Moreover, if her pay would at least cover her basic expenses, she would not have to work the second job. She plans therefore to argue that a pay raise would be cost-effective, since she could devote herself more fully to her primary job.

Demand levels could be feasibly lowered further by limiting work hours to 40 per week maximum and by having separate time devoted to her various duties. With these interventions, together with the above-mentioned elimination of night shift work, C.G. still faces very high demands, but Effort-Reward Imbalance is lowered. Within the framework of the Effort-Reward Model, the topic is broached of C.G.'s overly intense commitment to her work.

Another important safety valve would be facilitating taking time off when needed. Together with exploring strategies to better handle and triage those who attempt to interrupt her work, C.G. learns to say no.

Meaning and coherence are further bolstered by eliminating redundant administrative tasks to which C.G. "says no" and the hospital leadership accedes.

She is encouraged to monitor her own fatigue levels and to know when to stop before this becomes excessive. Part of this process is learning to delegate and share duties, rather than trying to do everything herself. Practical measures concerning sleep hygiene, including limiting caffeine intake are reviewed.

C.G. has a healthy social network outside work. With shorter work hours, a regular daytime work schedule and less fatiguing work conditions, she has the chance to nurture restorative, enjoyable activities. This is a viable countermeasure to her tendency to become overly involved in her work. C.G. is particularly encouraged to dance more frequently. The protective role of recreational physical activity with respect to breast cancer, weight control and overall health is emphasized.

With the implementation of the workplace changes summarized in Figure 10.2, together with more leisure time, C.G. begins to sleep better.

10.4 Comment

C.W. was referred by her oncologist who did not feel competent about advising on work-related questions. This is reportedly a very common problem regarding return-to-work issues that arise among patients with cancer [Tamminga *et al.*, 2011] [Tiedke *et al.*, 2011].

Further Reading

Sections 2.2.4.1, 2.5.3, 3.2.1.3, 3.4.2, 4.1.2.2, 4.2.3 and 4.3.1 are recommended as cross-references within part I of this book. Further references of particular relevance for this case study include:

[Åkerstedt *et al.*, 2007] [Fang *et al.*, 2012] [Gudbergsson *et al.*, 2006] [Gudbergsson *et al.*, 2009] [Miller *et al.*, 2006] [Rosenberg & Godhamri 2011] [Tamminga *et al.*, 2011] [Tiedke *et al.*, 2011] [Zee 2012].

	Underload	High Demand	Strictness	Time Pressure	Noxins	Threat avoidance	Conflict/ Uncertainty
Input						Avoid work with terminally ill patients	
Central Decision-Making							
Output/ Task Performance		• Separate time for carrying out physician orders, other aspects of patient care, supervising, addressing needs of families					• ↓ conflicting tasks (Carrying out physician orders, other aspects of patient care, supervising, addressing needs of families) • ↓ Interruptions from people
General	• Requests & receives pay raise →	• Eliminate night shift work • Quit 2nd job • Limit work hours to 40/week	• Facilitate taking time off from work when needed				• Eliminate redundant administrative tasks
Total	- 1 Underload = 3.5	- 6 High Demand = 26	- 1 Strictness = 6.5	Time pressure = 7	Noxious = 3	- 0.25 Threat avoidance = 14.75	-4 Conflict = 12

Figure 10.2 Summary of measures taken to lower OSI for C.G. Total OSI (85 – 12.25) = 72.75.

Chapter 11

Control Panel Worker with Paranoid Ideation: Fifth Clinical Case Study

T.S., in his late 40's monitors a control panel.

He has had major conflicts with his colleagues and supervisor, accusing them of misconduct.

He states that no one in his work organization can be trusted.

Total OSI = 80

Questions for reflection while reviewing this case:

- Is this a dangerously stressful work situation?
- Is the patient's work situation contributing to his disorder? *If so, how?*
- Could workplace modifications help improve the patient's clinical status? *If so, how?*

11.1 The Case: T.S. Mistrusts his Entire Work Collective

The difficulties for T.S. began about six months ago when he was obliged to testify in court about an accident involving a power outage. Since then, he has had increasing conflict with colleagues and staff and accuses them of misconduct. He states: "no one at work can be trusted and no one abides by the rules. They do not fulfil their work obligations, and thereby harm the work organization." He considers that there is no trust at work, and describes therefore feeling "under continuous psychological pressure." During the last month, he has approached the supervisor, general director and others in the hierarchy several times both verbally and in writing.

T.S. has demanded that the entire work collective be replaced because of the serious errors that they make. He doubts the quality of the equipment that is used. All the efforts of the supervisor as well as his colleagues to find a solution have been unsuccessful.

T.S. has completed vocational high school. He is married and has four children, the youngest of whom is in high school.

His wife states that over the past three months, T.S. has had outbursts of anger and has been acting belligerently. These bouts alternate with periods during which he is sulky and withdrawn. She says that he has had previous bouts of sulkiness from time to time, but that the aggressive behavior is completely unusual for T.S. She states that T.S. has been in generally good health, that he rarely drinks alcohol and does not smoke because he finds these habits "repulsive." He takes no medication. Review of systems is unremarkable. According to T.S.'s wife, family history is positive only for obesity and heart disease. T.S.'s wife is very worried about her husband and has taken him to their family physician, who referred T.S. for neuropsychiatric evaluation.

11.1.1 *Objective findings*

T.S. is an obese male who appears somewhat older than his stated age. Blood pressure is 130/85, pulse 85/minute. Other than obesity, the physical examination is entirely unremarkable. Except for borderline elevated triglycerides, biochemical, hematologic and endocrinologic laboratory findings are all within normal limits. BMI = 30.

- Neurological findings:

Unremarkable.

- Psychiatric findings:

Normal appearance, spontaneous behavior. Consciously experiences his surroundings appropriately, including persons in his surroundings, i.e. he is fully oriented in space and time. Verbal contact is well made and continuous. Attention is adequate, and maintained throughout the entire interview. Short-term and long-term memory are normal. Intellectual capacity is maintained. Intellectual level is appropriate for his level of education. Overall mood is subdued, and conveys a feeling of worriedness. During the interview, there were sudden episodes of anger. Anxiety is present. Motivation appears to be intact. Thought flow is formally intact. In the content, however, there are paranoid structured ideas, relations and interpretations. No perceptual abnormalities.

The interview with T.S., together with the data from the social worker and the workplace, and objective neuropsychiatric observations made in the outpatient setting, suggest that T.S. has social and behavioral deviations from the norms of his environment with suspected disorder of 1 to 2 mental functions. These are beyond his control. He has a lack of realistic assessment of himself and his environment. The pattern of findings is most consistent with Delusional Disorder (F22.0). This renders the patient socially dysfunctional. Additional diagnosis: overeating associated with other psychological disturbances (F50.4) [World Health Organization, 1993] (Appendix A, Section 1).

→Recommend thorough workup and treatment planning.

- Neuropsychological testing:

Right-handed, normal memory span, reaction time and attention.

- Psychiatric rating scale:

→Brief Psychiatric Rating Scale: Total score = 47

Prominent anxiety, emotional withdrawal and conceptual disorganization [Ventura *et al.*, 1993] [Shafer 2005].

- Neurophysiologic evaluation:

→Electroencephalographic findings:

Desynchronized EEG indicative of psychological tension.

→Auditory Event Related Potential Odd Ball Paradigm:

Somewhat diminished P300 amplitude, normal latency, consistent with the presence of psychotic symptoms or risk of such [d'Amato *et al.*, 1999] [Halford 2003] [Mathalon & Ford 2000].

11.2 T.S.'s Work Situation: Insights from the OSI

T.S. has been a control panel worker at a thermoelectric plant for twenty-two years, i.e. for his entire professional life. In Figure 11.1, each OSI stressor faced by T.S. is identified and categorized as either fixed or as modifiable.

- Underload:

We now have an example of work with a rather heavy intrinsic underload score, as seen in the left-most column of Fig. 11.1. Decision-making is also quite stereotypic, although some judgment is required. T.S. must continuously follow a low flow of homogeneous signals. The tasks he performs are also simple and monotonous. Very often he has nothing to do but sit and watch the display screen. Modifiable underload factors are quite inadequate pay and lack of recognition for work.

- High demand:

The above-described underload is combined with some elements of high demand. On the input level, there are a few information sources to follow almost simultaneously and the visual system is heavily burdened. T.S. must communicate information to colleagues from time to time. Although quite stereotypic, decisions must be made rapidly. Likewise, the simple, homogeneous tasks must be performed quickly and sometimes simultaneously. Besides these fixed high demand stressors, the modifiable factors include group piece rate, long work hours (four to five 12-hour shifts per week) and one to two night shifts per week. Moreover, since even during scheduled breaks, T.S. must still sit at the control panel and follow the situation on screen, he does not have true rest breaks.

> The job entails the UNHEALTHY COMBINATION OF HIGH DEMANDS AND HEAVY UNDERLOAD BURDEN. The latter includes lack of financial and emotional rewards:
>
> Some Effort-Reward Imbalance is present.

- Strictness:

The strictness burden is exceedingly heavy. While the fixed burden of these stressors is very high, over two-thirds are modifiable, including sedentary work in a confined, window-less workspace, very limited possibility to take time off from work and low influence over scheduling, tasks, work team and company policy. The sedentary fixed position during work is noteworthy particularly in light of obesity.

- Extrinsic time pressure:

The external factors creating time pressure are all inherent to the nature of the work performed by T.S.

This is a somewhat passive, yet also demanding job with extremely heavy strictness burden. Some job strain is present.

- Noxious exposures:

There is somewhat less than optimal heating and air-conditioning and noise not exceeding 90dB. Overall, exposure to noxious physical factors is fairly minimal for T.S.

- Threat Avoidant Vigilance:

Vigilance is the primary task of T.S. This, plus the knowledge that a wrong decision or lapse of attention could have serious consequences (power outages that are difficult and costly to rectify) creates a substantial TAV burden.

In addition, T.S. has occasionally heard about accidents. One of his colleagues committed suicide several years ago. He has also had to testify in court about an accident involving a power outage, as described earlier.

- Conflict and uncertainty:

The conflict burden is substantial. Much of this is modifiable, due to extrinsic problems related to computer glitches, a tense work atmosphere with possible violations of behavioral norms among those in leadership positions.

The thermoelectric plant is in financial crisis and layoffs have occurred as a result of downsizing, as noted. Not even those with seniority are free from the possibility of losing their jobs.

There is some TAV. The conflict burden is also substantial.

	Underload	High Demand	Strictness	Extrinsic Time Pressure	Aversiveness/ Noxious Exposures	Avoidance/ Symbolic Aversiveness	Conflict/ Uncertainty
Input	• Homogeneous signals • Low frequency of incoming signals	• A few info. sources • Heavy burden on visual system • Some communication needed	• Very strict requirements for signal detection	• No control over speed of incoming signals	• Noise (to 90dB)	• Vigilance is primary task • Occasionally hears about disturbing events (accidents)	Some: • Signal/noise conflict • Signal/signal conflict
Central Decision-Making	• Decisions fairly automatic but judgment required	• Rapid decision-making	• Fairly strict problem-solving strategy • Fairly strictly defined correct decision	• Decisions cannot be postponed		• Serious consequences of a wrong decision	Some: • Missing information needed for decision • Contradictory information • Often unexpected events change work plan
Output/ Task performance	• Homogenous tasks • Simple Tasks • Frequently nothing to do	• Occasional simultaneous task performance • Rapid task performance	• Work must meet a strictly-defined standard	• No control over rate of task performance			*Task performance hampered by*: • Extrinsic problems (computer glitches)
General	• Fairly inadequate pay • Lack of recognition of work	• Paid according to group performance • Long work hours • Lack of rest breaks • Night shift	• Fixed body position • Confined, window-less, workspace • Very limited in taking time off from work *Low influence over*: • Schedule • Tasks • Policy • With whom one works		Mild: • Heat • Cold	• Heard about colleague's suicide • Work-related litigation/Testifying in court (as a witness)	• Emotionally-charged work atmosphere • Some violations of behavior norms/abuses of power • Threat of job loss
	Fixed = 10.5 Modifiable= 3.5 Underload = 14	Fixed = 8.5 Modifiable= 6.75 High Demand = 15.25	Fixed = 6 Modifiable= 14.5 Strictness = 20.5	Fixed = 6 Extrinsic time pressure = 6	Modifiable = 3 Noxious exposures = 3	Fixed/past experience = 7.5 Threat Avoidance = 7.5	Fixed = 4.75 Modifiable= 9 Conflict= 13.75

Figure 11.1 Summary of the baseline OSI for T.S. Total OSI (Fixed = 43.25 + Modifiable = 36.75) = 80.

	Underload	High Demand	Strictness	Time Pressure	Noxins	Threat avoidance	Conflict/ Uncertainty
Input							
Central Decision-Making							
Output/ Task Perfor-mance	• *Explore possibilities for task alternation*						
General	• ↑ recognition of good work	• Eliminate night shift work • Limit work hours to 40/week • Regular, true rest breaks away from the control panel →	• Facilitate taking time off from work when needed • ↑ influence over with whom he works →	→	→	→	↓ emotional charge in work atmosphere
Total	-1.5 Underload = 12.5	- 5.75 High Demand = 9.5	- 3.5 Strictness = 17	Time pressure = 6	Noxious = 3	Threat avoidance = 7.5	-1 Conflict = 12.75

Figure 11.2 Summary of measures taken to lower OSI for T.S. Total OSI (80 – 11.75) = 68.25.

11.3 Intervention by the Occupational Neuropsychiatrist

T.S. was sent to a Rehabilitation Center for three weeks of rest and behavioral-cognitive therapy plus medication. He then met with the occupational neuropsychiatrist. After a few sessions, T.S. has progressively been able to distance himself from the delusions and thereby stopped articulating his accusations that the work collective and equipment were functioning improperly.

Four joint sessions with the occupational neuropsychiatrist were then held with the patient and his colleagues and the supervisors. The interventions are summarized in Fig. 11.2. These include elimination of night shift work, limitation of work hours, implementation of regular true rest breaks away from the control panel and strong encouragement by recognizing and affirming the good work performed by T.S. and his colleagues. These measures have also helped diminish the tension at work. Efforts are on-going to find alternative tasks to relieve the underload, without disrupting the work flow.

Recreational physical activity, especially swimming, is strongly recommended as a countermeasure for the vigilant, sedentary work. T.S. is referred to a dietician.

11.4 Further Thoughts and Comments

As discussed in Chapter 4, with rapid onset of psychosis and no prior history of this disorder, a substantial percentage of patients will fully recover. Paranoid or delusional disorders are considered a justifiable cause of disqualification from “safety-sensitive” jobs. There are, however, reports in the literature of successful maintenance of employment, even in sectors involving public safety despite several severe episodes of psychosis. In these cases, low dose medication, full disclosure to the employer and active support were vital [Teasdale & Deahl, 2007]. For persons recovering from delusional disorders or psychosis, finding workplaces where they feel encouraged and comfortable appears to be an important factor in vocational success [Woodside et al. 2006]. A realistic weight loss goal together within this framework can be an important step towards overall recovery [Mizock 2012].

Cross References

Sections 2.2.4.5, 2.4.2, 3.4.5, 4.1.6 and 5.1.1.2.1 (underload).

Chapter 12

Tram Driver with Post-traumatic Stress Disorder: Sixth Case Study

B.F. in his late 30s is a tram driver.

Subsequent to a serious work-related traffic accident,
he has had flashbacks, nightmares and frequent wakening.

He has withdrawn from family & friends and feels empty.

Total OSI = 110.5

Questions for reflection while reviewing this case:

- Is this a dangerously stressful work situation?
- Is the patient's work situation contributing to his disorder? *If so, how?*
- Could workplace modifications help improve the patient's clinical status? *If so, how?*

12.1 The Case: B.F. has Post-traumatic Stress Disorder

Six weeks ago, a child suddenly appeared on the track downhill in front of the tram which B.F. was driving. This was during the 2nd half of a split-shift, around sundown before the streetlights had been turned on. B.F. could not brake in time to avoid hitting the child, who incurred head trauma and was in a coma for several days.

Some of the passengers were slightly injured with the crash. When they saw the child, they fell silent. The ambulance arrived within minutes and took the child to the Emergency Center. The police came immediately thereafter and interrogated B.F intensively. An alcohol test was performed, the result of which was negative.

Although he did not incur any physical injuries, B.F. describes being "severely shaken" and could not "come back to himself." The first 2-3 days thereafter, he felt "numb." At the same time, he was completely preoccupied with the outcome of the child. He did not receive any debriefing. The local newspapers ran the accident as their lead story, with the headline: "tramway driver hits 5 year-old boy who is in critical condition."

B.F.'s professional license was suspended, pending the court hearing which took place three weeks later and lasted two weeks. The judge ruled that B.F. was not guilty. During this entire 5-week period, he did not receive any medical or psychological attention.

About two weeks after the accident, B.F. began to develop a fear of driving. This feeling worsened during the trial. Up until the accident, B.F. had had a perfect driving record, with which he had prided himself. He was "devastated by the loss of control and potential for disaster that this accident represented." He no longer felt confident that he could avoid an accident and began to question his professional competence.

He also has had flashbacks about the accident and sleep disturbances: trouble falling asleep and nightmares about driving. Since the accident, he has withdrawn from social contacts, avoiding communication with his friends and colleagues and even with his family.

B.F. has had high blood pressure for several years, treated with angiotensin-converting enzyme (ACE) inhibitors. Past medical history (including for previous mental illness) and review of systems are otherwise completely unremarkable. Family history is negative for hypertension and for mental illness.

He lives with his wife who is a nurse and their three children. B.F. has completed 3 years of university education which he discontinued for economic reasons. He became a tram driver because, at the time, it was a steady job which he needed to support his family.

B.F. occasionally smoked cigarettes as a student, usually around exam time. Since he began work as a tram driver, he has smoked about 10-15 cigarettes only on workdays, usually just before starting each shift, during the long period in between the split shifts, as well as during the very short breaks at the end of each tram route.

12.1.1 *Objective findings*

B.F. is an alert, anxious-appearing male who looks somewhat older than his stated age, blood pressure 160/100 mmHg after 5-minutes of rest, HR = 90/ min; slightly prolonged expiration with occasional wheezes. The remainder of the physical exam is normal. Body mass index = 25. Biochemical, hematologic and endocrinologic laboratory findings are all within normal limits.

- Neuropsychiatric findings:

Neurological: Symmetrical hyperreflexia and slight resting tremor.

Psychiatric: Recurrent intrusive recollections of accident with flashbacks, persistent symptoms of arousal (difficulty falling asleep and difficulty concentrating), avoidance of stimuli that arouse recollection of the accident and withdrawal from social interactions, all lasting over 1 month and not previously present.

Diagnosis:
Posttraumatic Stress Disorder with intrusive and avoidance symptoms (F43.1) [World Health Organization, 1993] (Appendix A, Section 1).

- Neuropsychological testing:

Right-handed, normal memory span, reaction time and attention.

- Questionnaire findings:

→Posttraumatic Cognitions Inventory [Foa *et al.*, 1999]
Negative cognition about self = 4.6 (high for PTSD)
Most noteworthy: "My life has been destroyed by the trauma."
Negative cognition about the world = 4.4 (below median for PTSD)
Most noteworthy: "I have to be on guard all the time."

Self-blame = 3.2 (median for PTSD)
Most noteworthy: "Somebody else would have stopped the event from happening."

→Impact of Events Scale (IES) [Horowitz *et al.*, 1979]
IES-Intrusions = 23 (high-average for PTSD males)
IES-Avoidance = 16 (high-average for PTSD males).

- Psychophysiologic and neurophysiologic evaluation

→Glare pressor test with electroencephalographic and polygraphic recording [Belkić, Ercegovac, Savić et al. 1992]:
Maximally desynchronized EEG during the resting and glare exposure periods, without habituation, after the 5th glare impulse, similar to that shown in Figure 3.14.
Diastolic BP increased by 7 mmHg after glare exposure 1 (G1) and 10 mmHg after glare exposure 5 (G5).
Strong psychogalvanic skin response to G1 and G5 similar to that of Figure 3.13 (Left panel).
The overall pattern is indicative of sustained central and autonomic hyperreactivity to glare suggesting increased sensitivity to glare exposure.

→Visual Event Related Go-NoGo CNV according to our protocol [Belkić, Savić, Djordjević et al. 1992], as shown in Figure 12.1.
In lead Cz:
Neutral: GO - CNV2 = -14μV, average GO-NOGO 12 μV difference.
Traffic: GO - CNV2 = -16μV, average GO-NOGO 14 μV difference.

This pattern is typical of professional drivers, especially those with arterial hypertension. Marked hyperreactivity is seen to imperative stimuli in both the neutral and explicitly traffic-related paradigms [Belkić, Savić *et al.*, 1992] [Emdad *et al.*, 1997].
This response is also consistent with the increased selective attention to trauma-related stimuli in patients with PTSD [Savić & Belkić 1995] [Clark *et al.*, 2009].

12.2 B.F.'s Work Situation: Insights from the OSI

B.F. has worked as a tram driver for fourteen years. In Figure 12.2, each OSI stressor for B.F. is identified and categorized as either fixed or as modifiable.

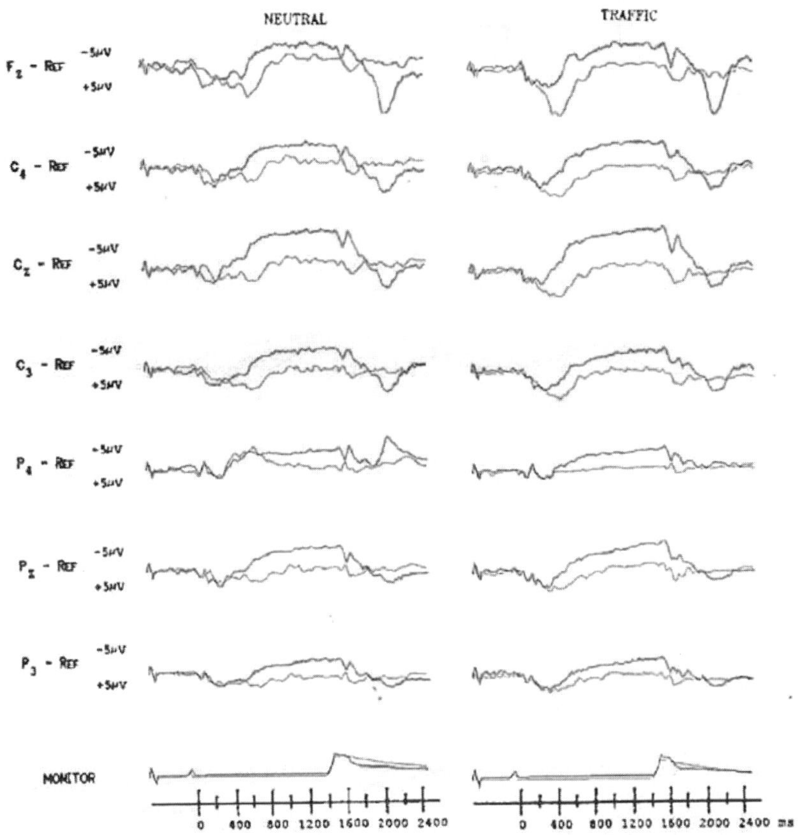

Figure 12.1 A markedly high CNV to the GO situation, with a large difference in the CNV between GO and NOGO situation, both for the neutral and for the explicit traffic avoidance paradigm.

- Underload:

For all professional driver profiles there is some intrinsic underload, as seen in the left-most column of Fig. 12.2. In addition, B.F. had been driving on the same tram route, so that incoming signals are quite homogeneous. Decision-making follows to some extent from the input, although judgment is obviously required. B.F. performs several tasks besides actual driving (checking and selling tickets, opening and closing the doors, giving information), but these are all relatively simple and quite monotonous. The long wait time between split shifts contributes to underload, since there is not enough time to go home nor is it possible to use the time for personal business. In addition, the pay is quite inadequate and good work (e.g. safe driving) is not recognized at all.

- High demand:

Urban mass transit operators all have exceedingly high demands on the input level. Although, as noted above, B.F. drove on the same route, he drove various vehicles, creating some heterogeneity which also contributed to input high demand. Drivers obviously are required to continuously make rapid decisions, and must carry out needed actions rapidly and often simultaneously. On the general level, modifiable elements include overtime (plus the actual long work day due to split shift) and night shift work, as well as lack of true rest breaks during actual worktime (the two split shifts). Due to heavy traffic, B.F. is usually behind schedule and obliged to continue almost immediately after arriving at the end station, in other words, without a real break. Facilities for hygiene are in poor condition and not easily assessable. To "keep himself going" under these conditions, he typically takes a couple of minutes for "a quick smoke," so he will be ready to face any impatient passengers.

> The combination of high demands plus underload indicates that EFFORT-REWARD IMBALANCE is present.

- Strictness:

The fixed strictness burden for B.F. is the highest we have seen thus far. The heaviest contribution is from the very stringent requirements for signal detection and fixed sedentary body position in a confined space. Law enforcement officers do monitor professional drivers' task performance, at least intermittently. Modifiable elements of strictness include lack of autonomous workspace (e.g. desk or locker), very limited possibility to take time off and low influence over scheduling, tasks and company policy. B.F. has no influence over who enters the tram.

- Extrinsic time pressure:

Besides the substantial fixed extrinsic time pressure burden, the need to adhere to an exceedingly tight schedule represents continuous deadline and speedup pressure.

> The total (high demands + extrinsic time pressure) score plus low decision-making latitude (high strictness scores) indicate that:
>
> JOB STRAIN is present.

- Noxious exposures:

Some glare and vibration exposure, as well as noise from traffic and from passengers are an intrinsic part of the urban mass transit operator's work environment. With poor shock absorbers in the trams, B.F. is exposed to additional whole-body vibration. Since the isolation, air-conditioning and heating systems are poor, he is also exposed to heat, cold and fumes.

- Threat Avoidant Vigilance:

This is the highest TAV burden we have encountered in all the cases presented thus far. Almost the entire TAV burden is an unmodifiable part of B.F.'s work as an urban transit operator. The very serious accident which precipitated B.F.'s current illness, together with having witnessed many fatal traffic accidents and testifying as a defendant with mass-media coverage are all part of his actual TAV experience.

- Conflict and uncertainty:

There is heavy conflict burden at the input and central levels inherent in the work of all professional drivers. The modifiable stressors are all on the task performance and general levels. These include vehicle breakdowns, disruptions or interruptions from passengers, as well as some abuse of power by those in high positions in the company. Due to budget cuts for public transportation, there is a threat of job loss. There are also positive elements, including quite healthy (though not ideal) interpersonal relations among colleagues and frequently positive interactions with passengers, contributing to the overall coherence of the job for B.F.

> The TAV burden is exceedingly high and is clearly a major CONTRIBUTOR to B.F.'s PSYCHOLOGICAL DISTRESS.
> Conflict-related stressors further contribute.
> Important buffers are also identified.

	Underload	High Demand	Strictness	Ext. Time P.	Noxious	TAV	Conflict/Uncertainty
Input	• Some homogeneous info. (drives on fixed route	• Several info. sources • Heavy burden on visual system • High info flow (City traffic) • 3 sensory modalities • Communication essential • Some heterogeneous info (different vehicles)	• Very strict requirements for signal detection	• No control over speed of incoming signals	• Glare • Noise	• Vigilance is primary task • Visually disturbing scenes (fatal accidents) • Hears about disturbing events (accidents & assaults)	• Signal/noise conflict (drives at night & in all weather conditions) • Some signal/signal conflict
Central Decision-Making	• Decisions fairly automatic but judgment required	• Rapid decision -making	• Fairly strict problem-solving strategy • Fairly strictly defined correct decision	• Decisions cannot be postponed		• Serious consequences of a wrong decision	• Missing information needed for decision • Contradictory information • Often unexpected events change work plan
Output/ Task performance	• Homogenous (though several) tasks • Simple Tasks • Nothing to do between split shifts	Task performance: • Simultaneous • Rapid	• Some task evaluation (law enforcement)	• Limited control over rate of task performance	• Vibration (poor shock absorbers)	• Hazards: (Threat of violence from passengers)	• Conflicting tasks in time/space *Task performance hampered by:* • Breakdowns • Interruptions from passengers
General	• Fixed pay • Fairly inadequate pay • Low chance for upgrade • Lack of recognition of work	• Long work hours • Lack of true rest breaks • Night shift • Called to fill in during vacation	• Fixed body position •Confined, workspace (+ inadequate ventilation) • Very limited in time off • No autonomous workspace *Low/no influence* • Schedule • Tasks • Policy • Who enters tram	• Deadline pressure •Speed-up	• Heat • Cold • Gases *Inadequate*: isolation, air-conditioning, heating system	• Has had a very serious accident • Witnessed many fatal accidents • Work-related litigation as a defendant • No system for emergencies	• Grievance procedure not confidential • Some violations of behavior norms/abuses of power • Threat of job loss
	Fixed = 4 Modifiable = 9 Underload = 13	Fixed = 15.5 Modifiable = 6.5 High Demand = 22	Fixed=10.5 Modifiable=10 Strictness = 20.5	Fixed = 5 Modifiable = 4 Ext. time p. = 9	Fixed = 4.5 Modifiable = 4.5 Noxious = 9	Fixed/past experience =16 Modifiable = 2 TAV = 18	Fixed = 9 Modifiable= 10 Conflict = 19

Figure 12.2 Summary of the baseline OSI for B.F. Total OSI (Fixed = 64.5 + Modifiable = 46) = 110.5.

12.3 Return to Healthier Work: The Process for B.F.

The total OSI score is above the acutely dangerous level. The accident together with the overall work stressor burden is the trigger of the Post Traumatic Stress Disorder. Given that urban mass transit operators are at very high risk for developing arterial hypertension [Ragland *et al.*, 1997] [Belkić, Savić, Theorell *et al.*, 1994] [Winkleby *et al.*, 1988], and given the inordinately high total OSI score, B.F. most likely has occupation-related hypertension. His response to the glare pressor test also corroborates that sensitization is present, with central and autonomic hyperreactivity and lack of habituation with repeated glare exposures. B.F.'s smoking pattern together with the documented relation between smoking intensity and total OSI scores among professional drivers [Belkić, Pavlović *et al.*, 1992] [Belkić *et al.*, 1996] [Emdad *et al.*, 1998b] strongly suggest that this dangerous habit is work-related in his case. B.F has never taken sick leave, which is a pattern seen among many professional drivers who are smokers [Belkić 1989]. He also frequently filled in when there was a driver shortage.

→B.F. is self-referred to the occupational neuropsychiatrist.
He wants to go back to work and proactively seeks help in order to do so. The case presentation up until this point recapitulates the initial workup performed by the occupational neuropsychiatrist.

B.F. is a competent, conscientious driver who appreciates the importance of his work, and finds coherence therein. He is motivated to return to work, and realizes that he needs help. B.F. himself immediately suggested some of the interventions outlined in Figure 12.3. In particular, he is keenly aware that the tram-line which he drives must be changed. B.F. states that he "could not bear the repeated reminder of the accident." However, he is concerned that the company, especially those in high positions, may view this request with askance, as if he were "seeking special privileges."

Cognitive behavioral psychotherapy and a short course of selective serotonin-reuptake inhibitors are initiated. A few sessions are required before B.F. feels sufficiently comfortable to reenact the accident, allowing himself to express his feelings. He experienced profound guilt about the child; this was exacerbated when he saw the newspaper headline and thereafter during the court trial. He realizes that he did everything he possibly could to avoid hitting the child. This theme helps segue to a deeper discussion about the toll of professional driving as a quintessential threat avoidant vigilant activity.

Within this framework, the importance of social support as a buffer is emphasized. B.F. recognizes that he needs to "reconnect" with family, friends and coworkers, and little by little reestablishes these links. He also begins to remember the many pleasant interactions that he has had with passengers. This bolsters his feelings of dignity and self-respect.

While B.F. has an overall appreciation of how difficult his work is, reviewing the OSI "brings it home for him." It also provides insights into the underlying factors that directly or indirectly may have contributed to the accident, as well as to his other health-related issues: arterial hypertension and smoking.

12.3.1 *Immediately implementable modifications in work conditions*

The next step is to define the modified work conditions needed for B.F. to actually be able to return to work (Figure 12.3). The occupational neuropsychiatrist fully agrees that the tramline should be changed and reassures B.F. that this is justified on clinical and scientific grounds. In other words, this modification would by no means be a "special privilege."

B.F. begins to admit to himself that he has been working under extremely unhealthy conditions. For example, the split-shift may seem to be "cost effective" for the company since thereby B.F. drives during the two rush hour periods when he is most needed. However, this creates a very long and fatiguing workday for him. Smoking has become an unhealthy response to the unproductive wait time in between shifts. Furthermore, the split shift is frequently associated with two blood pressure spikes per day [Uglješić, Belkić, Bošković *et al.*, 1992]. For these reasons, B.F. should not work the split shift.

As discussed in Chapters 2 and 3, night shift work is associated with fatigue as well as increased risk of accidents and cardiovascular disease among professional drivers. The realistic options for B.F are: 1) to work a regular day shift starting at mid-morning and ending with the afternoon rush hour or 2) to start with the morning rush hour and complete work in the early afternoon. B.F. is a "morning person" and therefore chooses the latter. This will give him a better chance to have true rest breaks after getting through the early morning rush hour. He also prefers avoiding the reminder of what happened when driving very late in the afternoon.

	Underload	High Demand	Strictness	Time Pressure	Noxins	Threat avoidance	Conflict/ Uncertainty
Input						• Δ to a different tram line to avoid repeat exposure to traumatic event • Debriefing, supportive discussion	
Central Decision-Making						• Recognition of the toll of driving as a 1° threat avoidant vigilant activity	
Output/ Task Performance	• No split-shift: no waiting time between shifts						
General	• ↑ recognition of good work	• Eliminate night shift work • Limit work hours to 40/week • True rest breaks away from the vehicle	• Facilitate taking time off from work when needed • ↑ influence over schedule				↓ emotional charge in work atmosphere ↑ help for work-related difficulties
Total	-1.5 Underload = 11.5	- 3.25 High Demand = 18.75	- 3.5 Strictness = 17	Time pressure = 9	Noxious = 9.0	- 0.5 + insight/support Threat avoidance= 17.5	- 0.5 Conflict = 18.5

Figure 12.3 Initial modifications in B.F.'s work situation integrated with cognitive-behavioral therapy: Total OSI (110.5 – 9.25) = 101.25.

As noted, B.F. frequently worked overtime to cover for driver shortages. The dangers of overtime work for professional drivers are emphasized. In particular, B.F. now realizes that he has an "emotional scar" from the accident. In order to heal properly, he must avoid exhaustion. He needs to learn to "say no" and the company "should be discouraged from relying upon the responsible, good drivers to compensate for driver shortages" [Belkić, Savić, Theorell *et al.*, 1994] (p.82).

The insights gleaned by B.F. can be redirected towards "*the positive*." He consciously appreciates that getting safely through each work day is an achievement worthy of recognition. B.F. is now determined to acknowledge this achievement for himself and his colleagues. B.F. also identifies the deleterious role of the press in sensationalizing the accident.

B.F. joins a smoking cessation group offered as part of a work-place health promotion program. He identifies work-related triggers of smoking. Several of these triggers will be eliminated with the modified work conditions. Among professional drivers, interventions directed at smoking have shown success when combined with improvements in working conditions [Emdad *et al.*, 1998][Uglješić, Belkić, Simeunović-Micković, Vukajlović 1992]. B.F. also learns that "smoking is a risk-behavior engendered by the need to regulate arousal and counteract unpleasant emotional-states" [Landsbergis, Schnall, *et al.*, 1998]. In other words, it is a maladaptive response to the stressors associated with professional driving. B.F. is well aware of the dangers of smoking. He demonstratively trashes the remaining cigarettes in his possession as an expression of his determination to quit smoking. He and his family take a short vacation and he does so. To bolster the maintenance phase and to counteract the anticipated challenges associated with professional driving, B.F. starts swimming regularly twice a week at the local swimming pool.

→ Clinical follow up after returning to work:

The therapy sessions included "reliving the trauma experience in a vivid manner that involves perceptual and emotional details" [Bryant *et al.*, 2008] (p.662). When these sessions were completed, B.F. returned to work with the modified conditions summarized in Figure 12.3. He did experience some fear initially. This diminished substantially as he adjusted to the new routine and began to enjoy the interactions with passengers. The IES intrusion and avoidance scores dropped to 8.8 and 7.9. The Post-traumatic Cognitive Inventory scores fell to 2.3, 4.0 and 1.8 for negative cognition of self, negative cognition of the world and self-blame.

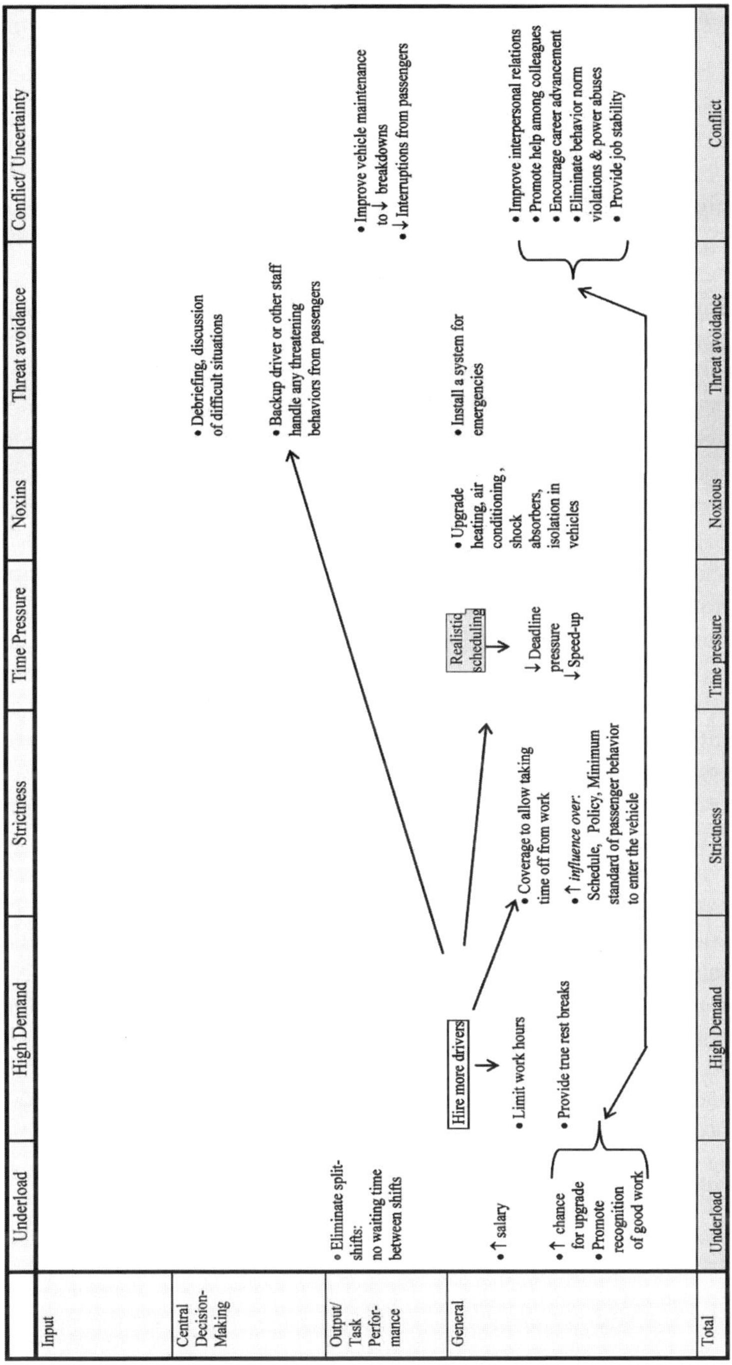

Figure 12.4 A comprehensive view of occupational stressors faced by B.F., that could be ameliorated by organizational measures.

12.3.2 *Outreach: Initial efforts towards improving work organization*

The clinical status of B.F. is markedly improved with the measures described in the subsection 12.3.1. Still, the work stressor burden is extremely high, with the total OSI score over 100. Even though B.F. had been overly conscientious, taking on a heavier than average load, most of his colleagues also have total OSI scores that exceeded 100. Now that the PTSD is more or less under control, B.F. is determined to help create a healthier work environment for himself and his colleagues. Figure 12.4 comprehensively summarizes the possible organizational measures that could be taken to lower the stressor burden for B.F and other tram drivers.

B.F. is now ready to talk about the accident with his colleagues. He decides to do this not to dwell on the negative, but rather to emphasize the need for a more positive image of urban mass transit operators within society at large. The good, responsible, courteous drivers deserve respect for performing this difficult job upon which the economy heavily relies. Sensationalistic news pieces should be discouraged. Instead, the media should be engaged as an ally to educate the public about the importance of traffic safety. This applies to all participants: passengers, bicyclists, pedestrians. Improved road conditions, proper lighting, separate lanes would also help. B.F. also decides to use some of his spare time to further study issues of accident analysis and prevention, with a view to interventions to improve traffic safety [Andersson & Menckel, 1995] [Greiner *et al.*, 1998] [Rajalin & Summala, 1997], including the use of mobile phones [Alm & Nilsson, 1995] that, in some countries, are still permitted while driving. He begins to collect materials such as a recent book written by a city mass transit driver who is also a journalist [Messing 2009]. He examines the literature about events such as person under train [Cotherau *et al.*, 2004] [Theorell *et al.*, 1992] [Theorell *et al.*, 1994], about the psychological and physiological consequences of city mass transit driving [Belkić, Savić, Theorell *et al.*, 1994] [Belkić & Schnall 2000] [Evans 1994] [Greiner *et al.*, 1997] and about interventions to improve the working conditions and health of professional drivers [Belkić, Savić *et al.*, 1995] [Emdad, *et al.*, 1998a] [Kompier & DiMartino 1995] [Kompier *et al.*, 2000] [Uglješić, Belkić, Simeunovic-Micković, Vukajlović, 1992]. His sense of purpose, competence and meaning broadens and deepens.

Suggested cross - references to other parts of this book

Sections 2.2.4.3, 2.5.1.2, 3.2.1.1, 3.2.2, 3.4.2, 3.5, 4.1.2, 4.3.2 and 4.4.1 are recommended as cross-references within part I of this book.

Chapter 13

Scientist with Bipolar Disorder: Seventh Clinical Case Study

Dr. A. in his early 30s is an assistant professor at a leading academic research institute.

He had been intensively involved in writing grant proposals, preparing manuscripts for publication, performing experimental work and supervising doctoral students.

He believed he needed only a few hours of sleep per night.

For the last 2 weeks, Dr. A. has had difficulty concentrating, has begun to doubt his abilities and has been in a sullen mood.

Total OSI = 104

Questions for reflection while reviewing this case:

- Is this a dangerously stressful work situation?
- Is the patient's work situation contributing to his disorder? *If so, how?*
- Could workplace modifications help improve the patient's clinical status? *If so, how?*

13.1 The Case: Dr. A. has Bipolar Disorder

For the past three months, up until the last two weeks, Dr. A. had been working more than 60 hours per week: writing grant proposals and manuscripts, performing experimental laboratory work (often during night hours) and supervising several doctoral students. He needed little sleep and managed to finish all these obligations, seemingly effortlessly. He describes himself as feeling as if he were always "driving in the fast lane." The situation changed dramatically when a submitted manuscript was rejected, with a caustically negative review. He also learned that one of the grants was turned down. Dr. A. became extremely dejected. For the past two weeks he has had difficulty concentrating on his work and has begun to think that he is "incapable of producing any worthwhile science." Upon repeated questioning, he admits that thoughts of suicide have crossed his mind, but denies that he has developed any plan or method.

Dr. A. describes having "always had strong mood oscillations." He would become very excited about his work, not being able to stop until he faced a setback or defeat. The latter would typically "overwhelm him," he would become sullen and "feel badly" about himself. But after some time, usually a few days, he would be "back on his feet" and then "into high gear" once again. He has recognized that these patterns could be consistent with manic-depressive disorder, especially given his family history. However, up until the most recent episode, he considered that he "could handle the mood swings" on his own.

Past medical history and review of systems are otherwise unremarkable. Dr. A. takes no medication.

One of his first cousins (maternal side) committed suicide at age 30. His paternal uncle was diagnosed with manic-depressive disorder.

Dr. A. is recently married; his wife is completing her doctorate and they do not yet have any children. His parents, who are secondary school teachers and his two siblings and their families live nearby and are in apparently good health.

As a student, Dr. A. was a volleyball champion. For the past two years, he has not been involved in this or any other physical activity due to "lack of time." He has been drinking 3-4 cups of coffee per day since he began his university studies at age 18.

Dr. A. graduated *magna cum laude* from a prestigious university. He earned his doctorate at the age of 28.

13.1.1 *Objective findings*

Dr. A. is an alert but subdued, well-developed male who looks his stated age, blood pressure 130/85 mmHg after 5-minutes of rest, HR = 65/ min; the physical exam is unremarkable. Body mass index = 23. Biochemical, hematologic and endocrinologic laboratory findings within normal limits.

- Neuropsychiatric findings:

Neurological examination: Unremarkable.

Psychiatric findings: Bipolar disorder, predominantly hypomania, current episode moderate depression (F31.3) with impaired social and occupational functioning [World Health Organization, 1993] (Appendix A, Section 1). Suicidal ideation present. Work-related stress is the likely trigger.

- Neuropsychological testing:

Right-handed, normal memory span, reaction time and attention.

- Questionnaire findings:

→Young Mania Rating Scale Score = 3.9 [Levy 2013] [Young *et al.*, 1978].
Answered according to his status immediately prior to the present depressive episode: hypomanic approaching manic levels.

→Hamilton Rating Scale for Depression [Hamilton 1960].
Score = 20 (moderate depression), based on current status.
Most noteworthy: Self-reproach, feels he has let people down, admits to suicidal ideas, decrease in actual time spent in activities with decreased productivity.

- Psychophysiologic and neurophysiologic evaluation:

→Quantitative EEG:
Eyes closed increased alpha band (7.5Hz to 14 Hz) asymmetry in the occipital region (O1 < O2) consistent with findings in early depression.

→Event-related potentials:
Standard GO-NOGO contingent negative variation (CNV) visual reaction time paradigm. Slightly attenuated GO CNV: CNV1 = –0.6 μV, CNV2 = – 4μV, CNV3 = + 3μV. Mean GO-NOGO difference = 5 μV.
Reaction time = 295 milliseconds, slightly below but within 1 standard deviation of the normative mean.

Findings within normal limits, but also seen in early depression [Savić & Belkić 1998].

13.2 Dr. A.'s Work Situation: Insights from the OSI

For the past two years, Dr. A. has been an assistant professor in a leading academic research institute. In Figure 13.1, each OSI stressor for Dr. A. is identified and categorized as either fixed or as modifiable.

- Underload:

The experimental work performed by Dr. A. sometimes requires him to carefully follow homogeneous and infrequent signals. However, most of the underload burden is related is potentially modifiable factors, as seen in the left-most column of Fig. 13.1. These include waiting time, mainly related to experiments, some monotonous administrative or technical tasks, inadequate pay, active opposition to career advancement and little recognition of good work. Dr. A.'s high-quality scientific work is not adequately appreciated. Some of his submitted manuscripts and grant proposals have been rejected by reviewers who either did not understand the work or were not objective. When Dr. A. has succeeded to publish or secure grants, this is often ignored due to jealousy amidst the competitive atmosphere in his department. Several of the professors in the department have actively opposed career advancement for Dr. A. and his colleagues.

- High demand:

Over half the demand burden is from stressors inherent in Dr. A.'s work. Scientific work clearly requires complex and complicated decision-making. Dr. A. supervises the work of graduate students and in relation to experiments he occasionally must make rapid decisions and perform several tasks quickly and simultaneously. In addition to his research, Dr. A. has teaching and administrative responsibilities. There is no special time set aside for the latter duties. Consequently, his work day usually is very long; he typically works over 60 hours per week. Rest breaks are frequently interrupted.

When performing experiments, several hours can elapse without having a chance to take a break. Dr. A. must perform these experiments when laboratory time is available; this is irregular and often at night. His pay is not fixed, rather it depends upon projects. In other words, he is working "on soft money." As mentioned above, his pay is inadequate; therefore Dr. A. has taken a second job "to make ends meet." His duties particularly grant applications and writing articles, require Dr. A. to work during formally-allocated vacation time.

JOB DEMANDS are EXCEEDINGLY HIGH and there is some underload, especially INSUFFICIENT REWARDS.

EFFORT-REWARD IMBALANCE is present.

- Strictness:

There is rigorous review of Dr. A.'s work from many sources. However, most of the strictness burden for Dr. A. is potentially modifiable. His workspace is confined, over-crowded and windowless. Due to severe space shortages even his own desk is not guaranteed. He has very limited possibilities to take time off from work and low influence over scheduling, work team, tasks and departmental policy.

- Extrinsic time pressure:

The major source of extrinsic time pressure is from incessant deadlines.

The EXCEEDINGLY HIGH DEMANDS together with together with HIGH STRICTNESS score indicate that:

JOB STRAIN is present.

- Noxious exposures:

Dr.A.'s work area is drafty and ventilation is poor. Noise up to 90 dB is sporadically present, more so recently due to nearby construction work. Dr. A.'s work area is dusty at times. Experimental work entails some exposure to chemicals. Overall, the noxious exposure load is thus not entirely inconsequential.

- Threat Avoidant Vigilance:

There is some need for vigilance because of accident risk associated with the experimental laboratory work. Dr. A. has heard about a colleague who suffered a major chemical burn in the laboratory, but he has never actually had or seen serious work-related accident. A graduate student working in the department committed suicide last year. Dr. A. has heard many other disturbing accounts about colleagues and students, related to career-blocking, lack of impartial review and consequent loss of funding, *inter alia*. He has talked with several graduate students and post-doctoral fellows whose frustration was so heavy that they decided to quit academic life altogether. There is no system in place at work to handle emergencies.

- Conflict and uncertainty:

This is the highest conflict score encountered thus far in all the cases. Over two-thirds of this burden could be ameliorated or even eliminated. The most egregious of these factors are on the general level. There is extreme emotional tension at work, very much related to intensive competition, so that colleagues undermine each other. This unhealthy atmosphere is due in large measure to abuses of power such as misappropriation of scientific results, as well as career blocking. The pointless tasks are of a technical/administrative nature. As noted earlier, Dr. A. relies upon "soft money" for his salary such that his employment status is tenuous. "Publish or perish" is the *modus vivendi.*

> The conflict burden is EXCEEDING HIGH and a likely CONTRIBUTOR to Dr. R's clinical status.
> The TAV burden is not negligible.

13.3 What are the Feasible Options for Dr. A. *vis-à-vis* the Work Environment?

The total OSI score for Dr. A. is above the acutely dangerous level and this is very likely to have contributed to his current clinical status. Specifically, the exceedingly high demands strongly reinforce hypomanic tendencies, whereas the lack of rewards/underload are a set-up for the depressive phase. The inordinately high conflict burden creates an atmosphere of emotional tension and destabilization.

→Dr. A. is self-referred to the occupational neuropsychiatrist. He realizes that his current situation is untenable and that his work is of pivotal importance to his well–being. The case presentation up until this point recapitulates the initial workup performed by the occupational neuropsychiatrist.

Dr. A. is a talented and dedicated researcher. Despite all the difficulties, he finds great satisfaction in scientific work. His self-esteem is closely linked to his career as a scientist.

In reviewing Dr. A.'s case, the occupational neuropsychiatrist is struck by the fact that he does not yet have a tenured position, even though he had been eligible for quite some time. Dr. A. admits that that this is probably due to his choice of a very prestigious academic center.

	Underload	High Demand	Strictness	Time Pressure	Noxins	Threat avoidance	Conflict/ Uncertainty
Input	Some with experiments: • Low frequency of incoming signals • Homogeneous information	Information: • Several sources • Heterogeneous • Heavy burden on visual system • Communication essential	• Some strict requirements for signal detection (laboratory experiments)		Sporadic: • Noise	• Some vigilance required ∝ lab • Listens to some emotionally-disturbing occurrences	Incoming information conflict: • Signal/signal • Signal/noise
Central Decision-Making		Decisions: • Complex • Complicated • Affect others (supervises) • Rapid decisions (occasional)		• Sometimes cannot postpone decisions		• Some serious consequences of wrong decision	Information: • Contradictory • Missing • Unforeseeable events require new plan: } Exacerbated by administrative actions
Output/ Task Perfor-mance	Some: • Waiting time: with experiments • Monotonous administrative tasks	Tasks: • Complex • Varied *Laboratory*: • Simultaneous • Rapid --Research + teaching + administration (no separate time)	• Work must meet a very strict standard (evaluation by reviewers, supervisors, students)	• Only partial control over rate of task performance		Hazards: • Laboratory	• Conflicting tasks (no time aside for research vs. teaching vs. administration) *Work hampered by* • Extrinsic problems • Interruptions from people
General	• Inadequate pay • Active opposition to career advancement • Little recognition of good work	• Pay depends on projects • >60 h/work week • Breaks often interrupted • Night shift/irregular work hours • 2nd job • Must work during "vacation time"	• Fixed body posi-tion (lab) • Confined, window-less workspace • Autonomous workspace not secure • Very limited in taking time off from work *Low influence over*: • Schedule • Tasks • Policy • Persons with whom he works	• Deadline pressure • Occasional speed-up (laboratory)	Mild: • Heat • Cold • Dust, chemicals (lab. work)	Past work exposures: • Heard about serious accident • Suicide occurrence • No system for emergencies	• Emotionally-charged work atmosphere • Little help with difficulties • Opposition to career advancement • Behavior norm violations, power abuses • No grievance redress • Some pointless tasks • Threat of job loss
Total	Fixed:1 Modifiable: 7.5 Underload = 8.5	Fixed: 20 Modifiable: 11.5 High Demand = 31.5	Fixed: 4 Modifiable: 13 Strictness = 17	Fixed: 2 Modifiable: 3 Time pressure = 5	Modifiable: 4 Noxious = 4	Fixed: 6 Modifiable: 3 Threat avoidance = 9	Fixed: 9 Modifiable: 20 Conflict = 29

Figure 13.1 Summary of the baseline OSI for Dr. A. Total OSI ((Fixed = 42) + (Modifiable = 62)) = 104.

In this setting, he had become so "caught up" in the immediate tasks surrounding grant proposals, experimental work, writing papers, teaching and administration, that he did not devote the needed time and energy to apply. He has seen several devastating episodes of career blocking among his colleagues. These further deterred him from proceeding with his application for the tenured position of associate professor.

→We now provide a scenario based upon the successful outcome of Dr.A.'s application for tenure. Unfortunately, all too often, this optimistic scenario does not take place in the academic world, even for those who are most deserving. In Section 13.4 we will explore the broader issues that need attention to create healthier work conditions for scientists.

The activity surrounding application for tenure helps Dr. A. to focus on a key goal-oriented task. The occupational neuropsychiatrist encourages him to make the "strongest possible arguments for his own case," as he has done so successfully in his scientific writing. Dr. A. shows his dossier to two eminent professors who agree to write letters in support of his application. In the face of a number of official complaints about lack of due process and fairness, in particular in relation to the graduate student who committed suicide, the department is now under scrutiny by the chancellor and advisory board of the university. Since Dr. A. is clearly qualified and deserving of tenure, the department expedites his case and approves his application.

A number of improvements in Dr. A.'s working conditions result from his new position. He is guaranteed a minimum salary, his pay is increased and he gets a small office of his own. While he does not have "absolute job security," he is no longer paid exclusively by "soft" money and his employment status is no longer tenuous.

Notwithstanding their importance, these tenure-related improvements in and of themselves will not be sufficient to protect Dr. A. from the extremes of bipolar disorder. Dr. A. is cognizant of this fact. He is also cognizant of the fact that without at least some support from those in leadership and from colleagues at the department, further improvements in the work situation will not be forthcoming. With his tenured status, Dr. A. is legally protected against discrimination. He decides to disclose the diagnosis of bipolar disorder to the human resources advisor for the university and ask for advice about whom to approach within the department.

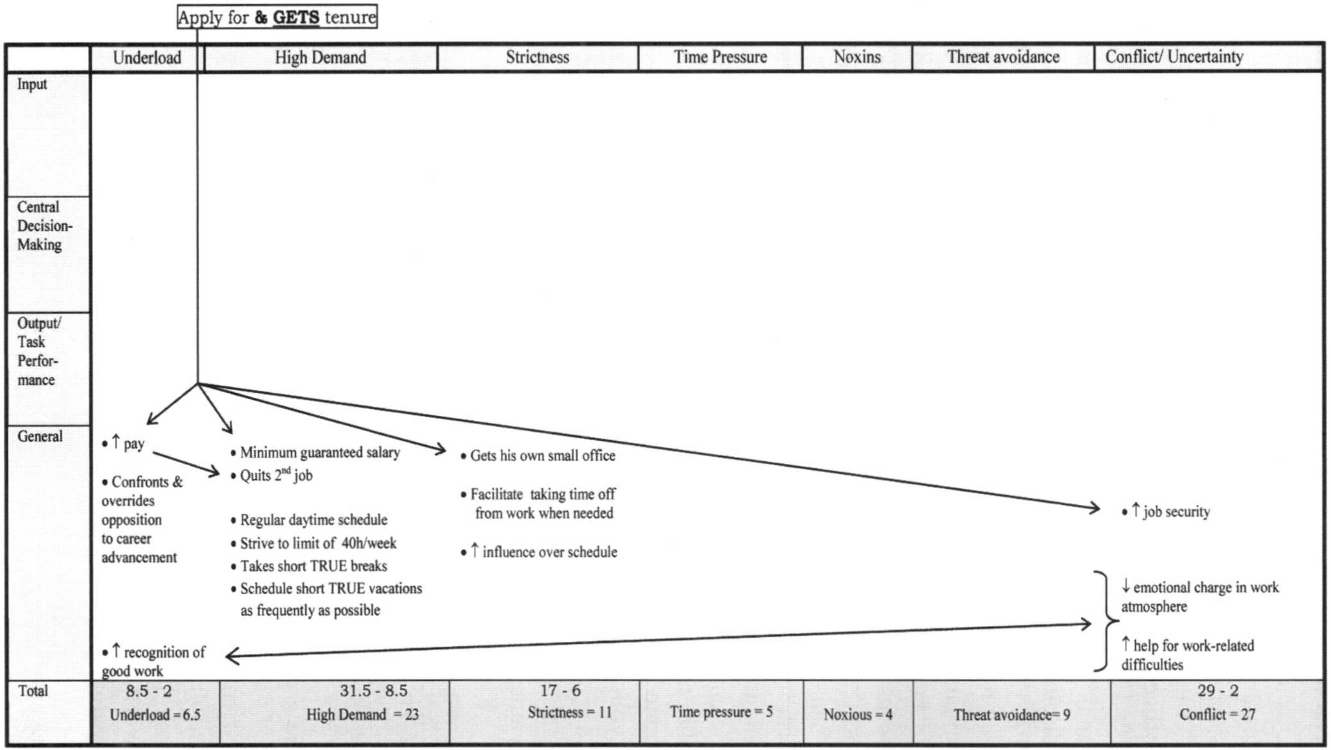

Figure 13.2 Immediate modifications in Dr. A.'s work situation integrated with cognitive-behavioral/pharmacologic therapy: Total OSI (104 – 18.5) = 85.5.

The needed workplace modifications that are realistically implementable are summarized in Figure 13.2. Dr. A. begins with those that are directly under his control. With the increased salary and a more secure job situation, he can quit his second job. He schedules regular short breaks during which he either closes his eyes and listens to calming music in his office or takes a brisk walk outside.

Limiting work hours and working a regular, daytime schedule are vital for stabilizing Dr. A.'s clinical status. Because he has agreed to disclosure, the occupational neuropsychiatrist can mandate these changes for Dr. A. The human resources advisor helps mediate this process, carefully selecting those in leadership who are most likely to facilitate a smooth transition.

Further therapeutic sessions with the occupational neuropsychiatrist focus upon reinforcing Dr. A.'s self-esteem, based upon his accomplishments achieved to date. A new behavior pattern, with "centeredness" at its core, is aimed at avoiding extremes. Dr. A. needs to learn how to work at a steady pace and to stop at the right time. Careful attention to sleep hygiene, including limitation of coffee-intake is vital. Scientific endeavor obviously consumes enormous cognitive resources; this must be recognized. Dr. A. begins to formulate counter-measures aimed at replenishment. These include resumption of team sport activity (volleyball), as well as music and walks in nature. Short vacations related to these activities are scheduled. He also consciously takes time to be with family and friends. A session is scheduled with his wife, who as a young scientist faces many of the same pressures as Dr. A.

Eventually, Dr. A. feels sufficiently strong and stable to reach out to colleagues at work. He starts by acknowledging and explicitly congratulating their success—often to their surprise, given the prevailing tension at work. Eventually, this tension is somewhat ameliorated, by Dr. A.'s efforts and the positive feedback from others.

13.4 Healthy Work for Scientists?

Scientific work has been characterized as "relaxed" according to the four-quadrant job strain model [Karasek & Theorell, 1990]. However, the working conditions of Dr. A., described by the OSI, are anything but relaxed. Such working conditions are not atypical. The implemented interventions were mainly directed to the underload, high demand and strictness aspects. The conflict burden was only minimally ameliorated.

Dr. A. was in the fortunate situation of being granted tenure, such that some job security, guarantees for at least part of his salary and other improvements were afforded him. A large number of scientists are not afforded these advantages and continue to work on "soft money" with short-term contracts and a highly uncertain future.

Peer review is intended to promote the scientific process in a constructive manner. Unfortunately, however, reviewers all too often "hide behind their anonymity" to display an appalling lack of collegiality, undermining the results of groups other than their own. This is particularly the case when competition is intense for scarce resources. Demoralization is a frequent concomitant of those on the receiving end of this process.

Scientists are increasingly bogged down with formal administrative tasks that drain their energies and talents. These tasks could be handled by others. Moreover, these processes could often be streamlined and coordinated, with reduction of tiresome redundancy.

The creative process which is seminal to scientific advancement may well attract individuals with a hypomanic proclivity [Goodwin & Jamison, 2007]. More awareness is needed of the warning signs of mental overload within the scientific milieu. Our recent results reveal that physicians with mental distress who are currently involved in scientific research are unlikely to seek needed help [Fridner *et al.*, 2012]. Supportive and healthy working conditions are imperative to protect the mental well-being of scientists.

Suggested cross - references to other parts of this book

Sections 2.2.4.4, 3.4.4 and 4.1.5, are recommended as cross-references within part I of this book.

Chapter 14

A Dysphoric Academic Physician near Formal Retirement Age: Concluding Case Study

Dr. L, an academic physician (adjunct professor), internist working in a leading training hospital is nearing formal retirement age.

He finds clinical work exhausting and yet is reluctant to abandon his primary professional domain.

He is fearful that retirement will signal a downward spiral for him. At times hc is overcome with feelings of sadness.

Current Total OSI = 85.75

Question for reflection while reviewing this case:

- How could the transition to retirement best maintain Dr. L.'s mental health and continued professional activity?

  Incorporate the OSI into your answer.

14.1 Dr. L. is Nearing Formal Retirement Age and is Dysphoric

Dr. L. has decided to consult his colleague, a neuropsychiatrist and trusted friend because of his uneasiness as he approaches retirement age. He perceives that colleagues have already begun to view him as "soon out the door." Notwithstanding, Dr. L. considers himself still capable of performing his clinical, research and pedagogical tasks. However, he admits that whenever he has outpatient clinic, he finds himself completely exhausted and "sitting idly" for up to several hours thereafter, incapable of any physical or intellectual work and avoiding contact with other people. He is particularly frustrated that due to these recurrent episodes of feeling "totally wasted," there is an ever-rising backlog of administrative tasks which looks to him "Sisyphusian." Recently, Dr. L. admits to displaying outbursts of anger at his wife, at younger colleagues, and hospital staff when they mention a topic or task which he would rather avoid. He subsequently feels ashamed for losing control over his behavior and withdraws further. He would like to get rid of these "lousy feelings" and to "stop being so morose," especially since these feelings are completely unusual for him.

The past history, review of systems, physical examination and laboratory findings are unremarkable. Body mass index is 26. Dr. L. has always been a non-smoker; he consumes 1-2 glasses of wine on Friday evenings. Up until his mid-forties, he had been an active basketball player.

Dr. L. has been married for nearly forty years; his wife is a music teacher. Their two grown children and three small grandchildren all live several hundred miles away, in Dr. L.'s hometown where his parents, in their late 80's and in good health, also live.

Dr. L. and his wife moved to their current residence twenty years ago, when he decided to accept a promising position which opened up at a leading university hospital. He admits that "the move was a big sacrifice." In many ways, he and his wife had to "start all over."

On the one hand, Dr. L. considers that he thrived in the more exciting ambience of academic medicine. Having secured major research grants, he and his group were able to publish some "landmark findings" that have been widely cited. On the other hand, he thinks that the cutthroat competition is "thoroughly disgusting." He and his wife find themselves feeling "quite lonely," since even after twenty years, they are still often seen as "outsiders."

Now, as Dr. L. approaches retirement age, this loneliness has become more acute. He knows that others are envious of his success, including, and perhaps even especially, since his salary is among the highest in the department. With retirement, not only will his income be lowered, but his entire status as a leading academic clinician is under threat. This makes him frightened and sad; he cannot help feeling that this is "the beginning of a downward spiral."

14.2 Dr.L.'s Work Situation: Insights from the OSI

In order to adequately approach Dr. L's upcoming retirement, we first need insight into his current work situation, as attending physician/adjunct professor. We will thereby use the OSI, and as with all the other cases, distinguish the fixed and modifiable stressors, in Figure 14.1.

- Underload:

While the total underload score is quite low, it is not entirely negligible. As seen in the left-most column of Fig. 14.1, Dr. L. performs some monotonous administrative tasks. He is a salaried employee of the university hospital with fixed pay. Even though there is external recognition via research grants and publications, among the colleagues and chair of his department, the competition and rivalry are such that good work is rarely acknowledged.

- High demand:

The total demand burden has been extremely high for Dr. L. Slightly more than half of this burden is from stressors inherent to his profile as attending physician specialist and his academic position, which entails research, teaching as well as administration. There is no special time set aside for the latter duties. Consequently, carrying out these varied obligations has led to long work hours, and he does a substantial amount of work at home. Dr. L. does try to take some breaks during the workday. However, these are frequently interrupted by colleagues and staff, as well as by patients who call him on his pager. He is also called at home quite often.

Dr. L. takes night call on two Thursdays per month; this entails work in the emergency room, and he is free on the Thursday dayshift and on most of the Friday dayshift thereafter. During night call and in relation to his inpatient responsibilities, Dr. L. performs a variety of invasive procedures.

He also teaches/supervises younger colleagues and students. He formally has 6 weeks of allotted vacation time. However, in his present position he has never taken more than 1-2 days without working: preparing lectures, writing scientific articles, performing editorial tasks and preparing grant applications, *inter alia.* Dr. L. has outpatient clinic twice and sometimes three times per week. Therein, between those who are scheduled and those who are unscheduled, he sees up to thirty patients, several of whom are new. Each of these patients requires substantial administrative work, particularly to ensure appropriate consultations and other needed triage, as well as fulfilling the formal obligations demanded by the university hospital clinic.

JOB DEMANDS have been extremely HIGH.
There are financial rewards,
but otherwise insufficient recognition of good work.
Some EFFORT-REWARD IMBALANCE has been present.

- Strictness:

The total strictness score is quite low compared to other physicians in a comparable setting: nearly a standard deviation below the mean for male academic physicians in the non-surgical specialties [Belkić & Nedić 2012]. Notably, Dr. L. has major control over his work schedule, such that the twice per month night call on Thursday evenings is by choice. He uses the daytime hours of Thursdays and Fridays for non-clinical work, and is quite satisfied with that arrangement. It is also his choice to take on non-clinical duties, and to perform various invasive procedures, upon the challenge of which he thrives. As a senior attending physician, his clinical judgment is rarely questioned. The most notable limitations are in taking time off and in deciding with whom he will work. He has some, albeit not major, influence over policy as his department and at the university hospital. As formal retirement age approaches, there is talk from the department chair about taking away his office space.

- Extrinsic time pressure:

The total extrinsic time pressure score for Dr. L. is slightly above the mean for male academic physicians in the non-surgical specialties [Belkić & Nedić 2012].

	Underload	High Demand	Strictness	Time Pressure	Noxins	Threat avoidance	Conflict/ Uncertainty
Input		Information: • Several sources • Heterogeneous • Communication essential • Rapid inflow (ER) • 3 sensory modalities • Visual burden (invasive procedures	• Strict requirements for detecting information --ER/ICU	• Limited control over speed of incoming information --Limited control of patient scheduling, # inpatients	Sporadic: •Noise (ER)	• Grave consequences of momentary lapse -ER/ICU • Visually-disturbing scenes (patients with end-stage disease) • Listens to emotionally-disturbing occurrences --Most severe patients	Incoming information conflict: • Signal/noise • Signal/signal
Central Decision-Making		Decisions: • Complex • Complicated • Affect others • Rapid --Supervises (several others) --ER/ICU	Somewhat strict: • Definition of correct decision	• Can't postpone decisions --ER/ICU		• Potentially fatal consequences of wrong decision	Information: •Contradictory •Missing --Can't get history, language barriers • Unforeseeable events require new plan -ER/ICU
Output/ Task Perfor-mance	• Some monotonous administrative tasks	Tasks quite: • Complex • Varied --Clinical, research, teaching, administration •Some simultaneous & rapid tasks: ER/ICU	• Somewhat strict evaluation of performance	• Limited control of performance rate --Limited control over # patients		• Hazardous tasks (infection)	• Some conflicting tasks no special time set aside for research, teaching or other non-clinical tasks) *Hampered by **some***: • Extrinsic problems • Interruptions from people
General	• Fixed pay • Little recognition of good work (competition & rivalry)	• >48 h/work week • Breaks often interrupted • Night shift 2x / month • Must work during "vacation time"	• Office space in jeopardy as formal retirement age approaches • Some limitations in taking time off from work *Somewhat limited influence over*: -With whom he works -Policy	• Deadline Pressure (research grants) • Speed-up		Past work exposures: • Needle-stick injuries • Witnessed serious accidents • Patient suicides • Work-related court testimony	*Some*: • Emotional tension among colleagues • Power abuses & violations of norms of behavior • Pointless tasks • Employment status in transition as formal retirement age approaches
Total	Modifiable: 4.5 Underload = 4.5	Fixed: 15.5 Modifiable: 14.5 High Demand = 30	Fixed: 4 Modifiable: 6.75 Strictness = 10.75	Fixed: 3.75 Modifiable: 4.75 Time pressure = 8.5	Modifiable: 0.5 Noxious =0.5	Fixed/past :12.5 Modifiable: 2 Threat avoidance = 14.5	Fixed: 8.5 Modifiable: 8.5 Conflict = 17

Figure 14.1 Summary of the baseline OSI for Dr. L. Total OSI = ((Fixed = 44.25) + (Modifiable = 41.5)) = 85.75.

Among the modifiable factors, due to limited control over outpatient scheduling and the overall number of patients he carries, the speed of incoming signals and task performance rate are substantially out of his control. Deadline pressure arises mainly in relation to research grants. Overall, he must speed up his work several times per week.

> This is an ACTIVE JOB with very high demands and substantial time pressure, but with some decision-making latitude.
>
> Full-blown job strain is not currently present.

- Noxious exposures:

Except for sporadic noise in the emergency room, exposure to noxious physical factors is minimal for Dr. L.

- Threat Avoidant Vigilance:

Dr. L. has a fairly heavy backlog of past exposures that contribute to the threat avoidant vigilance burden. This, together with caring for patients with end stage disease, and work in the ICU and ER contribute to high a TAV score, well over a standard deviation above the mean for male academic physicians in the non-surgical specialties [Belkić & Nedić 2012].

- Conflict and uncertainty:

The burden from conflict and uncertainty for Dr. L. is also well over a standard deviation above the mean for male academic physicians in the non-surgical specialties [Belkić & Nedić 2012]. Half of this burden is modifiable, with several general-level stressors. These include somewhat tense interpersonal relations, even though colleagues can count on each other for help with clinical difficulties. There are also violations of norms of behavior, mainly in the form of disrespectful, insensitive remarks made directly to colleagues by the department chair. Among the physicians with academic positions, there is a good deal of "backbiting." General level stressors also come from performing seemingly pointless administrative tasks, and for Dr. L., most acutely, because of uncertainty about his status in light of the approach of formal retirement age.

> The modifiable CONFLICT/UNCERTAINTY stressors appear to be contributing to Dr. L.'s dysphoria. The TAV burden, as cumulative exposure, should also be taken into account.

14.3 The Transition Process for Dr. L.

After the initial evaluation, as described in Section 14.1, Dr. L's friend and colleague suggests referral to an occupational neuropsychiatrist. Dr. L. agrees. He first completes the OSI for his current situation, as summarized in Section 14.2. Dr. L.'s answers to the open-ended questions are used as a springboard for guiding a plan of action.

On the one hand, it is clear that Dr. L. would like to continue working after formal retirement age. His work provides him with meaning, structure and satisfaction. He is highly competent; objectively speaking, his clinical, pedagogical and scientific contributions to his institution are invaluable. On the other hand, there are a substantial number of adverse conditions under which Dr. L. works. Many of these stressors could be ameliorated or eliminated entirely

A critical issue for this transition process is "navigation," through dialogue whenever possible, and with the backup of institutional policy, as well as the existing grievance procedure and legal protection of due process, as needed. Another vital consideration is that Dr. L. has clearly overextended himself in his work over the last twenty years at the university clinical hospital. This has been to the detriment of other dimensions of life: family and friends, cultural and recreational activity, as well as rest and introspection. His dysphoria, exhaustion and occasional outbursts of anger reflect this imbalance.

During the initial session with the occupational neuropsychiatrist, Dr. L. begins to work through some of these seemingly contradictory considerations. Thereafter, he concludes that he would like to continue with clinical work on a part-time basis. He sees an Emeritus Professorship as the best way for him to continue his research and pedagogical activity with somewhat attenuated intensity. In that capacity, he could offload some of the administrative work, which he finds so tiresome. In defining the scope of his clinical activity, he would like to minimize outpatient work, to at most one day per week. On the other hand, he is prepared to continue with most of the inpatient and ER work, including twice monthly Thursday night call, which he handles well and to which he is quite accustomed. Moreover, he realizes that this could be an important "bargaining point," since there is a shortage of physicians who are both competent and willing to take on night call and other types of emergency services.

Having defined a number of his objective goals and accompanying modification of work tasks, Dr. L. begins to broach the more sensitive topic of the interpersonal relations in the department. To his mind, these tensions are the *real* source of his demoralization, which have come to a head as he nears formal retirement age. He is particularly disturbed by the department chair, who sets a negative tone with his inappropriate behavior, and who appears to be particularly hostile to senior colleagues with high academic positions.

Dr. L. first needs to articulate and ventilate his frustration and anger. The occupational neuropsychiatrist has gained Dr. L's trust, so that he feels secure in so doing.

Next, they review the potential options. In going over the OSI questionnaire, the occupational neuropsychiatrist notes that there is a confidential grievance procedure in place at the university hospital, and that there is an explicit policy against age discrimination. Dr. L. has a legal right to continue to work after formal retirement age, and to be appropriately compensated. Dr. L. decides to proceed with a formal grievance, which will be treated confidentially, but can serve as an impetus for improving the climate at his department. He would like this to proceed in a constructive manner, whereby recognition of good work is promoted, together with an official "zero-tolerance" for harassment of any kind, whether based upon age, gender, ethnicity, handicaps, or just plain "envy."

In this connection, Dr. L. identifies the issue of his office as an important symbol. Within the grievance procedure, he explicitly requests a guarantee that his office will not be jeopardized.

Dr. L. starts thinking about what he would like his legacy to be. As much as he would like to be appreciated for his clinical acumen, research achievements and teaching, he would also like to know that he has contributed to creating a more collegial atmosphere in his department.

14.4 Comments and Further Thoughts

The actual outcome for Dr. L. is summarized in Figure 14.2, according to the OSI model. Viewed together with the concluding section of Chapter 2 (2.6), we can see a great potential for creating healthier work through a "bridging" solution [Zhan 2009], as formal retirement age approaches.

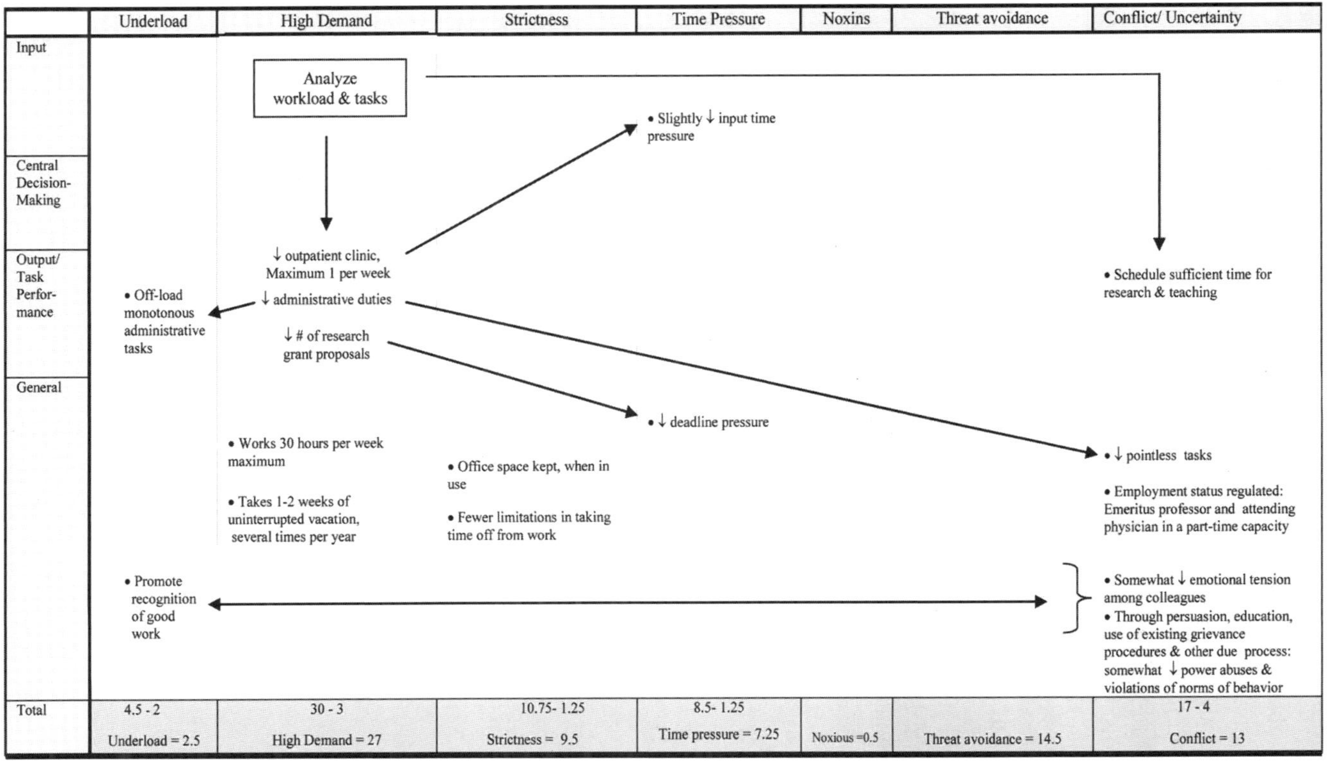

Figure 14.2 Summary of changes made in Dr. L's work conditions with transition to partial retirement: Total OSI (85.75 – 11.5) = 74.25.

We would also comment at this juncture, that Dr. L.'s case differs substantially from most of the other clinical case studies in that the proactive process has begun somewhat earlier. By that we mean: before neuropsychiatric pathology has become entrenched. In other words, this clinical case study thus focuses upon the pre-pathologic state, without a full-fledged diagnosis. As we have emphasized for other medical disciplines, this is when the chances for success are substantially better [Belkić, Savić, Theorell *et al.*, 1994] [Belkić, Savić *et al.*, 1995].

Further reading

Sections 2.2.4.1 and 2.6 are recommended as cross-references within part I of this book. Further references of particular relevance for this case study include:

[Coursolle *et al.*, 2010][Knežević 2011][Mezuk *et al.*, 2001][Saunders 2006][Zhan *et al.*, 2009].

Part III

A New Clinical Approach to Neuropsychiatry Focusing upon the Work Environment

Chapter 15

The Need for a New Subspecialty: Occupational Neuropsychiatry

A recent editorial in the British Journal of Psychiatry [Gilbody *et al.*, 2012] underscoring the link between the work environment and disorders such as depression, has emphasized the need for integrating occupational and mental health services. Within that framework, the authors call for implementation of interventions at the workplace.

This editorial is certainly a welcome development. Clearly, coordination between occupational medicine specialists and neuropsychiatrists would be a vast improvement over two potentially divergent clinical approaches that often leave working patients suffering from mental health disorders torn in between. Or worse yet, the role of the work environment as a potential source of the patient's psychological distress *as well as* a potential source of recovery may well remain underplayed or even ignored.

Nevertheless, just as our focus in Part II of this book was on the individual patient, we would also suggest that coordinated care might best be offered by an *individual* clinician with the needed multi-faceted expertise. Perhaps one of the most salient arguments in favor of such an approach is that, especially for patients suffering from mental health disorders, the establishment of trust and rapport with the clinician, based upon empathy is an essential prerequisite for effective care. Being shunted from one care-giver to another, especially when disclosing often painful and sensitive topics, is anathema for such patients.

At the same time, clinical training in psychiatry and neurology, as is true for most specialty training outside occupational medicine (with the noteworthy exception of pulmonary medicine, as discussed in section 4.3.5 of Chapter 4) has generally been quite bereft of attention to the work environment. Consequently, specialists in psychiatry and neurology generally lack the needed expertise to tackle work-related issues. On the other hand, specialists in occupational medicine do not usually have sufficient training in psychiatry and neurology to provide the needed care for patients with the more serious mental health disorders.

For most of the clinical case studies presented in Part II, it was the occupational neuropsychiatrist who provided the needed integrated care to navigate the process of return to *healthier* work for the patient. We mentioned in Chapter 6 that the appellation "occupational neuropsychiatrist" denoted a specialist in psychiatry and neurology, who also had expertise in occupational medicine and stress medicine. This combined clinical competence was essential.

When speaking of combined clinical competence another point should be emphasized. Namely, in some countries psychiatry and neurology are separate specialties. However, our experience and perspective would argue that their combination as neuropsychiatry is optimal. Clinical practice indicates that neurologic and psychiatric disturbances are very closely interrelated, and it is often impossible to clearly delineate these two entities. Moreover, primary neurologic disorders are almost inevitably accompanied by psychiatric manifestations. Most notably among the former are headaches and epilepsy, as illustrated in the 2nd and 3rd clinical cases, as well as degenerative disorders of the central nervous system, cerebrovascular disease, multiple sclerosis, brain tumors and head trauma, *inter alia.* Thus, the subspecialty for which we herein advocate would indeed be "occupational neuropsychiatry".

As reviewed in Chapter 2, work-related mental health disorders represent a problem of great magnitude. In light of the trends in working life [Gabriel & Liimatainen 2000] [Landsbergis, Cahill & Schnall, 1999] [Shirom 2011], if anything, these disorders are likely to become even more prevalent in the coming years. Given the enormous economic toll of work-related mental health disorders [Ahola *et al.*, 2011] [Belkić 2011][Guthrie *et al.*, 2010][Pro 2007], diminishing this burden would also be cost-effective [Leigh & Robbins 2004][Leigh 2006]. Subspecialists formally trained in psychiatry and neurology, as well as in occupational medicine and stress medicine, would be in the best position to tackle these problems from a clinical perspective.

Needless to say, as illustrated by the clinical case studies, the patient together with occupational neuropsychiatrist interact dynamically within a larger organizational setting. The need to incorporate a "social ecological" strategy, namely, one in which "supportive environmental conditions" are created to bolster efforts on the individual level has been highlighted [Stokols *et al.*, 1995] [Stokols *et al.*, 1996]. These concepts have been applied directly to the workplace. This is particularly important since focusing upon the outcome or "backend" of the stress process merely offers "damage limitation," instead of addressing the "sources of stress" in the organizational structure or nature of the workplace [Cartwright *et al.*, 1995]. Professor Stuart Donaldson [1995] points to one of the main criticisms of the current paradigm in work-site health promotion as the failure

> "to consider the system of work in which employee behavior is embedded" (p. 79-80).

15.1 An Occupational Neuropsychiatry Paradigm: Mental Health Disorders as Potential "Occupational Sentinel Health Events"

As outlined in detail in this book, there are a myriad of pathways by which work stressors can impact upon mental health. One of the roles of the occupational neuropsychiatrist would be to stay on the alert for the occurrence of unexpected patterns or clusters of mental health disorders in relation to the workplace. Historically, in other medical disciplines, the astute clinician has often been the one who identified occupationally-associated diseases, with resultant major changes in the work environment. A classic example is that of Professor Dr. Irving Selikoff and colleagues in the relation between asbestos exposure and mesothelioma, as well as pulmonary interstitial fibrosis (asbestosis), as noted in Chapter 4.

The concept of an "occupational sentinel health event" could be incorporated into the realm of neuropsychiatry. The fundamental role of the clinician for the implementation of the concept has been cogently summarized as follows:

> "The occupational sentinel health event concept conveys three important and related notions. First, it is useful as a heuristic device to allow health care providers and public health authorities to sort through health events of individuals and populations to determine *a priori* which health events and patterns of health events are most likely to be caused by occupation factors, given current knowledge. Second, the sentinel health event concept transforms the health problems of individuals into the potential health problems of populations. To recognize the diagnosis of an occupational disease in an individual as a sentinel health event facilitates the identification of others at the workplace who are also ill or who may become ill if exposure continues. Third, the occurrence of a sentinel health event may signify the failure of a system to control known occupational

> hazards and thereby to prevent cases of unnecessary occupational disease" (p. 20)[Markowitz 1998].

Clues concerning occupational sentinel health events can sometimes be obtained from the patient. This can include e.g. inquiries about other employees complaining of severe fatigue or being on sick-leave. Occurrences of suicide or suicide attempts at the workplace should be a particular warning sign. As noted, this query is incorporated into the Occupational Stressor Index.

More broadly, the total OSI score is an indicator of the total burden of job stressors. If the total OSI score is inordinately high, chances are that this is not an isolated occurrence. Rather, it is likely that dangerous conditions are present for others at the same workplace.

15.2 A Larger Framework for the Occupational Neuropsychiatrist

The clinical case studies of Part II, based upon the OSI, provide concrete examples of how the occupational neuropsychiatrist could actually function. However, a substantial gap exists between this new paradigm and established neuropsychiatric practice.

The pressing question then becomes how, in practice, to implement this paradigm? In the forthcoming, a public health approach to occupational neuropsychiatric practice is outlined, and schematically displayed in Figure 15.1.

There are a number of resource persons with whom to work, particularly social workers, occupational therapists and other members of the occupational health service team, including organizational psychologists, industrial hygienists and epidemiologists, if available. This team should then strive to work with key participants in the workplace, i.e. labor and management, in the process of hazard recognition and control.

The concepts and core methodology of Participatory Action Research (PAR) [Elden & Chisholm, 1993] [Schurman & Israel, 1995] provide a helpful framework for this process, which is of a cyclical nature, whereby

> "reflection and action in which the stakeholders (a) identify aspects of the system that they wish to change, (b) analyze 'causes' of system dysfunction, develop and implement action plans, create a plan to evaluate the effects of their actions" (p. 242).

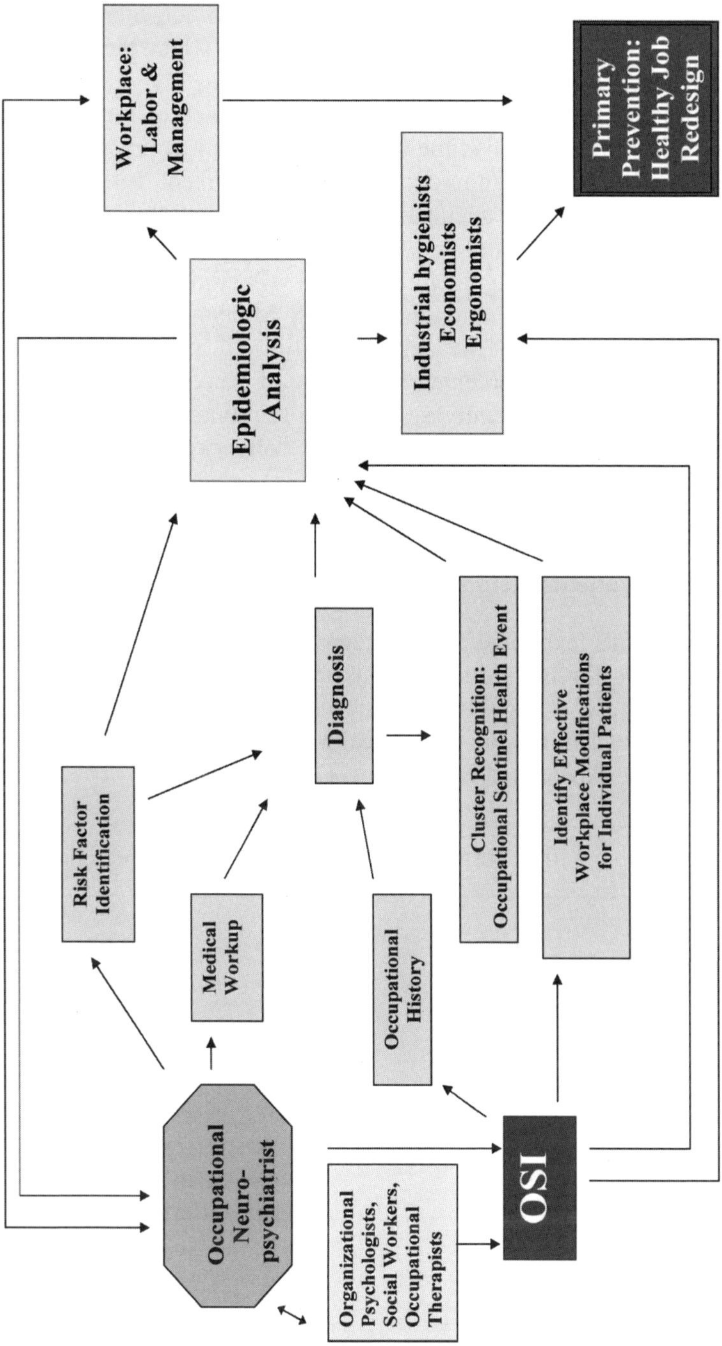

Figure 15.1 The Role of the Occupational Neuropsychiatrist and the OSI in the Larger Framework of Creating Healthy Workplaces. Adapted from Fisher J, Belkic K, A public health approach in clinical practice, Occupational Medicine: State of the Art Review 2000; 15: 245-253.

This PAR approach would be integrated with job-related monitoring feedback of workers' health [Karasek & Theorell, 1990], where the clinician's role would be of paramount importance.

Barriers to implementation may include: i) lack of training and skills in occupational health, ii) time limitations of clinical practice, iii) lack of access to the workplace/non-cooperative management, iv) fear on the part of management of the occupational relatedness of the neuropsychiatric disorders and the possibility of workers' compensation proceedings, v) employee fear of losing their jobs, and vi) clinician reluctance to get involved in possible litigation/depositions. Many of these barriers overlap with those obstructing the implementation of preventive services, in general. The lack of perceived legitimacy of preventive medicine and the concomitant lack of incentives, including reimbursement, *inter alia*, have been cited as major impediments to the delivery of preventive services [Maron *et al.*, 1998].

15.3 Can Workplace Modifications Suggested by the Clinician for Individual Patients Help Inform Workplace Intervention Trials?

The clinician's experience with regard to the efficacy of workplace modifications for individual patients also can be invaluable in a larger context. Those changes that clearly were effective for given patients could be extended into the public health realm, informing various levels of preventive workplace interventions [Fisher & Belkić, 2000].

This topic will be further developed in our concluding chapter.

Chapter 16

Perspectives towards a Humane Work Environment: A Clinical View

One of the abiding "take-home" messages of the last chapter, and indeed, of the entire book, is that the clinician, especially the occupational neuropsychiatrist, were that subspecialty to become fully established and developed, can make a vital contribution to the improvement of job conditions for individual patients with mental health disorders. Notwithstanding this pivotal role, the clinician cannot "work in a vacuum." A wider framework is needed. This is another "take-home" message of this book, one which we began to address in the previous chapter, especially via Figure 15.1.

Recapitulating Part II, it could certainly be concluded that the occupational neuropsychiatrist, working together with the patient, identified potentially-modifiable work stressors that may impact upon the patient's mental well-being. By ameliorating at least some of these, the overall job stressor burden, as quantitatively assessed via the OSI, was lowered. An iterative, constructive process was thereby begun, associated with improvement in the patient's clinical status. Thus, the third query posed for each of the case studies, would be answered in the affirmative.

The more challenging part of the third query, however, is "how?" How to implement these modifications in practice? In all the case studies, outreach was necessary, to e.g. colleagues, management within the work organization, the human resources advisor, *inter alia*. While this point was not belabored in the case presentations, the outreach process is delicate, complex and often fraught with difficulties.

In a number of the cases, the option of disclosure was chosen. Here, in particular, besides formal legal protection against discrimination, a climate of trust is necessary before most patients will feel sufficiently comfortable to reveal this sensitive information to others at their workplace. This is particularly true for mental health disorders, as well as for epilepsy, for which, as discussed, stigma persists, especially in relation to the workplace [Fisher, Vickrey *et al.*, 2000] [Jamison 2006] [Klimek 2011] [Manning & White1995] [Sudak *et al.*, 2008].

Critical to this entire process is empowerment, that the clinician's input would carry sufficient weight to actually have an impact upon the patient's working conditions. In some settings, this is already the case, but, in most cases, the clinician does not tread upon these issues that are generally considered outside his or her domain. In Chapter 15, we alluded to this and many other barriers hindering the implementation of clinician recommendations to promote healthier working conditions. This enters into the realm of public health policy, where legislative and related measures are needed.

At the same time, there is clearly a need for evidence-based clinical guidelines. Currently, such are still at a very early stage of development, with sparse data, some of which are contradictory. For example, a so-called "exposure-based" return to work program from the Netherlands developed by occupational physicians, in which patients sick-listed for common mental disorders were gradually exposed to more demanding work situations, resulted in a significantly *prolonged* return to work, compared to those receiving usual care. The study was cluster-randomized and controlled. On the basis of their results, the authors concluded that usual care was more appropriate for these patients than was the exposure-based RTW program [Noordik *et al.*, 2012].

On the other hand, as discussed in Chapter 4, on the basis of literature review and clinical research experience, Tse [2002] proposed some work-related guidelines for patients with bipolar disorders. These involved garnering support from workmates, managers, as well as the personal social network, advising the employers on provision of support systems within the actual workplace and liaising with government agencies to reinforce the client's aspiration to work. Broadly speaking, these recommendations are concordant with the outreach we envision. In Chapter 2, we cited the intervention study carried out among Japanese blue-collar workers [Kawakami *et al.*, 1997] for its corroboration of the role of occupational stressors in the etiology of depression. In the context of our present discussion, that study can also be viewed as an example of how improved work-conditions, namely:

- enhanced machine speed/performance with decreased need for overtime work,
- fewer checkpoints requiring starting and stopping the machines to lower psychological demands,

- on-the-job training to improve skill acquisition,
- bolstered supervisor training and availability for employees' needs,

are associated with a significantly diminished risk of depression, in comparison to those employees whose working conditions remained unchanged.

Concluding thoughts and questions

The reader may note that, unlike the rest of the book, this concluding chapter is left unstructured. This was intentional. At this juncture, we decided to be somewhat open-ended, to motivate further involvement and developments in this area, without predefining all the steps along the way. This coheres with a clinical approach, especially once a body of knowledge and expertise is acquired, and the needed tools are provided. We hope that juxtaposing Part I and Part II of this book will help in that process.

Can we envision a more humane work environment? For ourselves? For our patients?

These questions obviously imply the need to define a work environment which would promote mental health. Such a definition needs to be continuously refined and upgraded, based upon the examples we observe in our clinical experience, as well as more broadly, in daily life. The book entitled *Healthy Work* [Karasek & Theorell 1990] is now a classic and one which warrants particular attention in this context.

On the other hand, several of the clinical case studies presented in Part II of this book exemplify working conditions that are very the antithesis. With the aid of the Occupational Stressor Index, it was quite straight-forward to identify these "dangerously stressful working conditions" and to evaluate the extent to which these were contributing to the patient's clinical status. As discussed, whenever such inordinately high total OSI scores are encountered, the clinician needs to be on alert for occupational sentinel health events, including and especially those impacting upon mental health.

And yet, whenever the job stressor burden is successfully lowered and the patient's mental health status concomitantly improves, might we not also consider this a sentinel health event, but of a different nature?
→This time, a positive one, one that might inform multi-level preventive intervention trials.

An evidence-based strategy of this kind could potentially help protect not only patients who have already succumbed to psychiatric disorders, but also those with early, more easily treatable manifestations.

Successful clinical experience of this kind might also serve to inform primary prevention trials, aimed at creating more humane job conditions for working populations.

Appendices

Appendix A

Diagnostic Criteria for Selected Mental, Behavioral and Somatic Disorders

This Appendix is divided into three Sections. Section 1 is based upon the International Statistical Classification of Diseases and Related Health Problems (ICD-10) Classification of Mental and Behavioral Disorders [World Health Organization, 1993]. It should be noted that the ICD-10 is compatible with the Diagnostic and Statistical Manual of Mental Disorders (DSM-IV) [Bogenschutz 2000].

Emphasis is given to diagnoses that appear in Part II for the clinical cases. We also include some background diagnoses, particularly those that are discussed in Part I in relation to epidemiology, mechanisms and return to work.

In clinical practice, the ICD criteria for mental and behavioral disorders are often not followed strictly. Rather, experienced clinicians generally tend to match the patient's symptomatology to a mental prototype. This tendency is reflected to some extent with regard to the case presentations of Part II of this book. In developing the clinical guidelines for the upcoming ICD-11, the need for increased clinical utility and consistency has been emphasized [First 2012].

Section 2 provides definitions of somatic diseases that appear in the clinical cases of Part II, as well as some of the less well-known non-psychiatric entities discussed in Part I of this book. The ICD-10 classifications are used.

Section 3 includes mental, behavioral and somatic diagnoses pertaining to the clinical cases and to Part I but that have not yet made their way into the ICD-10. These diagnoses are directly or indirectly related to stressful working conditions.

Section 1 Diagnostic Criteria for Selected Mental and Behavioral Disorders based on the ICD-10

- **F17 Mental and behavioral disorders due to the use of tobacco**

F17.2 Tobacco dependence syndrome

Criteria:

Presence of ≥ 3 of the following manifestations occurring together for ≥ 1 month, or if these persist for < 1 month, have occurred repeatedly during 1 year:

(1) A strong desire or sense of compulsion to use tobacco;

(2) Difficulties to control the use of tobacco vis-à-vis starting, stopping or amount. This can be manifested by smoking more or for a longer period than intended or by a long-lasting desire or unsuccessful attempts to decrease or control the amount of smoking;

(3) A physiological withdrawal state* when tobacco use is diminished or stopped, manifested by a characteristic tobacco withdrawal syndrome or by the use of the same or very similar substances in order to relieve or avoid the withdrawal symptoms;

(4) Manifestations of tolerance to the effects of tobacco, such that there is a need for substantially increased amounts to achieve the desired effect or that there is a notably diminished effect with continued smoking of the same number of cigarettes;

(5) Preoccupation with smoking, e.g. that major alternative interests or pleasures are given up or reduced because of smoking;

(6) Continued smoking despite the person's awareness of the nature and extent of the harmful effects of smoking.

* Tobacco withdrawal symptoms (≥ 2) must be present:

(1) Craving for tobacco or other nicotine-containing substances;

(2) Weakness or malaise;

(3) Anxiety;

(4) Dysphoria;

(5) Irritability or restlessness;

(6) Insomnia;

(7) Increased appetite;

(8) Increased cough;

(9) Ulcerations in the mouth;

(10) Trouble concentrating.

- **F22 Persistent delusional disorders**

F22.0 Delusional disorder

Criteria:

A. Delusion(s) other than those typical for schizophrenia (i.e. with delusional disorder, these are not entirely impossible nor completely culturally inappropriate). The delusions may be related to perceived persecution, hypochondriasis, jealousy or grandiosity.

B. The delusion(s) from criterion A have been present for at least 3 months.

C. The general criteria for schizophrenia are not present.

D. No persistent hallucinations in any modality, except eventually transient or occasional auditory hallucinations that are not in the 3rd person or "giving a running commentary."

E. There may be intermittent depressive symptoms insofar as the delusions persist even when there is no mood disturbance.

F. No evidence of primary or secondary organic mental disorder or psychotic disorder due to psychoactive substance use.

- **F23 Acute and transient psychotic disorders**

G1. Acute onset of delusions, hallucinations, incomprehensible or incoherent speech, alone or in combination. No more than 2 weeks have elapsed between the first appearance of symptoms and the fully developed disorder.

G2. If there is perplexity, misidentification or impaired attention, these do not fulfill the criteria for organically-caused clouding of consciousness or attention.

G3. The disorder does not fulfill the symptom criteria for manic episode (F30.-), depressive episode (F32.-) or recurrent depression (F33.-).

G4. No evidence for recent use of psychoactive substances, dependence or withdrawal states, although moderate and unchanged level of use of alcohol or drugs does not necessarily rule out a diagnosis of F23.

G5. No organic mental disorder or major metabolic disturbances that could affect the central nervous system (childbirth is not included here).

- **F30 Manic episode**

F30.0 Hypomania

<u>Criteria</u>:

A. Elevated or irritable mood to an extent that is not normal for the individual and has lasted at least four consecutive days.

B. Presence of ≥ 3 of the following, with some interference in activities of daily living:

1) Increased activity or physical restlessness;
2) Increased loquaciousness;
3) Distractibility or trouble concentrating;
4) Decreased need for sleep;
5) Increased sexual energy;

6) Mild reckless or irresponsible behavior, such as spending money;

7) Increased sociability or over-familiarity.

C. The episode does not fulfill the criteria for mania with or without psychotic symptoms, anorexia nervosa, persistent mood disorder such as cyclothymia or dysthymia.

D. The episode is not attributable to psychoactive substance abuse, or to organic mental disorder.

F30.1 Mania without psychotic symptoms

Criteria:

A. Predominantly expansive, elevated or irritable mood that is not normal for the individual. Unless so severe as to require hospitalization, the mood change should have lasted at least for one week.

B. Presence of ≥ 3 of the following, with interference in activities of daily living:

1) Increased activity or physical restlessness;
2) Increased loquaciousness/pressured speech;
3) Flight of ideas or feeling that one's thoughts are racing;
4) Inappropriate behavior due to loss of social inhibitions;
5) Decreased need for sleep;
6) Exaggerated self-esteem or grandiosity;
7) Constant change in plans or activity and/or distractibility;
8) Reckless or irresponsible behavior that is not recognized as such by the individual, these may include spending sprees, reckless driving or engaging in foolish enterprises;
9) Sexual indiscretions or marked sexual energy.

C. No delusions or hallucinations, but perceptual changes may occur such as hyperacusis or heightened sensation of the vividness of colors.

D. Episode not attributable to substance abuse or organic mental disorder.

- **F31 Bipolar affective disorder**

Episodes are demarcated by a switch to the opposite or mixed polarity or by a remission. The episodes are not attributable to psychoactive substance use or to any organic mental disorder. There has been at least one affective episode in the past.

F31.0 Bipolar disorder, current episode hypomanic

F31.1 Bipolar disorder, current episode manic without psychotic symptoms

F31.3 Bipolar disorder, current episode moderate or mild depression.

- **F32 Depressive episode**

Criteria:

G1. The depressive episode should last for at least 2 weeks.

G2. No history of manic or hypomanic symptoms sufficient to fulfill the criteria for manic or hypomanic episodes.

G3. The episode is not attributable to psychoactive substance abuse, or to organic mental disorder.

Criterion B: Presence of ≥ 2 of the following symptoms:

1) Depressed mood to an extent that is not normal for the individual, lasting most of the day, nearly every day irrespective of external conditions;
2) Loss of interest or pleasure in activities that were usually enjoyable;
3) Loss of energy and increased fatigability.

Criterion C: Additional symptom(s) giving a total*

≥ 4 : mild depression **F32.0**

≥ 6 : moderate depression **F32.1** (without psychotic symptoms)

1) Loss of confidence or self-esteem,
2) Excessive or inappropriate feelings of self-reproach or guilt,
3) Recurrent thoughts of death or suicide or any suicidal behavior,
4) Diminished ability to concentrate or think, e.g. indecisiveness, vacillation,
5) Retardation or agitation of psychomotor activity,
6) Sleep disturbance,
7) Change in appetite with corresponding weight change.

(*The total number of symptoms is counted from Criterion B + Criterion C)

- **F40 Phobic anxiety disorders**

The symptoms are not due to delusions, hallucinations, or organic mental disorders, schizophrenia or related disorders, affective disorders or obsessive-compulsive disorder and are not due to cultural beliefs.

F40.0 Agoraphobia

Criteria:

A. Marked and consistent fear or avoidance of ≥ 2 of the following:
1) Crowds,
2) Public places,
3) Traveling alone,
4) Traveling away from home.

B. ≥ 2 simultaneous manifestations of anxiety in the feared situation(s) have occurred ≥ 1 time since the onset of this disorder, including ≥ 1 symptom(s) of autonomic arousal

Autonomic arousal symptoms:
1) Palpitations, rapid heart rate,

2) Sweating,
3) Shaking or trembling,
4) Dry mouth (not due to dehydration or to medication).

Chest and abdominal symptoms:

5) Difficulty in breathing,
6) Choking feeling,
7) Chest discomfort,
8) Nausea or other abdominal distress.

Mental/CNS symptoms:

9) Dizziness, light-headedness, feeling unsteady or as if about to faint,
10) Derealization (feeling that objects are unreal) or depersonalization (feeling that one is distant from oneself or "not really here"),
11) Fear of passing out, of losing control or of "going crazy,"
12) Fear of dying.

General symptoms:

13) Hot flushes or cold chills,
14) Numbness or tingling.

C. Avoidance or the anxiety symptoms cause emotional distress and the individual recognizes that these are excessive or irrational.

D. The symptoms are mainly in relation to the actual feared situation or thinking about it.

F40.0 Agoraphobia without panic disorder

F40.1 Agoraphobia with panic disorder

• F41 Other anxiety disorders

F41.0 Panic disorder (episodic, paroxysmal anxiety)

The symptoms are not due to a physical disorder or organic mental disorder, schizophrenia or related disorders, affective disorders or somatoform disorders.

Criteria:

A. Recurrent panic attacks that are not consistently related to a specific situation or object. These attacks are frequently spontaneous and unpredictable and not related to heavy physical exertion or to exposure to dangerous situations.

B. The panic attacks:

1) Are discrete episodes of intense fear,
2) Have an abrupt onset,
3) Reach their maximum intensity within a few minutes,
4) Must include ≥ 4 of the following symptoms, with ≥ 1 of the symptoms from items (a) to (d):

Autonomic arousal symptoms:

a) Palpitations, rapid heart rate,
b) Sweating,
c) Shaking or trembling,
d) Dry mouth (not due to dehydration or to medication).

Chest and abdominal symptoms:

e) Difficulty in breathing,
f) Choking feeling,
g) Chest discomfort,
h) Nausea or other abdominal distress.

Mental/CNS symptoms:

i) Dizziness, light-headedness, feeling unsteady or as if about to faint,

j) Derealization (feeling that objects are unreal) or depersonalization, (feeling that one is distant from oneself or "not really here"),

k) Fear of passing out, of losing control or of "going crazy,"

l) Fear of dying.

General symptoms:

m) Hot flushes or cold chills,

n) Numbness or tingling.

F41.1 Generalized anxiety disorder

The symptoms are not due to a physical disorder such as hyperthyroidism, or to organic mental disorders or to use of psychoactive substance-related disorder.

Criteria:

A. At least 6 months of prominent tension, worry and apprehension about everyday problems and occurrences.

B. Must include ≥ 4 of the following symptoms, with ≥ 1 of the symptoms from items (1) to (4):

Autonomic arousal symptoms:

1) Palpitations, rapid heart rate,

2) Sweating,

3) Shaking or trembling

4) Dry mouth (not due to dehydration or to medication).

Chest and abdominal symptoms:

5) Difficulty in breathing,

6) Choking feeling,

7) Chest discomfort

8) Nausea or other abdominal distress.

Mental/CNS symptoms:

9) Dizziness, light-headedness, feeling unsteady or as if about to faint,

10) Derealization (feeling that objects are unreal) or depersonalization (feeling that one is distant from oneself or "not really here"),

11) Fear of passing out, of losing control or of "going crazy,"

12) Fear of dying.

General symptoms:

13) Hot flushes or cold chills,

14) Numbness or tingling.

Tension-related symptoms:

15) Muscle tension or aches,

15) Inability to relax, restlessness,

16) Feeling on edge, keyed up/mentally tense,

17) Difficulty swallowing or sensation of a lump in the throat.

Other non-specific symptoms:

18) Exaggerated reaction to being startled or to minor unexpected events,

19) Trouble concentrating, mind goes blank due to worry,

20) Persistent irritability,

21) Trouble going to sleep due to worry.

C. This disorder does not fulfill the criteria for panic disorder, phobic anxiety disorder, obsessive-compulsive disorder or hypochondriacal disorder.

• F43 Reaction to severe stress and adjustment disorders

F43.0 Acute stress reaction

Criteria:

A. The patient has been exposed to an exceptional mental or physical stressor.

B. Symptoms occur within 1 hour after exposure to the stressor.

C. Two groups of symptoms on the basis of which the severity of the acute stress reactions is determined:

Mild (only criterion (1)) is fulfilled **F43.00**

Moderate (criterion (1) + ≥ 2 symptoms for criterion (2)) **F43.01**

Severe (criterion (1) + ≥ 2 symptoms for criterion (2)) **F43.02**
or the presence of dissociative stupor

Criterion (1): Criteria (B) and (C) and exclusion criteria are met for generalized anxiety disorder.

Criterion (2):

a. Withdrawal from social interaction,

b. Narrowed attention,

c. Disorientation,

d. Anger or verbal aggression,

e. Hopelessness or despair,

f. Hyperactivity which is without purpose or inappropriate,

g. Uncontrollable and excessive grief (according to the cultural milieu).

D. Insofar as the stressor is of a transient nature or can be ameliorated, the symptoms must begin to subside after 8 hours. Insofar as the exposure continues, the symptoms must begin to subside after 48 hours.

E. The reaction occurs without any concurrent mental or behavioral disorder from the ICD-10 except generalized anxiety disorder or personality disorders and does not occur within 3 months of the end of an episode of another mental or behavioral disorder.

F43.1 Posttraumatic stress disorder with intrusive and avoidance symptoms

Criteria:

A. The patient has been exposed to a stressful event or situation of extremely threatening or catastrophic nature, which would be likely to cause great distress to almost anyone.

B. The stressor is relived in persistent intrusive flashbacks, recurring dreams or distress when faced with events similar or related to the stressor.

C. The patient avoids or wishes to avoid situations similar or related to the stressor. This avoidance was not present prior to exposure to the stressor.

D. Either of the following:

1) Partial or complete inability to recall importance aspects of the period of exposure to the stressor,

2) Persistent symptoms of arousal or increased psychological sensitivity not present prior to exposure to the stressor -- two or more of the following:

a) Difficulty falling asleep or staying asleep,

b) Irritability or anger outbursts,

c) Trouble concentrating,

d) Hyper-vigilance,

e) Heightened startle response.

E. Criteria B, C and D must all be met within six months of the stressor or at the end of the stressful event, unless clearly specified otherwise.

F43.2 Adjustment disorders

Criteria:

A. Symptoms must occur within 1 month of the exposure to a recognizable psychosocial stressor which is not of catastrophic dimensions nor unusual.

B. The patient develops symptoms or shows disturbed behavior such as affective disorders (but no delusions or hallucinations), neurotic, stress-related or somatoform disturbances or conduct disturbances, but the criteria for any of these individual disorders are not fulfilled.

- **F50 Eating disorders**

F50.4 Overeating associated with other psychological disturbances

No specific criteria given by the ICD-10.

- **F51 Non-organic sleep disorders**

F51.0 Non-organic insomnia

A. Complaints of difficulty falling asleep, maintaining sleep or that sleep is non-refreshing.

B. Disturbed sleep ≥ 3 times per week for ≥ 1 month.

C. The disturbed sleep distresses the patient and/or interferes with daily life function.

D. No organic cause for the sleep disturbance, e.g. no neurological or other medical condition or use of medication or other psychoactive substance.

51.2 Non-organic disorder of the sleep-wake schedule

A. The sleep-wake pattern is out of synchrony with the desired sleep-wake schedule, the latter conforming to the demands of the environment and that to which others adhere in the patient's environment.

B. Due to disturbed sleep-wake schedule, the patient experiences insomnia during the main sleep period or hypersomnia during the waking period, nearly daily for ≥ 1month or repeatedly for shorter time periods.

C. The insufficient quantity, quality and timing of sleep distresses the patient and/or interferes with daily life function.

D. No organic cause for the disturbed sleep-wake pattern, e.g. no neurological or other medical condition or use of medication or other psychoactive substance.

F51.5 Nightmares

A. The patient awakens from nocturnal sleep or from naps with detailed, clear recall of extremely frightening dreams, usually with threats to survival, security or self-esteem. Usually the patient awakens during the second half of the sleep period, but may awaken at any time during the sleep period.

B. After awakening from the nightmares, the patient quickly becomes alert and oriented.

C. The dream itself and resulting sleep disturbance distress the patient.

D. No organic cause for the nightmare, e.g. no neurological or other medical condition or use of medication or other psychoactive substance.

Section 2 Classification based on the ICD-10 of Selected Somatic Disorders

- **Malignant neoplasms stated/presumed to be primary of specified sites C00-C75**

C45.0 and C45.1 Mesothelioma of the pleura and of the peritoneum

This is seen in asbestos industries and among utilizers of asbestos -- recognized as an occupationally-related cause of unnecessary disease and untimely death, related to exposure to asbestos. Preventive measures are warranted [Mullan & Murthy, 1991].

C50 Malignant neoplasm of the breast

This includes the connective tissue of the breast but excludes the skin of the breast.

- **Episodic/paroxysmal disorders of the nervous System G40-G47**

G40.3 Generalized idiopathic epilepsy and epileptic syndromes

This classification can include non-specific tonic-clonic epileptic seizures.

G43 Migraine headaches

G43.0 Migraine headaches without aura, otherwise known as common migraine.

G43.1 Migraine headaches with aura, otherwise known as classical migraine. The auras can be of various types, including acute-onset, prolonged aura, etc.

- **Lung diseases due to external agents J60-J70**

J60 Coal worker's pneumoconiosis

Seen among coal miners -- recognized as an occupationally-related cause of unnecessary disease and untimely death, related to exposure to coal dust. Preventive measures are warranted [Mullan & Murthy 1991].

J61 Pneumoconiosis due to asbestos and other mineral fibers -- Asbestosis

Seen in asbestos industries and among utilizers of asbestos -- recognized as an occupationally-related cause of unnecessary disease and untimely death, related to exposure to asbestos. Preventive measures are warranted [Mullan & Murthy 1991].

J66.0 Airway disease due to specific organic dust: cotton dust – Byssinosis

Seen in cotton industry workers -- recognized as an occupationally-related cause of unnecessary disease, disability and untimely death, related to exposure to cotton, flax, hemp and cotton-synthetic dusts. Preventive measures are warranted [Mullan & Murthy 1991].

Section 3 Description of Selected Mental, Behavioral and Somatic Disorders not yet included in the ICD-10

1 Burnout

According to Maslach and colleagues [2001], there are three dimensions to burnout, with exhaustion being the most central. The second dimension is cynicism: a distant attitude towards one's job, which reflects the person's attempt both cognitively and emotionally to distance him- or herself from work. This is considered to be a way to handle or cope with the work overload.

Lack of efficacy at work, with a diminished sense of personal accomplishment is the third dimension of burnout described by Maslach and colleagues [2001]. The Maslach Burnout Inventory [Maslach *et al.*, 1996] is widely used as a burnout assessment tool.

A drawback of the Maslach Burnout Inventory is that the queries concerning exhaustion and cynicism are phrased negatively, while items concerning professional efficacy are couched in positive terms. This may create a bias related to social desirability.

The Oldenburg Burnout Inventory (OLBI) is an alternative approach for evaluating burnout. In contrast to the Maslach Burnout Inventory, the OLBI includes positively and negatively framed queries that assess two core dimensions of burnout: exhaustion and disengagement from work.

The OLBI provides an assessment not only the affective aspects of exhaustion, but also of the physical and cognitive facets [Demerouti *et al.*, 2003]. We have used the OLBI among physicians in the clinical as well as the research setting. In our experience, the OLBI has very good face validity among our colleagues [Fridner *et al.*, 2012].

2 Shift work disorder

This refers to shift workers who experience insomnia and/or excessive sleepiness due to misalignment of the sleep-wake schedule. This disorder is usually diagnosed by history alone.

In order to make the diagnosis, these symptoms should last for at least one month and are not due to another sleep disorder, medications, or other medical/neurological disorder. The sleep-time misalignment can be demonstrated by a sleep log or activographic monitoring for at least one week [Rosenberg & Godhramji 2011] [Roth 2012].

3 *Karoshi*

Karoshi is defined as sudden death from ischemic heart disease or cerebrovascular disease due to overwork. This has been particularly attributed to long work hours and other heavy job demands [Shimomitsu & Levi, 1992].

Japan was the first country to identify *karoshi* and brought it to the attention of the world. With the 1996 revision of the Japanese Industrial Safety and Health Law, occupational physicians were empowered to act as direct advisors to employers regarding working conditions, with the aim of preventing *karoshi* and other occupational illnesses [Shimomitsu & Odagiri, 2000].

4 Masked Hypertension

Elevated awake ambulatory blood pressure but with normal clinic blood pressure has been labeled “masked,” “occult” or “hidden” hypertension. Masked hypertension is associated with increased cardiovascular risk. At least 10% and as many as 30% of adults with normal clinic blood pressure are reported to have masked hypertension [Pickering *et al.*, 2006].

Ambulatory blood pressure during waking hours (work and home) is more strongly associated with subsequent cardiovascular disease than the traditional measurement of casual clinic blood pressure. It is hypothesized that exposure to workplace stressors first elevates work blood pressure, but not clinic blood pressure. After chronic exposure to stressors, both daytime blood pressure as well as clinic blood pressure become elevated [Pickering *et al.*, 2006] [Belkić, Schnall, Landsbergis *et al.*, 2001][Landsbergis, Schnall, Belkić *et al.*, 2008].

The need to systematically apply ambulatory blood pressure monitoring among persons working in stressful occupations as a screening method has been underscored [Pickering *et al.*, 2006] [Belkić, Schnall, Landsbergis *et al.*, 2001][Landsbergis, Schnall, Belkić *et al.*, 2008][Nedić *et al.*, 2010][Uglješić, Belkić, Bošković *et al.*, 1992]. This would facilitate detection of masked hypertension before it progresses to fixed hypertension, with appropriate preventive measures instituted. Clusters of occult workplace hypertension within certain workplaces could be considered as a potential indicator of an occupational sentinel health event [Belkić, Schnall, Uglješić 2000] [Belkić, Schnall, Landsbergis *et al.*, 2001] [Mullan & Murthy 1991].

Appendix B

Completed Physician-Specific OSI Questionnaire and Score Sheet

A. Length and Location of Work

A.1 Current position: Ward physician specialist in neuropsychiatry

A.2 Years worked at your current position at the present site: 10 years

A.3 Type of employment:
a) Full time position
b) Part time position
c) Temporary capacity
d) Other capacity.

A.4 Total number of working years as a physician: 21 years

A.5 Total number of working years: 21 years

A.6 Work in other occupations besides as a physician? Yes No

Please answer the following questions for your working conditions in the past year for your main job as a physician, unless otherwise specified.

B. Type of Practice and Setting

B.1 Are you a specialist? Yes No

If yes, what is your specialty? Neuropsychiatry.

B.2 What is the setting of your practice?
a) Solo Private Practice/Consultant
b) Group Private Practice
c) Health maintenance organization (HMO)/private clinic or hospital
d) Public
e) Physician in training (intern)
f) Physician in specialty training (resident).

B.3 Percentage of inpatient work:
a) Less than 10%
b) Less than 50%, but at least 10%
c) 50% or more.

B.4 Percentage of patients with end-stage/incurable disease:
a) Less than 10%
b) Between 10 and 20%
c) Over 20% but less than 50%
d) 50% or more.

B.5 Percentage of emergency cases:
a) Less than 10%
b) Less than 50%, but at least 10%
c) 50% or more.

B.6 Number different institutions at which you work (including as a consultant)?
a) Only one
b) Two
c) Three or more.

C. Work Hours and Scheduling

C.1 How long is your ordinary workday? 8 hours

Do you ever work longer than that? Yes No

If yes, how many days per month (usually)? 8 to 10 days.

For how many hours per day? 1 to 2 hours, or if on-call 7 hours.

C.2. How many days do you usually work per week? 5-6 days, depending on when I am on-call.

C.3 Do you have a regular work schedule? Yes No

If yes, when do you usually begin work? 8:00 End work? 17:00.

C.4 Are you called at home during your free time regarding the clinical care of patients?

a) Never
b) Rarely
c) Occasionally
d) Frequently.

C.5 How many weeks of paid vacation per year? 6 weeks.

C.6 Do you work at another job outside your regular one? Yes No

If yes, what do you do?

Do you work at the other job throughout the year? Yes No

If yes:

How many hours per week do you work at the other job?

Do you work at the other job for extended periods? Yes No

If yes:

How many hours altogether do you work during extended periods?

C.7 Do you have the opportunity to take breaks during your workday?
a) Never
b) Rarely
c) Occasionally
d) Frequently.

C.8 If you do have some breaks, are these usually?
a) Short ones, mainly less than 15 minutes
b) Long breaks, mainly at least 30 minutes
c) Both short and long breaks.

C.9 If you have some breaks, are these true rest breaks so that you can completely be free from work obligations? Yes No

If no, why not:
There are always interruptions and there is no guaranteed relief.

C.10 How long do you typically work, without being able to take at least a short, 5 to 10 minute break? 3 to 4 hours.

C.11 Do you take night call? Yes No

If yes, do you work past midnight (late night shift)? Yes No

If yes, do you work the late night shift?
a) Constantly.
b) On a rotating basis.

If b, how many nightshifts do you usually work? 3 to 4 per month.

If you have night call, please answer the next 4 night shift related questions (C.12-C.15):

C.12 How much do you usually sleep during night call?
a) I usually get at least 4 to 5 hours per night.
b) Mainly between 2 and 4 hours, the rest of the time I'm busy.
c) At the most I get 2 hours of sleep; I'm busy most of the night.
d) Only a couple of hours; even if it's not busy, I am too agitated to sleep.

C.13 Are you obliged to be physically at the hospital during night call:
a) Yes
b) No, I am on pager, and only occasionally must come in.

C.14 What kind of free time adjacent to night call do you have? Please check all that apply
a) I come in for the night shift, having been free that day.
b) After the night shift, I go home in the morning.
c) I go on call after having worked that day, and must work at least part (if not all) of the next day.

If you answered (c):

C.15 Do you have guaranteed relief at a specified time after being on call?
a) Yes, I can go home and be certain that the patients under my responsibility are cared for by colleagues.
b) No, it can happen that I must stay on to be sure my patients are stable before I go home.

C.16 How difficult is it for you to take time off from work?
a) Not at all
b) A little
c) Somewhat
d) Very much.

C.17 How much say do you have about your work schedule?
a) Complete, it is entirely up to me.
b) To a large extent, I mainly decide on my work schedule.
c) A little, but mainly my schedule depends on others or is decided by others.
d) None, my schedule depends on or is decided by others. I have no say about it, whatsoever.

C.18 Do you perform work for your job at home?
a) Never
b) Rarely
c) Sometimes
d) Frequently.

If c or d, did you include that time in calculating your work hours for Questions B1and B2 above? Yes No

D. Salary, Possibilities for Advancement and Recognition

D.1 Upon what is your salary based?
a) Upon my own work: number of patients, interventions, hours worked.
b) Upon group work: number of patients, interventions, hours worked.
c) Fixed pay, irrespective of the amount of work.

D.2 My salary:
a) Covers substantially more than my basic needs and those of my family.
b) Covers a bit more than my basic needs and those of my family.
c) Just barely covers my basic needs and those of my family.
d) My salary is totally inadequate to meet my basic needs and those of my family.

D.3 Are there possibilities for you to upgrade your job title/advance your career? Yes No
Comment: The possibilities are limited.

If yes, do you receive support and encouragement to do so?
a) Definitely yes.
b) Yes, to some extent.
c) Not really, but there is no active opposition to such efforts.
d) No, there is active opposition to such efforts.

D.4 Is good work recognized at your workplace?
a) Definitely yes
b) Yes, to some extent
c) Not very much
d) Not at all.
Comment: The main focus at our department is on poor patient outcomes and errors by the physicians and nurses, not on good work.

E. Working Conditions and Exposures

E.1 Are you exposed to strong lights that create glare for you at work?
a) Never
b) Rarely
c) Occasionally, in the Operating Room or elsewhere
d) Frequently, in the Operating Room or elsewhere.

E.2 Do you encounter visually disturbing scenes, e.g. severe burns, trauma, grotesque dermatological pathology, at work?
a) Never
b) Rarely
c) Occasionally
d) Frequently.
Comment: Attempted and completed suicide, violence-related trauma.

E.3 Do you listen to accounts of emotionally disturbing occurrences?
a) Never
b) Rarely
c) Occasionally
d) Frequently.
Comment: Extremely frequently!

E.4 Do you perform heavy lifting during work?
a) Yes, I regularly must lift patients.
b) I do other heavy lifting, but not lifting patients.
c) No, I rarely do any heavy lifting during my workday.

E.5 Are you exposed to vibration during work?
a) Yes, I use vibrating hand tools (hours/week).
b) No, only very rarely or not at all.

E.6 Concerning heat exposure during work?
a) It rarely or never gets hotter than 25° C at work.
b) It rarely or never gets hotter than 30° C (86° F) at work.
c) It occasionally or often gets hotter than 30° C.

E.7 Concerning cold exposure during work?
a) It does not get colder than 20° C at work.
b) It rarely gets colder than 18° C (64° F) at work.
c) The heating system is poor, with temperatures <18° C.
Comment: Actually, this is extremely rare, but it does happen that the temperatures are below 20° C.

E.8 Are you exposed to gases, mists or dusts at work?
a) No, only very rarely or not at all.
b) Yes, at least occasionally.

E.9 Are you exposed to radiation during work? Yes No

If yes, do you wear a radiation badge? Yes No

E.10 Acute hazards at work: (please check all which are applicable)
a) Threat of violence from psychotic or otherwise dangerous patients.
b) Possible infection /close exposure to blood or other body fluids.
c) Work with flammable materials.
d) Other risk(s):
e) There are no special acute hazards where I work.

E.11 Workspace:
a) I have my own office.
b) I share an office with 1 colleague.

What is the approximate size of your office? 14 M^2
Does your workspace/office seem cramped/crowded to you? Yes No
Comment: Somewhat cramped.
If you share an office:
Do you have your own desk? Yes No

Must you sometimes look for an empty office in which to interview or examine patients? Yes No

What percent of your working day do you spend in your office? ~ 30 %.

E.12 Are there windows in the office in which you work?
a) Yes at my immediate workspace; I can look outside from where I work.
b) Yes, but not next to me, I can't look outside from where I am working.
c) No, I work in a windowless office.

E. 13 How is the ventilation in the area in which you work?
a) Adequate
b) Inadequate.

E.14 Is it drafty in the area in which you work? Yes No

F. Mishaps in Relation to Work

Please answer questions F1 through F6 for your entire work experience as a physician.

F.1 Have you suffered physical harm or injury at work? Yes No
If yes, was this a serious injury? Yes No

What happened?
These were actually minor injuries, from assaults by psychotic patients.

F.2 Have your colleagues/staff suffered physical harm or injury at work?
a) Yes, I witnessed such, with a fatal outcome.
b) Yes, I witnessed such, with a serious, but not fatal outcome.
c) I've heard about serious or fatal injury, but never witnessed it.
d) No, I have never witnessed or heard about serious injury at my work.

If a, b or c, please describe:
Fractures, head trauma from assaults by psychotic patients.

F.3 Has a patient under your care ever committed suicide?
a) Yes, this has happened on several occasions.
b) Yes, I have had one or two such patients.
c) No, but it has happened to colleague(s) with whom I work.
d) No, it has never happened to me or to colleague(s) with whom I work.
Comment:
Most recently, this could have been prevented if colleagues heeded my advice.

F. 4. Have you ever testified in court as a physician? Yes No

If yes, please mark all the following which apply:
a) I have testified as an expert witness about a patient.
b) I have been obliged to testify regarding a colleague or staff member.
c) I have been obliged to testify as a defendant in a malpractice case.
d) Other, please specify:

If yes:
F.5 Were the proceedings made public via the mass media? Yes No

F.6 Has an official complaint ever been made about your work? Yes No

Once again, please answer for your working conditions in the past year for your main job as a physician.

F.7 Is there a system in place at work for non-medical emergencies?
a) Yes, and I know that it functions properly.
b) Yes, but I do not know how well it actually functions.
c) No, there is no functioning system for non-medical emergencies.

G. Time Pressure

G.1 Are there deadlines by which a given job or task must be completed?
a) Never
b) Rarely
c) Occasionally
d) Frequently.

G.2 Are you obliged to speed-up your work tempo?
a) No, it happens only rarely or never.
b) Yes, during certain periods of the month or year.
c) Yes, at least weekly, but not daily.
d) Yes, every day.

G.3 With regard to your workload and time restrictions/constraints:
a) It is always possible to complete everything.
b) It is usually possible to complete everything.
c) Sometimes it is objectively impossible to complete everything, even with maximal effort.
d) Often it is objectively impossible to complete everything, even with maximal effort.

H. Problems, Restrictions/Constraints and Influence at Work

Please indicate the degree of influence do you have over:

	Major	Some	A Little	None
H.1 The number of patients under your care/ outpatient scheduling			x	
H.2 Which clinical tasks or procedures you perform			x	
H.3 Whether and how much you will take on other, non-clinical duties			x	
H.4 Which colleagues and staff you work with			x	
H.5 Planning and policy of your institution, including those regarding indications for medical procedures and for hospital admissions.			x	

H.6 Is your work overseen by others? Yes No

If yes, please check all which apply:
a) By more senior physicians,
b) By non-physician personnel e.g. administrators, nurses,
c) By physicians of your level or lower.

If yes,
H.7 Is your clinical judgment questioned?
a) Often
b) Sometimes
c) Rarely or never.

Please indicate the degree of strictness of rules and regulations regarding:

	Very strict	Somewhat strict	Flexible
H.8 Hospital admissions		x	
H.9 Patient scheduling		x	

H.10 Are there problems that directly hinder your providing adequate patient care?
a) Never
b) Rarely
c) Occasionally
d) Frequently.

If c or d, please check all problems which contribute to this hindrance:

a) Lack of needed supplies (including medications)
b) Lack of hospital beds
c) Understaffing
d) Administrative constraints to ordering needed supplies
e) Language barriers with patients (lack of translators)
f) Infra-structural problems (lack of elevators, power failures etc.)
g) Need for frequent patient transport under tenuous conditions
h) Delay or inability to obtain medical records
i) Difficulty in obtaining laboratory results
j) Limitations in ordering tests
k) Limitations on sending patients for consult
l) Other problems.

H.11 Do interruptions from other people (including work-related phone calls) prevent you from proceeding with your work?
a) Never
b) Rarely
c) Occasionally
d) Frequently
Comment:
This often occurs at critical moments!

I. Interpersonal Interactions and Social Climate

I.1 Can you get help for difficult cases and/or clinical dilemmas?
a) Yes, I can almost always count on such help.
b) Yes, more often than not.
c) I can't count on getting such help.
d) Rarely or never do I get the help I need.

I.2 In general, how is the social climate at your workplace?
a) Excellent, we get along very well; misunderstandings are very rare.
b) Good, most the time we get along well, with few misunderstandings and tensions.
c) Fair, we have our ups-and-downs; there are misunderstandings and tensions.
d) Poor, there is a great deal of tension and conflict.

I.3 When obliged to display knowledge and/or skills in front of colleagues and/or supervisors (e.g. during rounds, journal club, other presentations):
a) The atmosphere is constructive and conducive to growth and learning.
b) There is some tension. Oversights and/or lack of knowledge will be noticed and commented upon. If these are of major importance, there may be adverse consequences for me.
c) These occasions are highly unpleasant. Event the slightest oversight or lack of knowledge inevitably becomes a point of ridicule and/or chastisement.

I.4 Are there abuses of power or violations of norms of behavior at work?
a) Never
b) Rarely
c) Occasionally
d) Frequently.

If yes, please describe:
→Career blocking, demeaning comments from some colleagues and from persons in supervisory positions.
→Clinical assessment and recommendations are often ignored.
→There is also manipulation of scheduling procedures.

I.5 Can work-related grievances be taken to a responsible body for resolution?
a) Yes, this can be done in an efficient and confidential manner.
b) In principle, yes, but this is not effective and/or cannot be done confidentially.
c) No, there is no possibility to redress grievances at work.

J. Workload and Activities

Please indicate how often you handle patients who are:

	Frequently	Occasionally	Rarely/ Never
J.1 Severely disturbed	x		
J.2 Cannot provide a history	x		

J.3 How many inpatients are usually under your direct care at one time?
a) None
b) One to five
c) <u>Six to ten</u>
d) Eleven to twenty
e) Over twenty.

J.4 How many of these are in intensive care (including CCU)?
a) None
b) One to two
c) <u>Three to five</u>
d) Six to ten
e) Over ten.

J.5 How many outpatients do you usually see during one work shift?
a) None
b) One to ten
c) <u>Eleven to twenty</u>
d) Twenty-one to thirty
e) Thirty-one to forty
f) Over forty.

If you answered b-f, how many of these are new patients?
<u>One to two new outpatients per work shift</u>.

J.6 How many patients do you admit to the hospital during a shift?
a) None
b) <u>One to five</u>
c) Six to ten
d) Eleven to twenty
e) Over twenty.

If you admit patients to the hospital (b-e):

J.7 Are you obliged to care for these newly-admitted patients, or do you transfer them to other colleagues?
a) I must care for all the patients whom I admit during a given shift.
b) I must care for some of the patients whom I admit during a given shift.
c) The patients whom I admit are nearly always transferred fairly rapidly to other colleagues.

J.8 Does it happen during your workday that several people seek your attention at the same time? (Including people on the telephone)
a) Yes, many times each day.
b) Yes, a few times each day.
c) Yes, but only once or twice each day.
d) No, rarely or never.

J.9 If people simultaneously seek your attention, how many do so?
a) Rarely more than two.
b) Usually two, but sometimes more.
c) Usually three or more.

J.10 Does it occur that during your work hours, you must be physically at work, but there is nothing to do?
a) Never
b) Rarely
c) Occasionally
d) Frequently
Comment:
This is due to waiting time, especially during night call after midnight because of delays before an announced patient arrives. Since I am awakened by the call and am expecting the patient any minute, I cannot sleep or even relax.

J.11 Do you oversee or supervise the work of:
Check all which apply
a) Physicians at your level of training or higher
b) Physicians with less training than yourself
c) Medical students
d) Other health professionals
e) Others.

J.12 Number of persons other than yourself, for whose work you must take responsibility: I take partial responsibility for the work of 1-2 younger colleagues.

J.13 Besides clinical work, other major work activities include:
Please check all which apply:
a) Teaching in small groups (students and residents)
b) Lecturing to larger groups
c) Research
d) Administrative duties
e) Other:

J.14. If you have other major work activities, is there special time set aside for these? Yes No

If no, please check all that apply:
a) I perform these duties simultaneously with my clinical work.
b) I work after normal work hours to complete these activities.

J.15. Are you under pressure to publish/present new findings or results at Congresses/meetings outside your Institution?
a) Yes, if I fail to do so in sufficient quantity, my career will suffer and I may even lose my position
b) Yes, but there are no major adverse consequences if I fail to do so.
c) No, such activity is entirely up to my own initiative and choice.

Which of the following do you perform on a regular basis?
J.16 Non-invasive diagnostic procedures: Yes No EEG

J.17 Invasive procedures: Yes No
Lumbar puncture, occasionally

J.18 Surgical interventions: Yes No

J.19 Tasks outside the realm of a physician: Yes No
Administrative

J.20 Are there work tasks that you are obliged to perform that you consider pointless? Yes No
Completing redundant forms.

J.21 Do you use a computer as part of your clinical work? Yes No

If yes, please check all of the uses you have for the computer

a) To obtain data (lab, medical records, etc.) about my patients.

b) For patient write-ups, e.g. discharge summaries.

c) For help in triaging to other departments and other institutions.

d) For statistical analyses that would be for clinical purposes.

e) For electronic communication with colleagues (consults).

f) For electronic communication with patients.

g) For searching the medical literature to elucidate a clinical question.

h) Other:

In which of the above circumstances is the computer most helpful?
Searching the literature.

In which of the above circumstances is the computer more of a burden?
When it gets stuck!

K. Recent Changes at Work

Please answer the following questions for the last 6 months

	Yes	No
K.1 Has there been an increase in the length of your workday?	x	
K.2 Has there been increased time pressure/number of deadlines?	x	
K.3) Have you had an increase in work responsibility?	x	
K.4 Have you been promoted?		x
K.5 Have you been demoted (lowered position)		x
K.6 Has your pay been cut?		x
K.7 Is there a threat that you will be laid off?		x

L. Other Questions about Your Workplace:

	Yes	No
L.1 Is there a trade union at your workplace?	x	
L.2 Is there an explicit policy at your workplace to provide equal opportunity to those who have been underrepresented in medicine? If yes:		x
Is this policy explicitly addressed to women?		
Is this policy explicitly addressed to ethnic minorities?		
Is this policy explicitly addressed to other underrepresented groups?		
L.3 Is there a pension-plan available at your workplace?	x	
L.4 Is any health-care program provided by your workplace?	x	

M. Open-ended Questions about Your Current Work

M.1 What is the best part(s) about your present work?

- Satisfaction when patient care yields a good outcome.

M.2 What is the hardest part of being a physician of your profile?

- Exhausting night call
- Low pay
- Few possibilities for advanced training
- Patient suicides, especially when I know this could be prevented.

M.3 What do you think could be done to make that difficulty less of a burden?

- Better distribution of patient care responsibility.

M.4 What do you think could be done to improve work as a physician of your profile?

a. Immediate, very feasible:

- Have two physicians on-call together
- Increased pay.

b. More long-range changes requiring organizational modifications:

- Advanced training in other major medical centers.
- Better organization
- Improved medical facilities.

c. What would be the most important immediate change to improve work as a physician of your profile?

- Diminish night-call duty.

M.5 If attempts were made to improve the conditions for your job, what would you suggest to preserve the good aspects of your work as it now stands?

- Keep the regular clinical and organizational meetings.

Score Sheet: OSI for Physicians

OSI Aspect #1 – Underload

IU1: Homogeneous information
• **0** = Fixed feature for MD's: Heterogeneous information.

IU2: Low flow of new information
• **0** = Fixed feature for MD's: Either high flow of information or flow is under the physician's control.

IU3: No need for communication
• **0** = Fixed feature for MD's: Works with others.

Input Underload Total: IU1 + IU2 + IU3 = 0

CUT: Automatic decision-making
• **0** = Fixed feature for MD's: Decisions not automatic.

Central Underload Total: CUT= 0

OU1: Homogeneous tasks
• **0** = Fixed feature for MD's: Tasks are heterogeneous.

OU2: Simple tasks
• **0** = Fixed feature for MD's: Tasks are not simple.

OU3: Nothing to do
0 J.10 = a Always something to do.
0.5 J.10 = b Rarely nothing to do.
• **1** J.10 = c <u>Occasionally nothing to do</u> <u>Waiting for patients: night call</u>.
2 J.10 = d Frequently nothing to do.

Output Underload Total: OU1 + OU2 + OU3 = 1.0

GU1: Fixed pay
0 D.1 = a or b Paid by individual or group work.
• **2** D.1 = c <u>Fixed pay</u>.

GU2: Inadequate pay
0 D.2 = a Pay covers substantially more than basic needs.
0.5 D.2 = b Pay covers a bit more than basic needs.
1 D.2 = c Pay just barely covers expenses.
• **2** D.2 = d Pay is totally inadequate.

GU3: Lack of promotion prospects
0 D.3 = Yes, there are possibilities for job upgrade, no active opposition.
• **1** D.3 = Yes + d: There are upgrade possibilities, but active opposition.
2 D.3 = No promotion prospects.

GU4: Lack of recognition of good work
0 D.4 = a Good work definitely recognized.
0.5 D.4 = b Good work recognized to some extent.
• **1.5** D.4 = c Not very much recognition of good work.
2 D.4 = d Good work not recognized at all.

General Underload Total: GU1+ GU2 + GU3 + GU4 = 6.5

7.5 = Total Underload Score

OSI Aspect # 2 – High Demand

IH1: Three or more information sources simultaneously
• **1.75** Range = 1 → 2 Based on ER work: B.5 and number of people seeking attention: J.8–J.9.

IH2: Heterogeneous information
• **1.75** Range = 1.5 → 2 Based on tasks: J.13, J.16 – J. 19
Teaching, administration, research plus clinical duties, including diagnostic procedures (EEG, lumbar puncture).

IH3: Heavy burden on visual system
• **0.5** B.1 = Primary care, psychiatrist, non-invasive cardiologist
1 B.1 = Surgeon, radiologist, pathologist, dermatologist or performs many procedures: J.16–J.18.

IH4: More than five new signals per minute
• **1.5** Range = 1 → 2 Based on burden: ER work: B.5, workload: J.3–J.6, J.11–J.13 and on control over workload: H.1–H.3.

IH5: Three sensory modalities simultaneously
0 B.1 = Pathologist, radiologist.
• **1** B.1 = Clinician, not surgeon or anesthesiologist and few invasive procedures: J.17 – J.18.
2 B.1 = Surgeon, anesthesiologist or invasive procedures: J.17 – J.18.

IH6: Communication necessary for work
1 B.1 = Pathologist, radiologist.
• **2** B.1 = Physician involved in patient care.

Input High Demand Total: IH1 + IH2 + IH3 + IH4 + IH5 + IH6 = 8.5

CH1: Complex decisions/interrelated elements
• **2** = Fixed feature for MD's: Decisions are complex.

CH2: Complicated decisions/many elements
• **2** = Fixed feature for MD's: Decisions are complicated.

CH3: Decisions affect the work of others
1 J.11–J.12 = No explicit supervision, but some implicit.
• **1.5** J.11–J.12 = Supervises 1 to 2 others, at least partially.
2 J.11–J.12 = Supervises 3 or more others.

CH4: Rapid decisions
1.5 B.3, B.5, J.4 = Mainly outpatient work.
• **2** B.3, B.5, J.4 = Substantial ER and/or inpatient and/or ICU work.

Central High Demand Total: CH1 + CH2 + CH3 + CH4 = 7.5

OH1: Heterogeneous tasks
• **1.75** Range= 1→ 2 Based on tasks: J.13, J.16–J.19.

OH2: Simultaneous task performance
0 B.5=a and J.4=a and J.8=c or d
1 B.5=b or J.4=b or J.8=b
• **2** B.5=c or J.4=c-e or J.8=a
Based on ER work, ICU patients, simultaneous attention sought, add 0.5 if J.7=a or b, cares for patients newly-admitted on work shift.

OH3: Complex tasks

- **1.5** Range = 1 → 2 Based on profile B.1 and tasks: J.13, J.16 – J.19.

OH4: Rapid task execution

- **1.25** Range = 0.5 → 2 Based on ER, ICU, invasive procedures: B.5, J.4, J.17–J.18

Output High Demand Total: OHI + OH2 + OH3 + OH4 = 6.5

GH1: Piece rate

- **0** D.1 = c Fixed pay.
  1 D.1 = b Pay based on the group's work.
  2 D.1 = a Pay based on individual work.

GH2: Long work hours

0 Works not more than 40 hours per week.
0.5 Works 40 to 42 hours per week.
1 Frequently > 42 hours /week or occasionally >48hours/week.
- **2** Frequently > 48 hours/week or occasionally > 60hours/week.

  Calculate from C.1–C.3, add 0.5 points if called at home C.4 = c, d or works at home C.18 = c, d and hours not included, to 2 maximum.

GH3: Two or more jobs

- **0** C.6 = Works at one job only.
  2 C.6 = Works at two or more jobs.

GH4: Lack of rest breaks

0 C.7 = d Frequently has rest breaks.
1 C.7 = c Occasionally has rest breaks.
1.5 C.7 = b Rarely has rest breaks.
2 C.7 = a Never has rest breaks.

- **2** Add 0.5 points if only short breaks C.8 = a, if breaks interrupted C.9 = no, or if over 2 hours without a break C.10, to maximum 2 points.

GH5: Night shift work

0 C.3 = Regular work schedule and C.11 = no night shift work.
0.5 C.3 = Irregular work schedule and C.11 = no night shift work.
1 C.11 = Yes + a: night shift only.

1.5 C.11 = Yes + b Rotating night shift, up to four night shifts/month.
1.75 C.11 = Yes + b Rotating night shift ≥ once/week, not > q 4th night.
2 C.11 = Yes + b Rotating night shift ≥ every third night.

- **2** Add 0.5 points if < 24 free time after working a rotating night shift C.14, or if irregular schedule C.3 = no, or no guaranteed relief C.15 = b, to maximum 2 points.

GH6: Insufficient paid vacation

- **0** C.5 = Over four weeks paid vacation.

1 C.5 = Three to four weeks paid vacation.
1.5 C.5 = Two weeks paid vacation.
2 C.5 = Less than two weeks of paid vacation.

General High Demand Total: GHI + GH2 + GH3 + GH4 +GH5 +GH6 = 6

28.5 = Total High Demand Score

OSI Aspect # 3 – Strictness Aspect

IST: Strict requirements for signal detection

Range = 1.5→ 2, based on B.1, B.5, J.4, J.17–18.

1.5 Minimal ER work, no ICU patients, no invasive procedures.

- **1.75** Not a surgeon or anesthesiologist, some ER or ICU patients and a few or no invasive procedures.

2 Surgeon or anesthesiologist, ≥ 50% ER work and/or many invasive procedures.

Input Strictness Total: IST = 1.75

CS1: Strict problem solving strategy

- **0.5** Range = 0→ 1 Based on H.5 and H.8–H.9, maximum 1 if very strict rules and regulations.

CS2: Strictly defined correct decision

- **1.25** Range= 1→ 1.5, based on H.5 – H.9, maximum 1.5 if very strict rules and regulations and/or overseen, with judgment often questioned.

Central Strictness Total: CS1 + CS2 = 1.75

OST: Strict evaluation of performance

- **1.5** Range = 1 → 2, based on H.6 and I.3, maximum 2, if overseen and slightest oversight noted.

Output Strictness Total: OST = 1.5

GS1: Fixed Posture

0.5 B.1, E.11, J.5, J.16–19: Fairly mobile, very little work time in office.

- **1** B.1, E.11, J.5, J.16–19: Mainly single posture, but free to move, substantial outpatient work in office.

1.5 B.1, E.11, J.16–19 Lots of procedures, anesthesiologists.

2 B.1, E.11, J.16–19 Surgeons performing long operations.

GS2: Confined, windowless, poorly ventilated work area

0 Works in >1 location, E.11 part IV: minimal time in office.

0.5 Over 50% of time in non-confined work area, with a direct window E12 = a, and E11 indicates non-confined work area.

1 Spends over 50% of time in a non-confined work area, with an indirect window E12 = b and non-confined work area E11.

- **1.5** Windowless office, shared with 1 colleague E11, E12 = c; or confined/crowded space, shares office with two or more colleagues, has an indirect window E11, E12 = b.

2 Windowless office, confined/crowded space, shares office with two or more colleagues, E11, E12 = c.

Add 0.5 points to 2 maximum, if inadequate ventilation E13 = no.

GS3: Lack of autonomous workspace

0 E.11 Has own desk/workspace and has own office.

1 E.11 Has own desk or workspace but shares an office.

2 E.11 No autonomous workspace.

Add 1 point to 2 maximum, if must seek free office space to talk with

- **2** or examine patients.

GS4: Limited chance to take time off from work

0 C.16 = a No problem to take time off.

1 C.16 = b A little difficult to take time off.

1.5 C.16 = c Somewhat difficult to take time off.

- **2** C.16 = d Very difficult to take time off.

GS5: Limited influence over work schedule

0 C.17 = a Complete influence.

0.5 C.17 = b Major influence.

• **1** C.17 = c A little influence.

2 C.17 = d No influence.

GS6: Limited influence over deciding with whom he or she works

0 B.1 = Pathologist or radiologist and H.4 = major influence.

1 B.1 = Patient care, H.1, H.4 = major influence, H9 = flexible.

1.5 B.1 = Patient care, H.1, H.4 = some influence, H9 = rather strict.

• **2** B.1 = Patient care profile, H.1, H.4 = little influence H9 = very strict. If combined answers, choose worst profile

GS7: Limited influence over what work tasks will be

1 H2 clinical and H3 non-clinical tasks: major influence.

1.25 H2 clinical and H3 non-clinical tasks: some influence.

1.5 H2 clinical and H3 non-clinical tasks: a little influence.

2 H2 clinical and H3 non-clinical tasks: no influence.

• **2** If pressure to publish, present findings at congresses, J.15 = a or b, add 0.5 points, to maximum 2.

GS8: Limited influence over policy

0 H.5 = Major influence.

0.5 H.5 = Some influence.

• **1.5** H.5 = A little influence.

2 H.5 = No influence.

General Strictness Total:GS1+GS2+GS3+GS4+GS5+GS6+GS7+GS8=13

18 = Total Strictness Score

OSI Aspect # 4 – Extrinsic Time Pressure

IEPT: Control of incoming signals

• **2** Range = 1→ 2 Based on profile B.1, control of number of patients under his/her care and of outpatient scheduling, H.1, H.9
Direct patient care, little control of number of patients under care and of outpatient scheduling.

Input Extrinsic Time Pressure Total: IEPT= 2

CEPT: Decisions cannot be postponed

1 B.1, B.3, B.5, J.4 = Mainly outpatient or non-clinical work, minimal emergency work and no ICU patients.

• **1.5** B.5, J.4 = 10 – 50% emergency patients, some ICU patients.

2 B.5, J.4 = Mainly emergency patients or many ICU patients.

Central Extrinsic Time Pressure Total: CEPT = 1.5

OEPT: Control of task performance rate

1 H.1 – H.3 = Major control over # patients, clinical tasks, other duties.

1.5 H.1 – H.3 = Some control over # patients, clinical tasks, other duties.

• **2** H.1 – H.3 = Little or no control over number of patients, clinical tasks, other duties.

Output Extrinsic Time Pressure Total: OEPT = 2

GEP1: Deadline pressure

0 G1 = a Never faces deadline pressure.

0.5 G1 = b Rarely faces deadline pressure.

1 G1 = c Occasionally faces deadline pressure.

• **2** G1 = d Frequently faces deadline pressure.

GEP2: Speedup

0 G2 = a Rarely or never must speed up work tempo.

1 G2 = b Speed up at certain periods of the month or year.

1.5 G2 = c At least weekly speed up, but not daily.

• **2** G2 = d Daily must speed up work tempo.

Add 0.5 points to 2 maximum, if B.5=c, if mainly emergency work.

General Extrinsic Time Pressure Total: GEP1 + GEP2 = 4

9.5 = Total Extrinsic Time Pressure Score

OSI Aspect # 5: Aversiveness/ noxious exposures

INOX1: Glare

• **0** E1 = a Never exposed to glare.

0.5 E1 = b Rarely exposed to glare.

1 E1 = c Occasionally exposed to glare.

2 E1 = d Frequently exposed to glare.

INOX2: Noise
• **0.25** Range = 0 → 0.5 Maximum if working primarily in the ER, B.5.

Input Noxious Exposure Total: INOX1 + INOX2 = 0.25

ONOX1: Isometric lifting
• **0** E.4 = c No lifting.
1 E.4 = b Lifts less than 50 kg.
2 E.4 = a or b Lifts patients or otherwise over 50 kg regularly.

ONOX2: Vibration exposure
• **0** E.5 = b No vibration exposure.
0.5 E.5 = a Uses vibrating hand tools up to 5 hours per week.
1 E.5 = a Uses vibrating hand tools over 5 hours per week.

Output Noxious Exposure Total: ONOX1 + ONOX2 = 0

GNOX1: Heat exposure
0 E.6 = a Temperatures do not exceed 25° C.
• **0. 5** E.6 = b Temperatures can exceed 25° C, up to 30° C.
1 E.6 = c Temperatures can 30° to 40° C°.
Add 0.5 points, if E.13 = b inadequate ventilation.

GNOX2: Cold exposure
0 E7 = a Temperatures always at least 20° C.
0.5 E7 = b Temperatures always at least 18° C.
1 E7 = c Temperatures can be between 10° and 18° C.
• **0.25** Temperatures usually, but not always at least 20° C.
Add 0.5 points, if E.14 = yes, drafty.

GNOX3: Exposure to fumes, gases and/or dusts
• **0** E.8 = a No exposure to fumes, gases or dusts.
1 E.8 = b Occasional exposure to fumes, gases or dusts.

General Noxious Exposure Total: GNOX1 + GNOX2 + GNOX3 = 0.75

1.0 = Total Noxious Exposure Score

OSI Aspect # 6: Threat Avoidance/ Symbolic Aversiveness/ Disaster Potential

IAVOI1: Need for sustained alertness to avoid serious consequences
1 B.1 = Pathologist or other area without patient contact.
1.5 B.3, B.5 = a Mainly non-emergency, outpatient work.
• **2** B.3, B.5 = b or c Substantial emergency and/or inpatient work.

IAVOI2: Visually disturbing scenes
0 E.2 = a Never.
0.5 E.2 = b Rarely.
• **1** E.2 = c Occasionally: Completed or attempted suicide, trauma.
2 E.2 = d Frequently.

IAVOI3: Listen to accounts of emotionally disturbing occurrences
0 E3 = a Never.
0.5 E3 = b Rarely.
1 E3 = c Occasionally.
• **2** E3 = d Frequently.
Add 1 point if B4 = c, d Large % patients with end-stage or incurable disease, 0.5 points if B4 = b, add 1 point if F.3 = a, b patient suicide, add 0.5 if F.3 = c, heard about patient suicide, to maximum 2 points.

Input Symbolic Aversiveness Total = IAVOI1 + IAVOI2 + IAVOI3 = 5

CAVOIT: Serious consequences of wrong decisions
• **2** Fixed feature for MD's: Potential injury or fatality from error.

Central Symbolic Aversiveness Total: CAVOIT = 2

OAVOIT: Hazardous task performance
1 E.10 = e No acute hazards reported.
• **2** E.10 = a – d Acute hazards present: Infection, threat of violence.
Add 1 point to maximum 2, for radiation exposure, E.9.

Output Symbolic Aversiveness Total : OAVOIT = 2

GAVOI1: Experienced physical harm/injury at work
0 F.1 = No.
• **1** F.1 = Yes, but not serious physical harm.
2 F.1 = Yes, if serious physical harm.

GAVOI2: Witnessed physical harm or injury at work
0 F.2 = d Never heard about or witnessed a serious accident at work.
0.5 F.2 = c Heard about but never witnessed a serious accident at work.
• **1** F.2 = b Witnessed serious accident at work.
2 F.2 = a Witnessed fatal accident at work.

GAVOI3: Patient suicide
0 F.3 = d Not to respondent nor to colleagues with whom he/she works.
1 F.3 = c Has happened to colleagues, but not to respondent.
1.5 F.3 = b One or two of respondent's patients have committed suicide.
• **2** F.3 = a Several of respondent's patients have committed suicide.

GAVOI4: Litigation/testifying in court/official complaints about work
0 F.4 = No
1 F.4 = Yes, a As expert witness, only.
• **1.5** F.4 = Yes, b Testified about a colleague or staff member or official complaint to workplace, F.6.
2 F.4 = Yes, c Defendant in a malpractice case.
Add 0.5 points if proceedings made public F.5, to maximum 2 points.

GAVOI5: Lack of functioning emergency system
0 F.7 = a Yes and knows that it functions properly.
1 F.7 = b Yes, but does not know whether it functions properly.
• **2** F.7 = c No functioning system for non-medical emergencies.

General Symbolic Aversiveness Total =
GAVOI1 + GAVOI2 + GAVOI3 + GAVOI4+ GAVOI5 = 7.5

16.5 = Total Symbolic Aversiveness Score

OSI Aspect # 7: Conflict/Uncertainty

ICNFL1: Signal/noise conflict
• **2** Fixed feature for MD's: Frequent signal/noise conflict.

ICNFL2: Signal/signal conflict
• **2** Fixed feature for MD's: Frequent signal/signal conflict.

Input Conflict Total: ICNFL1 + ICNFL2 = 4

CCNFL1: Missing information needed for decision-making
- **2** H.10 = e, h, i Language barriers, delayed medical records, difficulty in getting lab, J.1, J.2 frequently disturbed patient or can't get history.

1.5 Otherwise.

CCNFL2: Contradictory information
- **2** Fixed feature for MD's: Contradictory information.

CCNFL3: Unforeseeable events require new plan
- **2** B.5 = c >50% ER work or J.4 = c-e, 3 or more ICU patients.

1.5 B.5 = b 10-50% ER or J.4 = b, one or two ICU patients.

1 Otherwise, minimum for MD's.

Central Conflict Total: CCNFL1 + CCNFL2 + CCNFL3 = 6

OCNFL1: Conflicting demands in time and space

0 G.3 = a It is always possible to complete everything.

0.5 G.3 = b It is usually possible to complete everything.

1 G.3 = c Occasionally objectively impossible to complete everything.

2 G.3 = d Frequently impossible to complete everything.

Add 0.5 points each: J.14 = no special time set aside for non-clinical tasks, J.7 = a, b cares for newly admitted patients during shift to a
- **2** maximum of 2 points.

OCNFL2: External conditions hamper task performance

0 H.10 = a Never.

0.5 H.10 = b Rarely.

1 H.10 = c Occasionally.
- **2** H.10 = d Frequently.

OCNFL3: Interruptions from people hamper task performance

0 H.11 = a Never.

0.5 H.11 = b Rarely.

1 H.11 = c Occasionally.
- **2** H.11 = d Frequently.

Output Conflict Total: OCNFL1 + OCNFL2 + OCNFL3 = 6

GCNFL1: Emotionally-charged work atmosphere
0 I.2 = a Colleagues and staff get along well.
0.5 I.2 = b Minimal tension among colleagues and staff.
1 I.2 = c Some tension among colleagues and staff.
2 I.2 = d Great deal of tension and conflict among colleagues and staff.
• **1.5** Add 0.5 points if I.3 = b some tension with display of knowledge; add 1 point if I.3 = c high tension with display of knowledge, to maximum of 2 points.

GCNFL2: Help with difficulties
0 I.1 = a Can count on help.
0.5 I.1 = b Usually can count on help.
• **1.5** I.1 = c Can't count on help.
2 I.1 = d Rarely or never gets help which is needed.

GCNFL3: Opposition to career advancement
0 D.3 = Yes + a or b: Support for advancement, or no possibilities.
1 D.3 = Yes and c: No support, but no active opposition.
• **2** D.3 = Yes and d: Active opposition to career advancement.

GCNFL4: Violations of behavior norms/abuses of power
0 I.4 = a Never.
0.5 I.4 = b Rarely.
1.5 I.4 = c Occasionally.
• **2** I.4 = d Frequently.

GCNFL5: Lack of redress of grievances
0 I.5 = a Redress can be done and is efficient and confidential.
• **1** I.5 = b Redress in principle, but not effective or not confidential.
2 I.5 = c No possibility to redress grievances.

GCNFL6: Threat of job loss
• **0** A.3 = a, b K.7 = no Stable position, no threat of job loss.
1 A3 = c K.7 = no Temporary work, but no threat of job loss.
2 K.7 = Yes Threat of job loss present.
If K.7 = no and A.3 = d, evaluate whether this is temporary versus stable employment.
Add 0.5 points to a maximum of 2 points if J.15 = a: Could lose position if fails to publish or present results at conferences.

GCNFL7: Job lacks coherence

0 J.20 = No performance of pointless tasks.

• **1** J.20 = Performs pointless tasks Redundant administration.

General Conflict Total = GCNFL1 + GCNFL2 + GCNFL3 + GCNFL4 + GCNFL5 + GCNFL6 + GCNFL7 = 9

25 = Total Conflict Score

$$\sum_{\text{Aspect } k=1}^{k=7} = \textbf{Total OSI Score} = \textbf{106}$$

Bibliography

Aasland, O.G., Ekeberg, O. and Schweder, T. (2001). Suicide rates from 1960 to 1989 in Norwegian physicians compared with other educational groups, Soc. Sci. Med., 52, pp. 259–265.

Aboa-Éboulé, C., Brisson, C., Maunsell, E., Masse, B., Bourbonnais, R., Vezina, M., Milot, A., Theroux, P. and Dagenais, G. (2007). Job strain and risk of acute recurrent coronary heart disease events. JAMA, 298, pp. 1652–1660.

Adami, H-O., Hunter, D., and Trichopoulos, D. (2002). *Textbook of Cancer Epidemiology* (Oxford University Press, Oxford).

Adams, S., Roxe, D., Weiss, J., Zhang, F. and Rosenthal, J. (1998). Ambulatory blood pressure and Holter monitoring of emergency physicians before, during, and after a night shift, Acad. Emergency Med. 5, pp. 871– 877.

Aftanas, L.I. and Golocheikine, S.A. (2001). Human anterior and frontal midline theta and lower alpha reflect emotionally positive state and internal attention: high-resolution EEG investigation of meditation, Neurosci. Lett., 310, pp. 57 – 60.

Ahlberg-Hulten, G.K., Theorell, T., and Sigala, F. (1995). Social support, job strain and musculoskeletal pain among female health care personnel, Scand. J. Work Environ. Health, 21, pp. 435–439.

Ahola, K., Virtanen, M., Honkonen, T., Isometsä, E., Aromaa, A. and Lönnqvist J. (2011). Common mental disorders and subsequent work disability: A population-based Health 2000 Study, J. Affect. Disord., 134, pp. 365–372.

Akben, S., Subasi, A. and Tuncel, D. (2011). Analysis of EEG signals under flash stimulation for migraine and epileptic patients, J. Med. Syst. 35, pp. 437 – 443.

Åkerstedt, T. (1990). Psychological and psychophysiological effects of shift work, Scand. J. Work. Environ. Health, 16 (suppl 1), pp. 67–73.

Åkerstedt, T. (2003). Shift work and disturbed sleep/wakefulness, Occup. Med., 53, pp. 89–94.

Åkerstedt, T., Peters, T., Anund, A. and Kecklund, G. (2005). Impaired alertness and performance while driving home from the night shift—a driving simulator study, J. Sleep Res., 14, pp. 17–20.

Åkerstedt, T., Kecklund, G. and Gillberg, M. (2007). Sleep and sleepiness in relation to stress and displaced work hours, Physiol. Behav., 92, pp. 250–255.

Alfredsson, L., Hammar, N., and Hogstedt, C. (1993). Incidence of myocardial infarction and mortality from specific causes among bus drivers in Sweden, Int. J. Epidemiol., 22, pp. 57–61.

Alm, H. and Nilsson, L. (1995). The effects of a mobile telephone task on driver behaviour in a car following situation, Accid. Anal. Prev., 27, pp. 707–715.

Ambrosini, A., Magis, D. and Schoenen, J. (2010). Migraine - clinical neurophysiology, Handb. Clin. Neurol. 97, pp. 275–293.

Aminoff M.J. (1998). *Harrison's Principles of Internal Medicine,* 14th Ed., eds. Fauci, A., Martin, J., Braunwald, E., Kasper, D., Isselbacher, K., Hauser, D., Wilson, J.,

Longo, D. and Jameson J., Chapter 361 "Electrophysiologic studies of the central and peripheral nervous systems," (McGraw-Hill, New York) pp. 2282 – 2287.

Andersen, K. Hawgood, J., Klieve, H., Kõlves, K. and De Leo, D. (2010). Suicide in selected occupations in Queensland: evidence from the State suicide register, Aust. New Zeal. J. Psychiatry, 44, pp. 243–249.

Andersen, M.F., Nielsen, K.M. and Brinkmann, S. (2012). Meta-synthesis of qualitative research on return to work among employees with common mental disorders, Scand. J. Work Environ. Health, 38, pp. 93 – 104.

Andersson, R. and Menckel, E. (1995). On the prevention of accidents and injuries: A comparative analysis of conceptual frameworks, Accid. Anal. Prev., 27, pp. 757–768.

Andre, C., Lelord, F., Legeron, P., Reignier, A., and Delattre, A. (1997). Controlled study of outcome after 6 months to early intervention of bus driver victims of aggression, Encephale, 23, pp. 65–71.

Angelakis, E., Lubar, J.F., Stathopoulou, S. and Kounios, J. (2004). Peak alpha frequency: an electroencephalographic measure of cognitive preparedness, Clin. Neurophysiol., 115, pp. 887–897.

Antonovsky, A. (1991). *Health, Stress and Coping*, (Jossey Bass, San Francisco).

Araki, S. and Murata, K. (1993). Determination of evoked potentials in occupational and environmental medicine: A review, Environ. Res. 63, pp. 133–147.

Araki, T., Kasai, K., Yamasue, H., Kato, N., Kudo, N., Ohtani, T., Nakagome, K., Kirihara, K., Yamada, H., Abe, O., and Iwanami, A. (2005). Association between lower P300 amplitude and smaller anterior cingulated volume in patients with posttraumatic stress disorder: a study of victims of Tokyo subway sarin attack, Neuroimage, 25, pp. 43–50.

Arigoni, F., Bovier, P.A. and Sappino, A.P. (2010). Trend of burnout among Swiss doctors, Swiss Med. Wkly., 140:w13070.

Aronoff, G.M., Erdil, M. and Hartenbaum, N.P. (2005). *A Physician's Guide to Return to Work* eds. Talmage, J.B, Melhorn, J.M. and Hyman, M., Chapter 10 "Medications, driving and work.," (American Medical Association Press, Chicago) pp. 133–162.

Ashton, C., Golding, J., Marsh, V., Thompson, J., Hassanyeh, F. and Tyrer, S. (1988) Cortical evoked potentials and clinical rating scales as measures of depressive illness, Psychol. Med., 18, pp. 305–317.

Ashton, C., Marshall, E., Hassanyeh, F. and Marsh, V. (1994). Biological correlates of deliberate self-harm behavior: a study of electroencephalographic, biochemical and psychological variables in parasuicide, Acta Psychiatr. Scand., 90, pp. 316–323.

Astbury, C., and Southgate, J.L, (2007). *Fitness for Work: The Medical Aspects* 4th Ed., eds. Palmer, K.T., Cox, R.A.F., and Brown, I., Chapter 14 "Gastrointestinal and liver disorders," (Oxford University Press, Oxford) pp. 311–344.

Bachneff, S.A., and Engelsmann, F., (1980). Contingent negative variation, postimperative negative variation and psychopathology, Biol. Psychiatry, 15, pp. 323–328.

Backman, A.L. (1983). Health survey of professional drivers, Scand. J. Work Environ. Health, 9, pp. 30–35.

Badawy, R.A.B. and Jackson, G.D. (2012). Cortical excitability in migraine and epilepsy: A common feature? J. Clin. Neurophysiol. 29, pp. 244–249.

Bakker, A.B., Killmer, C.H., Siegrist, J., and Schaufeli, W.B. (2000). Effort-reward imbalance and burnout among nurses, J. Adv. Nursing, 31, pp. 884–891.

Balch, C.M. and Shanafelt, T. (2010). Combating stress and burnout in surgical practice: A review, Adv. Surg., 44, pp. 29–47.

Baldwin, D.S., and Rudge, S.E., (1995). *Health Risks To The Health Care Professional.* ed. Litchfield P. Chapter, "Depression and suicide in doctors and medical students," (Royal College of Physicians of London, London) pp.77–89.

Balmes, J.R., Speizer, F.E. (2011). *Harrison's Principles of Internal Medicine* 18th Ed., eds. Longo D.L., Fauci A., Kasper D., Hauser S., Jameson J., Joseph Loscalzo J.. Chapter 256 "Environmental lung disease," (McGraw Hill, New York) electronic version.

Bara, A-C. and Arber, S. (2009). Working shifts and mental health—findings from the British Hoursehold Panel Survey (1995-2005), Scand. J. Work Environ. Health, 35, pp. 361–367.

Barrett, K., McCallum, W.C. and Pocock, P.V. (1986). Brain indicators of altered attention and information processing in schizophrenics, Br. J. Psychiatry, 148, pp. 414– 420.

Bartley, M. (1994). Unemployment and ill-health: understanding the relationships, J. Epidemiol. Community Health, 48, pp. 333–337.

Basar, E., Schurmann, M. and Sakowitz, O. (2001). The selectively distributed theta system: functions, Int. J. Psychophysiol., 39, pp. 197–212.

Basini, S.G., and Hurley, J.J. (1994). Hierarchy and the meaning of working, Eur. Work. Organizational Psychology, 4, pp. 51–64.

Becker, D.R., Bebout, R.R. and Drake, R.E. (1998). Job preferences of people with severe mental illness: A replication, Psychiatric Rehabil. J., 22, pp. 46–50.

Becker, D.R., Drake, R.E. and Concord, N.H. (1994). Individual placement and support: a community mental health centre approach to rehabilitation, Community Ment. Health J., 30, pp. 193– 206.

Begleiter, H., Porjesz, B., Chou, C.L., and Aunon, J.I. (1983). P3 and stimulus incentive value, Psychophysiology, 20, pp. 95– 101.

Belkić, Dž. and Belkić, K. (2002a). A paradigm change in the spectral analysis of time signals for cardiovascular regulation, *3rd Int. Conf. Work Environment & Cardiovascular Diseases—ICOH.*

Belkić, Dž. and Belkić, K. (2010). *Signal Processing in Magnetic Resonance Spectroscopy with Biomedical Applications* (Taylor & Francis Group, London).

Belkić, K. (1984). Methodology for detecting individuals at high risk for developing the acquired cardiovascular disorders, Master's Thesis, University of Belgrade Center for Multidisciplinary Studies, 138 p.

Belkić, K. (1986). Light stress and the cardiovascular system: The glare pressor test, Ergonomics, 29, pp. 563–568.

Belkić, K. (1989). Neural Mechanisms and Risk of Sudden Cardiac Death – An Epidemiologic Approach, PhD Thesis, University of Belgrade Center for Multidisciplinary Studies, 276 p.

Belkić, K. (1995a). Unpublished field observations and semi-structured interviews among commercial pilots.

Belkić, K. (1995b). Psychosocial factors and myocardial ischemia among women. (Report to the Swedish Medical Research Council, Stockholm).

Belkić, K. (2003). *The Occupational Stress Index: An Approach Derived from Cognitive Ergonomics and Brain Research for Clinical Practice* (Cambridge International Science Publishing, Cambridge).

Belkić, K. (2009). Physicians' working conditions and health: Insights and strategies informed by the Occupational Stressor Index (Seminar to the Department of Oncology, Karolinska University Hospital, Stockholm).

Belkić, K. (2011). *A Physician's Guide to Return to Work,* eds. Talmage, J.B, Melhorn, J.M. and Hyman, M., Chapter 24 "Return-to-Work in Scandinavia: Experience and Insights with a Focus on Sweden," (American Medical Association Press, Chicago) pp. 465–472.

Belkić, K. and Belkić, Dž. (2002b). Spectral Analysis of interacting time signals for cardiovascular regulation: clinical relevance. *Conf. Computational & Mathematical Methods in Science & Engineering*, pp. 372–374.

Belkić, K., Belkić, Dž. and Savić, C. (2002). Dynamics of working life and heart rate variability: Potential applications of an econeurocardiologic model among physicians as a heavily burdened occupational group, *3rd Int. Conf. Work Environment & Cardiovascular Diseases—ICOH.*

Belkić, K., Emdad, R., Theorell, T., Cizinsky, S., Wennberg, A., Hagman, M., Johansson, L., Savić, C. and Olsson, K., (1996). *Neurocardiac Mechanisms of Heart Disease Risk among Professional Drivers* (Swedish Working Life Council, Stockholm).

Belkic, K., Emdad, R., and Theorell, T. (1998). Occupational profile and cardiac risk: possible mechanisms and implications for professional drivers, Int. J. Occup. Med. Environ. Health, 11, pp. 37–57.

Belkić, K., Ercegovac, D., Savić, C., Panić, B., Djordjević, M. and Savić, S. (1992). EEG arousal and cardiovascular reactivity in professional drivers: The glare pressor test, Eur. Heart J. 13, pp. 304 – 309.

Belkić, K., Jelić, V., Djordjević, M., Micković, Lj. and Uglješić, M. (1991). Rhythm disturbances in apparently healthy professional drivers, Kardiologija, 12, pp. 167–170.

Belkić, K., Landsbergis, P., Schnall, P., Baker, D., Theorell, T., Siegrist, J., Peter, R., and Karasek, R., (2000). Psychosocial factors: review of the empirical data among men. Occup. Med. State of the Art Reviews, 15, pp. 24–49.

Belkić, K., Landsbergis, P., Schnall, P. and Baker, D. (2004). Is job strain a major source of cardiovascular disease risk? Scand. J. Work Environ. Health, 30, pp. 85–128.

Belkić, K., Micković, Lj., Milić, B. and Savić, S. (1987). Blood pressure and electrocardiographic changes elicited by he glare pressor test, Arch. Environ. Health, 42, pp. 37–43.

Belkić, K. and Nedić, O. (2007). Workplace stressors and lifestyle-related cancer risk factors among female physicians: Assessment using the Occupational Stress Index, J. Occup. Health, 49, pp. 61–71.

Belkić, K. and Nedić, O. (2012). Night work, total occupational burden and cancer/cardiovascular risk factors in physicians Med. Pregl., 65, pp.461–469.

Belkić, K., Pavlović, S., Djordjević, M, Uglješić, M. and Micković, Lj. (1992). Determinants of cardiac risk in professional drivers, Kardiologija, 13, pp. 145–149.

Belkić, K., Peruničić, J., Bošković, D. and Djordjević, M. (1992). Preliminary results of standard, behavioral and occupational risk factors in patients forty years old or younger suffering from acute myocardial infarction, *Yug. Cong. Cardiology*.

Belkić, K. and Savić, Č. (2000). Dehumanization versus humanization of work: Insights from cognitive ergonomics and brain research, Occup. Med. State of the Art Reviews, 15, pp. 87– 94.

Belkić, K. and Savić, Č. (2008). The occupational stress index: An approach derived from cognitive ergonomics applicable to clinical practice, Scand. J. Work. Environ. Health, Suppl 6, pp. 169 –175.

Belkić, K., Savić, Č., Djordjević, M., Uglješić, M. and Micković, Lj., (1992). Event-related potentials in professional city drivers: heightened sensitivity to cognitively relevant visual signals, Physiol. Behav. 52, pp. 423– 427.

Belkić, K., Savić, C., Micković, Lj. and Uglješić, M. (1992). Behavioral measures for prevention of cardiovascular disease in professional drivers, Rev. Rada, 22, pp. 22–27.

Belkić, K., Savić, Č., Theorell, T., Rakić, Lj., Ercegovac, D., and Djordjević, M. (1994). Mechanisms of cardiac risk among professional drivers, Scand. J. Work. Environ. Health, 20, pp. 73–86.

Belkić, K., Savić, C., Theorell, T., and Cizinsky, S. (1995). *Work Stressors and Cardiovascular Risk: Assessment for Clinical Practice. Stress Research Reports. Report Number: 256.* (National Institute for Psychosocial Factors and Health. Section for Stress Research, Karolinska Institute, WHO Psychosocial Center; Stockholm).

Belkić, K. and Schnall, P. (2000) On a San Francisco public transport line: burden and consequences upon the human operator. The Job Stress Network Website: Center For Social Epidemiology (www.workhealth.org).

Belkić, K., Schnall, P., Landsbergis, P. and Baker, D. (2000). The workplace and cardiovascular health: Conclusions and thoughts for a future agenda, Occup. Med. State of the Art Reviews, 15, pp. 307–321.

Belkić, K. Schnall, P., Landsbergis, P., Schwartz, J., Gerber, L., Baker, D. and Pickering, T.G. (2001). Hypertension at the Workplace—An occult disease? The need for work site surveillance, Adv. Psychosom. Med., 22, pp. 116–138.

Belkić K, Schnall P, Baker D, Uglješić M. (2002). How do we move from epidemiological evidence to prevention-oriented clinical practice? The Need for Occupational Cardiology, *3rd Int. Conf. Work Environment & Cardiovascular Diseases—ICOH.*

Belkić, K. Schnall, P., Savić, C. and Landsbergis, P. (2000). Multiple exposures: Towards a model of total occupational burden, Occup. Med. State of the Art Reviews, 15, pp. 94–105.

Belkić, K., Schnall, P. and Uglješić, M. (2000). Cardiovascular evaluation of the worker and workplace: A practical guide for clinicians, Occup. Med. State of the Art Reviews, 15, pp. 213 – 222.

Belkić, K., Schwartz, J., Schnall, P., Pickering, T.G., Steptoe, A., Marmot, M., Theorell, T., Fossum, E., Høieggen, A., Moan, A., Rostrup, M. and Kjeldsen S.E. (2000). Evidence for mediating econeurocardiologic mechanisms. Occup. Med. State of the Art Reviews, 15, pp. 117–162.

Bender, A. and Farvolden, P. (2008). Depression and the workplace: a progress report. Curr. Psychiatry Rep., 10, pp. 73–79.

Berg, A.T. and Shinnar, S. (1991). The risk of seizure recurrence following a first unprovoked seizure: a quantitative review. Neurology, 41, pp. 965–972.

Besken, E., Pothmann, R. and Sartory, G. (1993). Contingent negative variation in childhood migraine, Cephalgia, 13, pp. 42 –43.

Bigert, C., Gustavsson, P., Hallqvist, J., Hogstedt, C., Lewne, M., Plato, N., Reuterwall, C. and Scheele, P. (2002). Myocardial infarction among professional drivers—A population-based case-referent study. *3rd Int. Conf. Work Environment & Cardiovascular Diseases—ICOH.*

Bigert, C., Gustavsson, P., Hallqvist, J., Hogstedt, C., Lewne, M., Plato, N., Reuterwall, C., and Scheele, P. (2003). Myocardial infarction among professional drivers, Epidemiology, 14, pp. 333–339

Böcker, K.B., Timsit-Berthier, M., Schoenen, J. and Brunia, C.H. (1990). Contingent negative variation in migraine, Headache, 30, pp. 604–609.

Bocquillon, P., Dujardin, K., Betrouni, N., Phalempin, V., Houdayer, E., Bourriez, J-L., Derambure, P. and Szurhaj, W. (2009). Attention impairment in temporal lobe epilepsy: a neurophysiological approach via analysis of the P300 wave, Hum. Brain Mapp., 30, pp. 2267–2277.

Bogenschutz M.P. and Nurnberg, H.G. (2000). *Kaplan & Sadock's Comprehensive Textbook of Psychiatry* 7th Ed., eds. Sadock, B.J. and Sadock, V.A. Chapter 9 "Classification of Mental Disorders," (Lippincott Williams & Wilkins, Philadelphia), pp.824–839.

Bøggild, H., and Knutsson, A. (1999). Shift work, risk factors and cardiovascular disease, Scand. J. Work. Environ. Health, 25, pp. 85–99.

Bohle, P., Quinlan, M., and Mayhew, C. (2001). The health and safety effects of job insecurity: An evaluation of the evidence, Econ. Labour Relat. Rev., 12, pp. 32–60.

Boissel, J-P and Haugh, M.C. (1993) The iceberg phenomenon and publication bias: the Editors' fault? Clin. Trials. Met. Anal., 28, pp. 309–315.

Boksem, M.A.S., Meijman, T.F. and Lorist M.M. (2005). Effects of mental fatigue on attention: An ERP study, Cognit. Brain Res., 25, pp. 107 – 116.

Bond, N.W. (1979). Conditioned suppression, heart rate and pulse volume: effects of instructions on extinction, Physiol. Behav. 23, pp. 838 – 843.

Bonde, J., Hansen, J., Kolstad, H., Mikkelsen, S., Olsen, J., Blask, D., Härmä, M., Kjuus, H., de Koning, H., Olsen, J., Møller, M., Schernhammer, E., Stevens, R. and Åkerstedt T. (2012). Work at night and breast cancer – report on evidence-based options for preventive actions, Scand. J. Work Environ. Health, 38, pp. 380–390.

Bourbonnais, R., Comeau, M., Vezina, M., and Dion, G. (1998). Job strain, psychological distress, and burnout in nurses, Am. J. Industrial Med., 34, pp. 20–28.

Boxer, P.A., and Wild, M.S. (1993). Psychological distress and alcohol use among fire fighters. Scand. J. Work Environ. Health, 19, pp. 121–125.

Boxer, P.A., Burnett, C., and Swanson, N. (1995). Suicide and occupation: A review of the literature, JOEM, 37, pp. 442–452.

Boyce, P. (1974). Sinus arrhythmias as a measure of mental load, Ergonomics, 17, pp. 177–183.

Braby, C.D., Harris, D. and Muir, H.C. (1993). A psychophysiological approach to the assessment of work underload, Ergonomics, 36, pp. 1035–1042.

Braunwald, E., Fauci, A., Kasper, D., Hauser, S., Longo, D. and Jameson, J. (2002). *Harrison's Principles of Internal Medicine* 15th Ed. (McGraw-Hill, New York).

Brisson, C. (2000).Women, work and CVD, Occup. Med. State of the Art Reviews, 15, pp. 49–57.

Brooker, A-S. and Eakin, J.M. (2001). Gender, class, work-related stress and health: Toward a power-centred approach, J. Community Appl. Soc. Psychol., 11, pp. 97–109.

Brown, D.E., James, G.D., Nordloh, L., and Jones, A.A. (2003). Job strain and physiological stress responses in nurses and nurse's aides: predictors of daily blood pressure variability, Blood Press. Monit., 8, pp. 237–242.

Brown, G.W. and Moran, P.M. (1997) Single mothers, poverty and depression, Psychol. Med., 27, pp. 21–23, 1997.

Brown, I. and Prevett, M.C. (2007). *Fitness for Work: The Medical Aspects* 4th Ed., eds. Palmer, K.T., Cox, R.A.F., and Brown, I., Chapter 8 "Epilepsy," (Oxford University Press, Oxford) pp. 169–188.

Brown, I.D. (1994). Driver fatigue, Human Factors, 36, pp. 298– 314.

Bruder, G.E. (1992). P300 findings for depressive and anxiety disorders, Ann. N.Y. Acad. Sci., 658, pp. 205–222.

Brunet, A., Boyer, R., Brillon, P., Ehrensaft, E, and Stephenson, R. (1998). Lifetime exposure to traumatic events among a sample of city bus drivers, Psychol. Rep., 83, pp. 1155–1160.

Bryant, B., Mastrodomenico, M., Kim, L., Felmingham, K., Hopwood, S., Kenny, L., Kandris, E., Cahill, C. and Creamer, M. (2008). Treatment of acute stress disorder: A randomized controlled trial, Arch. Gen. Psychiatry, 65, pp. 659–667.

Buckley, T.C., Blanchard, E.B. and Neill, W.T. (2000). Information processing and PTSD: a review of the empirical literature, Clin. Psychol. Rev., 20, pp. 1041–1065.

Campbell, J., Prochaszka, A.V., Yamashita, T. and Gopal, R. (2010). Predictors of persistent burnout in internal medical residents: A prospective cohort study, Acad. Med. 85, pp. 1630–1634.

Cannon, W.B. (1914). The emergency function of the adrenal medulla in pain and the major emotions, Am. J. Physiol., 33, pp. 356–372.

Caples, S.M., Gami, A.S. and Somers, V.K. (2005). Obstructive sleep apnea, Ann. Intern. Med., 142, pp. 187–197.

Carayon, P., Smith, M.J., and Haims, M.C., (1999). Work organization, job stress, and work-related musculoskeletal disorders, Human Factors, 41, pp. 644–663.

Carlton, O.H. and Cook, C.C.H. (2007). *Fitness for Work: The Medical Aspects* 4th Ed., eds. Palmer, K.T., Cox, R.A.F., and Brown, I., Chapter 24 "Alcohol and drug misuse," (Oxford University Press, Oxford) pp. 527–545.

Carpenter, L.M., Swerdlow, A.J., Fear, N.T. (1997). Mortality of doctors in different specialties: findings from a cohort of 20 000 NHS hospital consultants, Occup. Environ. Med. 54, pp. 388–395.

Carter, J.T., (2007). *Fitness for Work: The Medical Aspects* 4th Ed., eds. Palmer, K.T., Cox, R.A.F., and Brown, I., Chapter 18 "Seafarer fitness," (Oxford University Press, Oxford) pp. 629–632.

Carter, J.T., Major, H.G., Erlam, A.R., Janvrin, S.B., (2007). *Fitness for Work: The Medical Aspects* 4th Ed., eds. Palmer, K.T., Cox, R.A.F., and Brown, I., Chapter 28 " Health and transport safety: fitness to drive," (Oxford University Press, Oxford) pp. 605–612.

Cartwright, S., Cooper, C.L. and Murphy, L.R. (1995) *Job Stress Interventions* eds. In: Murphy, L.R., Hurrell, J.J., Sauter, S.L. Puryear Keita, G. Chapter 15 "Diagnosing a Health Organization: A proactive approach to stress at the workplace," (American Psychological Association, Washington, D.C., 1995) pp. 217–233.

Cavallo, A., Ris, M.D. and Succop, P. (2003). The night float paradigm to decrease sleep deprivation: good solution or a new problem? Ergonomics, 46, pp. 653 – 663.

Center, C., Davis, M., Detre, T., Ford, D.E., Hansbrough, W., Hendin, H., Laszlo, J., Litts, D.A., Mann, J., Mansky, P.A., Michels, R., Miles, S.H., Proujansky, R., Reynolds, C.F. 3rd and Silverman, M.M. (2003). Confronting depression and suicide in physicians: a consensus statement. J. Am Med. Assoc., 289, pp. 3161–3166.

Centor, R., Morrow, R., Poses, R. and Vega, C. (2012). Doc burnout—worse than other workers. Nov 13, 2012, www.medscape.com.

Chalernvanichakorn, T., Sithisarankul, P., and Hiransuthikul, N. (2008). Shift work and type 2 diabetic patients' health, J. Med. Assoc. Thai., 91, pp. 1093–1096.

Chambers, R., and Belcher, J. (1994). Predicting mental health problems in general practitioners. Occup. Med., 44, pp. 212–216.

Charney, D.S., Deutch, A., Southwick, S.M. and Krystal, J.H. (1995). *Neurobiological and Clinical Consequences of Stress: From Normal Adaptation to Post-Traumatic Stress Disorder* eds. Friedman, M.J., Charney, D.S. and Deutch, A. Chapter 15, "Neural circuits and mechanisms of post-traumatic stress disorder," (Lippincott-Raven Publishers, Philadelphia) pp. 271–287.

Chattopadahyay, P, Cocce, E., Toone, B. and Lader, M. (1980). Habituation of physiological responses in anxiety, Biol. Psychiatry, 15, pp. 711–721.

Chen, W., Shen, X., Liu, X., Luo, B., Liu, Y., Yu, R., Sun, G., Shen, M. and Wang, W. (2007). Passive paradigm single-tone-elicted ERPS in tension-type headaches and migraine, Cephalalgia, 27, pp. 139–144.

Cheng, Y., Guo, Y.L. and Yeh, W.Y. (2001). A national survey of psychosocial job stressors and their implications for health among working people in Taiwan. Int. Arch. Occup. Environ. Health, 74, pp. 495–504.

Cherny, N. (2010). Taxonomy distress: including spiritual suffering and demoralization, J. Support. Oncol., 8, pp. 13–14.

Chiappa, K.H. (1989). *Evoked Potentials in Clinical Neurology*, 2nd Ed. (Raven Press, New York).

Ciganek, L. (1961). Theta-discharges in the middle-line: EEG symptom of temporal lobe epilepsy, Electroencephalogr. Clin. Neurophysiol. 13, pp. 669 – 673.

Clark, C.R., McFarlane, A.C., Weber, D.L. and Battersby, M. (1996). Enlarged frontal P300 to stimulus change in panic disorder, Biol. Psychiatry, 15, pp. 845 – 856.

Clark, C.R., Galletly, C.A., Ash, D.J., Moores, K.A., Penrose, R.A., McFarlane and A.C. (2009). Evidence-based medicine evaluation of electrophysiological studies of anxiety disorders, Clin. EEG Neurosci., 40, pp. 84–112.

Claverie, B., Brun, A., Nizard, A., Brenot, P. and Paty, J. (1984). Multiparametric outlines with CNV. Application to depressive syndromes Ann. N.Y. Acad. Sci., 425, pp. 556 – 569.

Cobb, S., Rose, and R.M., (1973). Hypertension, peptic ulcer disease and diabetes in air traffic controllers, JAMA, 224, pp. 489 – 492.

Cohen, S. (1980). After-effects of stress on human performance and social behavior, Psych. Bulletin, 88, pp. 82–108.

Cole, P. and Rodu B. (2001). *Cancer Principles and Practice of Oncology*, 6th Ed., eds. DeVita, V., Hellman, S. and Rosenberg, S. Chapter 14.2 "Descriptive epidemiology: Cancer statistics," (Lippincott Williams & Wilkins, Philadelphia) pp. 228–241.

Coles, G.H., Gratton, G. and Fabiani, M. (1990). *Principles of psychophysiology: Physical, Social and Inferential Elements*, eds. Cacioppo, J.T. and Tassinary L.G. Chapter 13 "Event-related potentials." (Cambridge University Press, Cambridge) pp. 413–455.

Compton, M., Carrera, J.S. and Frank, E. (2008). Stress and depressive symptoms/dysphoria among U.S. medical students: results from a large, nationally-representative survey, J. Nerv. Ment. Dis., 196, pp. 891–897.

Connor, M.J. and Walton, J.A. (2011). Demoralization and remoralization: a review of these constructs in the healthcare literature, Nurs. Inq., 18, pp. 2–11.

Coomber, S.E.L., and Harris, P.A. (2007). *Fitness for Work: The Medical Aspects* 4th Ed., eds. Palmer, K.T., Cox, R.A.F., and Brown, I., Chapter 20 "Women at work," (Oxford University Press, Oxford) pp. 445 – 466.

Cooper, C.L., and Marshal, J. (1976). Occupational sources of stress: A review of the literature related to coronary heart disease and mental ill health, J. Occup. Psychol., 49, pp. 11–28.

Cooper, R., Osselton, J.W. and Shaw, J.C. (1980). *EEG Technology*, 3rd Ed. (Butterworth's, London).

Corbin, W.R., McNair, L.D. and Carter, J. (1996). Self-esteem and problem driving among male and female college students, J. Alcohol Drug Educ., 42, pp. 1 – 14.

Cornell Index N-4, (1985). Validated version from the Serbian Psychologists Association, (Philip Višnić, Belgrade).

Costa, G. (2003). Shift work and occupational medicine: an overview, Occup. Med. (London), 53, pp. 83 – 88.

Cothereau, C., de Beaurepaire, C., Payan, C., Cambou, J.P., Rouillon, F. and Conso, F. (2004). Professional and medical outcomes for French train drivers after 'person under train' accidents: three year follow up study, Occup. Environ. Med., 61, pp. 488 – 494.

Coursolle, K., Sweeney, M., Raymo, J. and Ho J-H. (2010). The association between retirement and emotional well-being: does prior work-family conflict matter? J. Gerontology, 65, pp. 609–620.

Cox, R.A.F. and Nugent, I.M. (2007). *Fitness for Work: The Medical Aspects* 4th Ed., eds. Palmer, K.T., Cox, R.A.F., and Brown, I., Chapter 12 "Orthopaedics and trauma of the limbs," (Oxford University Press, Oxford) pp. 261 – 291.

Cropley, M., Steptoe, A. and Joekes, K., (1999). Job strain and psychiatric morbidity, Psychosom. Med., 29, pp. 1411–1466.

Dababneh, A.J., Swanson, N., and Shell, R.L., (2001). Impact of added rest breaks on the productivity and well being of workers, Ergonomics, 44, pp. 164–174.

Dalrymple, J. and Appleby, J. (2000). Cross section study of reporting of epileptic seizures to general practitioners, BMJ, 320, pp. 94 – 97.

d'Amato, T., Karoumi, B., Rosenfeld, F., Saoud, M., Brunon, A. and Dalery J. (1999). Vulnerability to schizophrenia: II. Familial status of auditory evoked potential abnormailities, Encephale, 25, pp. 288 – 295.

D'arcy, E., Gawryluk, J., Beyea, S., Hajra, S., Feindel, K. and Clarke, D. (2011). Tracking cognitive changes in new-onset epilepsy: functional imaging challenges, Epilepsia, 52 (suppl 4), pp. 43 – 46

Dark, S.J. (1987). Characteristics of medically disqualified airman applicants in calendar years 1982 and 1983, Aviat. Space Environ. Med., 58, pp. 452 – 460.

Dasgupta, A.K., Saunders, M., and Dick, D.J. (1982). Epilepsy in the British Steel Corporation: an evaluation of sickness, accidents and work records, Br. J. Ind. Med., 39, pp. 146 – 148.

Dasinger, L.K., Krause, N., Thompson, P.J., Brand, R.J. and Rudolph, L.(2001). Doctor pro-active communication, return-to-work recommendation, and duration of disability after a workers' compensation low back injury, J. Occup. Environ. Med., 43, pp. 515 – 525.

Davies, E., Hall, S. and Clarke, C. (2003). Two year survival after malignant cerebral glioma: patient and relative reports of handicap, psychiatric symptoms and rehabilitation, Disab. Rehab., 25, pp. 259 –266.

Decety, J., Wang, C-Y. and Cheng, Y. (2010). Physicians down-regulate their pain empathy response: An event-related brain potential study. Neuroimage, 50, pp.1676 – 1682.

De Gaudemaris, R. (2000). Clinical issues: Return to work and public safety Occup. Med. State of the Art Reviews, 15, pp. 223 – 230.

Demarquay, G., Caclin, A., Brudon, F., Fischer, C. and Morlet, D. (2011). Exacerbated attention orient to auditory stimulation in migraine patients, Clin. Neurophysiol., 122, pp. 1755 – 1763.

Demerouti, E., Nachreiner, F., Bakker, A.B. and Shaufeli, W.B. (2001). The job demands resources model of burnout, J. Appl. Psychol., 86, pp. 499 – 512.

Demerouti, E., Bakker, A.B., Vardakou, I. and Kantas, A. (2003). The convergent validity of two burnout instruments: A multitrait-multimethod analysis, Eur. J. Psychol. Assess., 19, pp. 12 – 23.

Detaille, S.I., Heerkens, Y.F., Engels, J.A., van der Gulden, J.W.J. and van Dijk, F.J.H. (2009). Common prognostic factors of work disability among employees with a chronic somatic disease: a systematic review of cohort studies, Scand. J. Work Environ. Health, 35, pp. 261 – 281.

Diamond, H. (1998). Vocational decision making in a psychiatric outpatient program, Occup. Therapy Mental Health, 14, pp. 67 – 80.

Djindjić, N., Jovanović, J., Djindjić, B., Jovanović, M. and Jovanović, J.J. (2012). Associations between the Occupational Stress Index and hypertension, Type 2 diabetes mellitus, and lipid disorders in middle-aged men and women, Ann. Occup. Hyg., 56, pp. 1051 – 1062.

Donaldson, S.I. (1995). *Job Stress Interventions.* eds. In: Murphy, L.R., Hurrell, J.J., Sauter, S.L. Puryear Keita, G., Chapter 6 "Worksite health promotion: A theory-driven, empirically based perspective," (American Psychological Association, Washington, D.C., 1995) pp. 73 – 90.

Donchin, E., Hefley, E., Hillyard, S.A., Loveless, N., Maltzman, I., Ohman, A., Rösler, F., Ruchkin, D. and Siddle, D. (1984). Cognition and event-related potentials: II. The orienting reflex and P300, Ann. N. Y. Acad. Sci., 425, pp. 39 – 57.

Dongier, M. (1973). Clinical applications of the CNV: a review. Electroenceph. Clin. Neurophysiol Suppl. 33, pp. 309 – 315.

Drake, M.E., Pakalnis, A., Phillips, B, Padamadan, H., and Hietter, S.A. (1991). Auditory evoked potentials in anxiety disorder, Clin Electroencephalogr., 22, pp. 97 – 101.

Driesen, K., Jansen, N., van Amelsvoort, L. and Kant, I. (2011). The mutual relationship between shift work and depressive complaints—a prospective cohort study, Scand. J. Work Environ. Health, 37, pp. 402–410.

Dubrovsky, B., Solyom, L. and Barbas, H.(1978). Characteristics of the Contingent Negative Variation in Patients Suffering from Specific Phobias, Biol. Psychiatry, 13, pp. 531 – 540.

Duffy, C.A. and Mc Goldrick, A.E. (1990). Stress and the bus driver in the UK transport industry, Work & Stress, 4, pp. 17–27.

Duncan, C.C., Mirsky, A.F., Lovelace, C.T. and Theodore, W.H. (2009). Assessment of the attention impairment in absence epilepsy: Comparison of visual and auditory P300, Int. J. Psychophysiol., 73, pp. 118 – 122.

Duncan-Johnson, C.G. and Donchin, E. (1977). On quantifying surprise: the variation of event-related potentials with subjective probability, Psychophysiology, 16, pp. 53 – 55.

Dupre, M., George, L., Liu, G. and Peterson, E. (2012). The cumulative effect of unemployment on risks for acute myocardial infarction, Arch. Intern. Med., doi:10.1001/2013.jamainternmed.447.

Eaker, E., Sullivan, L., Kelly-Hayes, M., D'Agostino, R. and Benjamin, E. (2004). Does job strain increase the risk for coronary heart disease or death in men and women? The Framingham offspring study, Am. J. Epidemiol. 159, pp. 950–958.

Eaton, W.W., Anthony, J.C., Mandel, W. and Garrison, R. (1990). Occupations and the prevalence of major depressive disorder, J. Occup. Med., 32, pp. 1079–1087.

Ehlers, C.L., Havstad, J.W., Garfinkel, A. and Kupfer, D.J. (1991). Nonlinear analysis of EEG sleep states, Neuropsychopharmacology, 5, pp. 167 – 176.

Ekstedt, M., Söderström, M., Åkerstedt, T., Nilsson, J., Sondergaard, H-P. and Perski, A. (2006). Disturbed sleep and fatigue in occupational burnout, Scand. J. Work Environ. Health, 32, pp. 121 – 131.

Elden, M. and Chisholm, R. (1993). Emerging varieties of action research: Introduction to the special issue, Hum. Relations, 46, pp. 121 – 142.

Eliot, R.S. (1974). *Stress and the Heart.* (Futura Publishing Co., Mt. Kisco).

Eliot, R.S. (1979). Stress and the Major Cardiovascular Disorders.: (Futura Publishing Co: Mount Kisco).

Elton M. (1984). A longitudinal investigation of event-related potentials in depression, Biol. Psychiatry, 19, pp. 1635 – 1649.

Emdad, R. (1997). An integrative approach to neurocardiologic mechanisms of heart disease risk in professional drivers: Application of neuropsychophysiologic and work environment models, PhD Thesis, Karolinska Institute, 94 p.

Emdad, R., Belkić, K., Theorell, T., Wennberg, A., Hagman, M., Johansson, L., Savić, Č. and Cizinsky, S. (1996). Electrocortical responses to ecologically relevant visual stimuli among professional drivers with and without cardiovascular disease, Integ. Physiol. Behav., 31, pp. 96 – 111.

Emdad, R., Belkić, K., Theorell, T., Cizinsky, S., Savić, Č. and Olsson, K. (1997). Work environment, neurophysiologic and psychophysiologic models among professional drivers with and without cardiovascular disease: Seeking an integrative neurocardiologic approach, Stress Med., 13, pp. 7 – 21.

Emdad, R., Belkić, K., Theorell, T. and Cizinsky, S. (1998a). What prevents professional drivers from following physicians' cardiologic advice? Psychoth. Psychosom., 67, pp. 226–240.

Emdad, R., Belkić, K., Theorell, T., Cizinsky, S., Savić, Č. and Olsson, K. (1998b). Psychophysiologic sensitization to headlight glare among professional drivers with and without cardiovascular disease, J. Occup. Health Psychol. 3, pp. 147 – 160.

Engström, L.G. and Janson, S. (2007). Stress-related sickness absence and return to labour market in Sweden,. Disab. Rehab., 29, pp. 411 – 416.

Ercegovac, D. (1971). General considerations regarding the physiology and pathophysiology of sleep, Anal. Zavod. Mental. Zdravlje, 3, pp. 7 – 24.

Ercegovac, D. and Savić, Č. (1982). Circadian rhythm and the cardiovascular system, Psihijatr. Danas, 2 – 3, pp. 163 – 178.

Evanoff, B., Wolf, L., Aton, E., Canos, J. and Collins, J. (2003). Reduction in injury rates in nursing personnel through introduction of mechanical lists in the workplace, Am. J. Ind. Med., 44, pp.451–457.

Evans, G.W. (1994). Working on the hot seat: urban bus operators, Accid. Anal. Prev., 22, pp.181–193.

Evans, G.W., Carrere, S. and Johansson, G. (1989). A multivariate perspective on environmental stress, Arch. Complex Environ. Studies, 1, pp. 1– 5.

Evans, O. and Steptoe, A. (2002). The contribution of gender-role orientation, work factors and home stressors to psychological well-being and sickness absence in male- and female-dominated occupational groups, Soc. Sci. Med., 54, pp. 481–492.

Fabian, E., Waterworth, A. and Ripke, B. (1993). Reasonable accommodations for workers with serious mental illness: Type, frequency, and associated outcomes, Psychosoc. Rehab. J. 17, pp. 163 – 172.

Fang, F., Fall, K., Mittle, M., Sparén, P., Ye, W., Adami, H-O. and Valdimarsdóttir, U. (2012). Suicide and cardiovascular death after a cancer diagnosis, N. Engl. J. Med., 366, pp. 1310 – 1318.

Ferrie, J.E., Head, J., Shipley, M.J., Vahtera, J., Marmot, M.G. and Kivimäki, M. (2006). Injustice at work and incidence of psychiatric morbidity: the Whitehall II study, Occup. Environ. Med. 63, pp. 443-450.

Fialho, G., Cavichio, L., Povoa, R. and Pimenta J. (2006). Effects of 24-h shift work in the emergency room on ambulatory blood pressure monitoring values of medical residents, Am. J. Hypertens., 19, pp. 1005–1009.

Fifield, J., Reisine, S.T. and Grady, K. (1991). work disability and the experience of pain and depression in rheumatoid arthritis, Soc. Sci. Med. 33, pp. 579 – 585.

Fine, L. (2000a). Chemical and physical factors, Occup. Med. State of the Art Reviews, 15, pp. 18 – 24.

Fine, L. (2000b). Chemical and physical exposure regulations in the U.S., Occup. Med. State of the Art Reviews, 15, pp. 273 – 275.

First, M.B. (2012). A practical prototypic system for psychiatric diagnosis. the ICD-11 clinical descriptions and diagnostic guidelines, World Psychiatry, 11 pp. 24 – 25.

Fisher, J. and Belkić, K, A public health approach in clinical practice, Occup. Med. State of the Art Reviews, 15, pp. 245 – 253.

Fisher, R.S., Vickrey, B.G., Gibson, P., Hermann, B., Penovich, P., Scherer, A. and Walker, S. (2000). The impact of epilepsy from the patient's perspective I. Descriptions and subjective perceptions, Epilepsy Res., 41, pp. 39 –51.

Flach, P., Groothoff, J., Krol, B. and Bültmann, U. (2011). Factors associated with first return to work and sick leave durations in workers with common mental disorders, Eur. J. Public Health, 22, pp. 440 – 445.

Foa, E., Ehlers, A., Clark, D., Tolin, D. and Orsillo, S. (1999). The Postraumatic Cognitions Inventory (PTCI): development and validation, Psychol.Assess. 11, pp. 303 – 314.

Folkow, B. (1994) *Textbook of Hypertension.* ed. Swales, J.D. Chapter 21 "Autonomic nervous system in hypertension," (Blackwell Scientific Publications, London) pp.427-438.

Folkow, B. (1988). Stress, hypothalamic function and neuroendocrine consequences Acta Med. Scand., 723, pp. 61–69.

Forcella, L., De Donato, A., Reversi, S., Fattorini, E. and Boscolo, P. (2009). Occupational stress, job insecurity and perception of the health status in Italian teachers with stable or temporary employment, J. Biol. Regul. Homeostatic Agents, 23, pp. 85–93.

Ford, J.M., Mathalon, D.H., Kalba, S., Marsh, L. and Pfefferbaum, A. (2001). N1 and P300 abnormalities in patients with schizophrenia, epilepsy, and epilepsy with schizophrenialike features, Biol. Psychiatry, 49, pp. 848 – 860.

Ford, J., Pfefferbaum, A. and Roth, W. (1992). P3 and schizophrenia, Ann, NY Acad. Sci., 658, pp. 146 – 163.

Frank, E., Carrera, J.S., Stratton, T., Bickel, J. and Nora, L.M. (2006). Experiences of belittlement and harassment and their correlates among medical students in the United States: longitudinal survey, BMJ., 333, pp. 682– 687.

Frank, E. and Dingle, A.D. (1999). Self-reported depression and suicide attempts among U.S. women physicians, Am. J. Psychiatry, 156, pp. 1887–1894.

Frankenhaeuser, M. and Gardell, B. (1976). Underload and overload in working life: Outline of a multidisciplinary approach, J. Human Stress, 2, pp. 35–46.

Frankenhaeuser, M., and Johansson, G. (1986). Stress at work: Psychobiological and psychosocial aspects, Int. Rev. Appl. Psych., 35, pp. 287 – 299.

Frankl, V.E. (1963-2007). *Man's Search for Meaning: An Introduction to Logotherapy.* (Beacon Press, Boston).

French, S.E., Lenton, R., Walters, V. and Eyles, J. (2000). An empirical evaluation of an expanded Nursing Stress Scale, J. Nurs. Meas. 8, pp. 161–178.

Fretska, E., Bauer, H., Leodolter, M., and Leodolter, L. (1999). Loss of control and negative emotions: a cortical slow potential topography study, Int. J. Psychophysiology, 33, pp. 127 – 141.

Fridberg, D., Hetrick, W., Brenner, C., Shekhar, A., Steffen, A., Malloy, F. and O'Donnell, B. (2009). Relationships between auditory event-relataed potentials and mood state, medication and comorbid psychiatric illness in patients with bipolar disorder, Bipolar Dis., 11, pp. 857 – 866.

Fridner, A., Belkić, K., Marini, M., Minucci, D., Pavan, L. and Schenck-Gustafsson, K. (2009). Recent suicidal ideation among female university hospital physicians in Sweden and Italy (The HOUPE Study): Cross-sectional associations with work stressors, Gender Med., 6, pp. 314–328.

Fridner, A., Belkić, K., Minucci, D., Pavan, L., Marini, M., Pingel, B., Putoto, G., Simonato, P., Løvseth, L.T. and Schenck-Gustafsson, K. (2011). The work environment and recent suicidal thoughts among male university hospital physicians in Sweden and Italy (the HOUPE study). Gender Med., 8, pp. 269–279.

Fridner, A., Belkić, K., Marini, M., Gustafsson-Sendén, M. and Schenck-Gustafsson, K. (2012). Why don't Academic Physicians Seek Needed Professional Help for Psychological Distress? Swiss Med. Wkly., 142, w13626 (8 pp.).

Friedman, D., Nessler, D., Kulik, J. and Hamberger, M. (2011). The brain's orienting response (novelty P3) in patients with unilateral temporal lobe resections, Neuropsychologia, 49, pp. 3474 – 3483.

Fuller, R. (1984). A conceptualization of driving behaviour as threat avoidance, Ergonomics, 27, pp. 1139–1155.

Gabel, S. (2012). Demoralization in mental health organizations: leadership and social support help, Psychiatr. Q., 83, pp. 489-96.

Gabriel , P. and Liimatainen, M-R., (2000). *Mental Health in the Workplace*, (International Labor Organization, Geneva).

Gaillard, A.W.K. (1993). Comparing the concepts of mental load and stress, Ergonomics, 36, pp. 991 – 1005.

Galfalvy, H.C., Oquendo, M.A. and Mann, J.J. (2008). Evaluation of clinical prognostic models for suicide attempts after a major depressive episode, Acta Psychiatr. Scand., 117, pp. 244–252.

Gamble, J.F. (2000). Low-level hydrocarbon solvent exposure and neurobehavioural effects, Occup. Med., 50, pp. 81 – 102.

Gardell, B. (1987). *Work Organization and Human Nature.* (The Swedish Work Environment Fund, Stockholm).

Gardell, B., Aronsson, G. and Barklof, K. (1983). *The Working Environment for Local Public Transport Personnel*, (The Swedish Work Environment Fund, Stockholm).

Georges, E., Wear, M. and Mueller, W. (1992). Body fat distribution and job stress in Mexican-American men of the Hispanic Health and Nutrition Examination Survey. Am. J. Human Biol., 4, pp. 657–667.

Gerdle, B. and Hedberg, G. (1988). Alcohol consumption and complaints from the musculoskeletal system among engine drivers--An epidemiological study, Scand. J. Soc. Med., 16, pp. 105–109.

Geurts, S.A., and Sonnentag, S. (2006). Recovery as an explanatory mechanism in the relation between acute stress reactions and chronic health impairment, Scand. J. Work Environ. Health, 32, pp. 482 – 492.

Giedke, H. and Bolz, J. (1980). Pre- and postimperative negative variation (CNV and PINV) under different conditions of controllability in depressed patients and healthy controls. Prog. Brain Res., 54, pp. 579 – 582.

Gilbody, S., Bower, P. and Rick, J. (2012) Better care for depression in the workplace: integrating occupational and mental health services, Br. J. Psychiatry, 200, pp. 442 – 443.

Glanzman, P., and Froehlich, W.D. (1984). Anxiety, stress, and contingent negative variation reconsidered. Ann. N. Y. Acad. Sci., 425, pp. 578 – 584.

Godin, I., Kittel, F., Coppieters, Y. and Siegrist, J., (2005). A prospective study of cumulative job stress in relation to mental health, BMC Public Health, 5, pp. 67–76.

Gold, K.J., Sen, A. and Schwenk, T. L. (2012). Details on suicide among US physicians: data from the National Violent Death Report System, Gen. Hosp. Psychiatry, http://dx.doi.org/10.1016/j.genhosppsych.2012.08.005.

González-Morales, M.G., Rodríguez, I. and Peiró, J.M. (2010). A longitudinal study of coping and gender in a female-dominated occupation: Predicting teachers' burnout, J. Occup. Health Psychol., 15, pp. 29–44.

Goodwin, F.K. and Jamison, K.R. (2007). *Manic-depressive illness: Bipolar Disorders and Recurrent Depression*. 2nd Ed. (Oxford University Press, Oxford).

Gorman, J.M. (2000). *Kaplan & Sadock's Comprehensive Textbook of Pyschiatry*. 7th Ed., eds. Sadock, B.J. and Sadock, V.A., Chapter 15.1 "Anxiety disorders: Introduction and overview," (Lippincott Williams & Wilkins, Philadelphia) pp.1441–1444.

Grassi, L. and Magnani, K. (2000). Psychiatric morbidity and burnout in the medical profession: An Italian study of general practitioners and hospital physicians, Psychother. Psychosom. 69, pp. 329–334.

Green, R.G., Muir, H., James, M., Gradwell, D. and Green, R.L. (1991). *Human Factors for Pilots*. (Avebury Technical, Hampshire).

Greiner, B.A. and Krause, N. (2000). Expert-observer assessment of job characteristics, Occup. Med. State of the Art Reviews, 15, pp. 175 – 183.

Greiner, B.A., Krause, N., Ragland, D.R. and Fisher, J.M. (1998), Objective stress factors, accidents, and absenteeism in transit operators: A theoretical framework and empirical evidence, J. Occup. Health Psychol., 3, pp. 130 – 146.

Greiner, B.A., Ragland, D.R., Krause, N., Syme, S.L. and Fisher, J.M., (1997). Objective measurement of occupational stress factors—An example with San Francisco urban transit operations, J. Occup. Health Psychol., 2, pp. 325–342.

Grey Walter, W., Cooper, R., Aldridge, V.J., McCallum, W. and Winter, A.L. (1964). Contingent negative variation: An electric sign of sensorimotor association and expectancy in man, Nature, 203, pp. 380 – 384.

Griffin, J.M., Fuhrer, R., Stansfeld, S.A. and Marmot, M. (2002). The importance of low control at work and home on depression and anxiety: do these effects vary by gender and social class? Soc. Sci. Med., 54, pp. 783 –798.

Grin-Yatsenko, V., Baas, I., Ponomarev, V. and Kropotov, J. (2009). EEG power spectra at early stages of depressive disorders, J. Clin. Nuerophysiol. 26, pp. 401 – 406.

Grossi, G. (1999). The stress of unemployment—coping patterns, psychological and physiological responses and implications for health, PhD Thesis, Stockholm University, 135 p.

Grossi, G. and Santell, B. (2009). Quasi-experimental evaluation of a stress management programme for female county and municipal employees on long-term sick leave due to work-related psychological complaints, J. Rehabil. Med. 41, pp. 632 – 638.

Grynderup, M.B., Mors, O., Hansen, Å.M., Andersen, J.H., Bonde, J.P., Kaergaard, A., Kaerlev, L., Mikkelsen, S., Rugulies, R., Thomsen, J.F. and Kolstad, H.A. (2012). A two-year follow-up study of risk of depression according to work-unit measures of psychological demands and decision latitude, Scand. J. Work Environ. Health, 38, pp. 527 – 536.

Gudbergsson, S.B. (2007). Life after cancer: work experiences, living conditions and impact of cancer in tumour-free cancer survivors, PhD Thesis, University of Oslo, Faculty of Medicine, 73 p.

Gudbergsson, S.B., Fosså, S.D., Borgeraas, E. and Dahl, A.A. (2006). A comparative study of living conditions in cancer patients who have returned to work after curative treatment, Support. Care Cancer, 14, pp. 1020 – 1029.

Gudbergsson, S.B., Fosså, S.D., Lindbohm M-L. and Dahl A.A. (2009). Received and needed social support at the workplace in Norwegian and Finnish stage 1 breast cancer survivors: A study from the Nordic Study Group of Cancer and Work (NOCWO), Acta Oncol., 48, pp. 67 – 75.

Gunnarsdottír, H. and Rafnsson, V. (1995) Mortality among Icelandic nurses, Scand. J. Work Environ. Health, 21, pp. 24 – 29.

Gunter, T.C., Van der Zande, R.D., Wiethoff, M., Mulder, G. and Mulder, L.J.M. (1987). Visual selective attention during meaningful noise and after sleep deprivation, Current Trends in Event-Related Potential Research, Supplement 40, pp. 99 – 107.

Gustavsen, B. (1990). *Vägen till bättre arbetsliv. Strategier och arbetsformer i ett utvecklingsarbete* (Arbetslivscentrum, Stockholm).

Gustavsson, P., Alfredsson, L., Brunnberg, I., Hammar, N., Jakobsson, R., Reuterwall, C. and Ostlin, P. (1996). Myocardial infarction among male bus, taxi, and lorry drivers in middle Sweden, Occup. Environ. Med., 53, pp. 235 – 240.

Guthrie, R., Ciccarelli, M. and Babic, A. (2010). Work-related stress in Australia: The effects of legislative interventions and the cost of treatment, Int. J. Law Psychiatry, 33, pp. 101 – 115.

Gyorffy, Z., Adám, S., Csoboth, C. and Kopp, M. (2005). The prevalence of suicide ideas and their psychosocial backgrounds among physicians, Psychiatr. Hung. 20, pp. 370–379.

Habermas, J. (1981). *Theorie des kommunikativen Handelns* (SuhrkampVerlag, Frankfurt am Main).

Halford, J.J. (2003). Neurophysiologic correlates of psychiatric disorders and potential applications in epilepsy. Epilepsy Behav., 4, pp. 375 – 385.

Hamilton, M. (1960). A rating scale for depression, J. Neurol Neurosurg Psychiatry, 23, pp. 56 – 62.

Hammar, N., Alfredsson, L., Smedberg, M. and Ahlbom, A. (1992). Differences in the incidence of myocardial infarction among occupational groups, Scand. J. Work Environ. Health, 18, pp. 178 – 185.

Hansen, E.S. (1993). A follow-up study on mortality of truck drivers, Am. J. Indust. Med., 23, pp. 811 – 821.

Hansen, J. (2001). Increased breast cancer risk among women who work predominantly at night, Epidemiology, 12, pp. 74 –77.

Hansenne, M., Pitchot, W., Moreno, A., Zaldua, I. and Ansseau M. (1996). Suicidal behavior in depressive disorder: an event-related potential study, Biol. Psychiatry, 40, pp.116 – 122.

Hara, K., Ohta, K., Miyajima, M., Hara, M., Iino, K., Matsuda, A., Watanae, S., Matsushima, E., Maehara, T. and Matsuura, M. (2012). Mismatch negativity for speech sounds in temporal lobe epilepsy, Epilepsy Behav., 23, pp. 335 – 341.

Harrington, J.M. (1972). Mortality from coronary artery disease of English and Hamburg sea pilots, Trans. Soc. Occup. Med., 22, pp. 19–23.

Hawton, K., Agerbo, E., Simkin, S., Platt, B. and Mellanby, R.J. (2011). Risk of suicide in medical and related occupational groups: A national study based on Danish case population-based registers, J. Affective Disorders, 134, pp. 320–326.

Hebb, D.O. (1960). *A Textbook of Psychology* (Saunders, Philadelphia).

Hedberg G.E. (1988). The period prevalence of musculoskeletal complaints among Swedish professional drivers, Scand. J. Soc. Med., 16, pp. 5–13.

Hees, H., de Vries, G., Koeter, M. and Schene, A. (2012). Adjuvant occupational therapy improves long-tern depression recovery and return-to-work in good health in sick liested employees with major depression: results of a randomised controlled trial, Occup. Environ. Med., 9 pages doi:10.1136/oemed-2012:100789.

Hees, H., Koeter, M. and Schene, A. (2012). Predictors of long-term return to work and symptom remission in sick-listed patients with major depression, J Clin Psychiatry, 73, pp. e1048-e1055.

Heimberg, D., Naber, G., Hemmeter, U., Zechner, S., Witzke, W., Gerhard, U., Dittmann, V., Holsboer-Trachsler, E. and Hobi, V. (1999). Contingent negative variation and attention in schizophrenic and depressed patients, Neuropsychobiology, 39, pp. 131 – 140.

Heinrichs, M., Wagner, D., Schoch, W., Soravia, L.M., Hellhammer, D.H. and Ehlert U. (2005). Predicting posttraumatic stress symptoms from pretraumatic risk factors: a 2-year prospective follow-up study in firefighters. Am. J. Psychiatry, 162, pp. 2276–2286.

Hellerstedt, W.L. and Jeffery, R.W. (1997). The association of job strain and health behaviours in men and women. Int. J. Epidemiol., 26, pp. 575–583.

Hem, E., Grønvold, N.T., Aasland, O.G. and Ekeberg, O. (2000). The prevalence of suicidal ideation and suicidal attempts among Norwegian physicians. Results from a cross-sectional survey of a nationwide sample, Eur. Psychiatry, 15, pp. 183–189.

Henry, J.P. (1982). The relation of social to biological processes in disease, Soc. Sci. Med., 16, pp. 369–380.

Henry, J.P. (1992). Biological basis of the stress response, Integ. Physiol Behav Sci. 27, pp. 66–83.

Henry, J. (1994) *Textbook of Hypertension*. ed. Swales, J.D., Chapter 32 "Psychosocial stress and hypertension," The relevance of animal studies. (Blackwell Scientific Publications, London) pp. 633–639.

Hernberg, S. (1980). Evaluation of epidemiologic studies in assessing the long-term effects of occupational noxious agents, Scand. J. Work Environ. Health, 6, pp. 163–169.

Hernberg, S. (1981). Negative results in cohort studies-How to recognize fallacies, Scand. J. Work Environ. Health, 7 Suppl. 4, pp. 121–126.

Hernberg, S. (1984). Work related disease-Some problems in study design, Scand. J. Work Environ. Health, 10, pp. 3267–372.

Herner, B. (1993). High frequency of suicide among younger physicians. Unsatisfactory working situations should be addressed, Läkartidningen, 90, pp. 3449–3452.

Hiebert, F.R., Skovron, M.L. and Nordin, M. (2003). Work restrictions and outcome of non-specific low back pain, Spine, 28, pp. 722 – 728.

Hixson, J.D., Balcer, L.J., Glosser, G. and French, J.A. (2006). Fear sensitivity and the psychological profile of patients with psychogenic nonepileptic seizures, Epilepsy Behav., 9, pp. 587 – 592.

Himani, A., Tandon, O.P. and Bhatia, M.S. (1999). Study of P300-event related potentials in patients with major depression. Indian J. Physiol. Pharmacol., 43, pp. 367 – 372.

Hochschild, A. and Machung, A. (1989). *The Second Shift: Working Parents and the Revolution at Home* (Viking Press, New York).

Hockey, G.R.L. (1997). Compensatory control in the regulation of human performance under stress and high workload: A cognitive-energetical framework, Biol. Psychol., 45, pp. 73 – 93.

Hohnsbein, J., Falkenstein, M. and Hoormann, J. (1995). Effects of attention and time-pressure on P300 subcomponents and implications for mental workload research, Biol. Psychol., 40, pp. 73 – 81.

Holland, P., Lane, S., Whitehead, M., Marson, A. and Jacoby, A. (2009). Labor market participation following onset of seizures and early epilepsy: Findings from a UK cohort, Epilepsia, 50, pp. 1039 – 1039.

Holmgren, K. and Dahlin Ivanoff, S. (2004). Women on sickness absence—views of possibilities and obstacles for returning to work, Disab. Rehab., 26, pp. 213 – 222.

Hon, E.H. and Lee, S. (1963). Electronic evaluation of the fetal heart rate. VIII. Patterns preceding fetal death, further observations, Am. J. Obstet. Gynecol., 87, pp. 814 – 826.

Horowitz, M., Wilner, N. and Alvarez, W. (1979). The Impact of Event Scale: a measure of subjective stress, Psychosom, Med, 41, pp. 209 – 218.

Horwath E. and Weissman, M. (2000). *Kaplan & Sadock's Comprehensive Textbook of Psychiatry.* 7th Ed., eds. Sadock, B.J. and Sadock, V.A., Chapter 15.2, "Anxiety disorders: Epidemiology," (Lippincott Williams & Wilkins, Philadelphia) pp. 1444–1450.

Houston, R.J., Bauer, L.O. and Hesselbrock, V.M. (2004). P300: evidence of cognitive inflexibility in female adolescents at risk for recurrent depression. Progr. Neuropsychopharmacol. Biol. Psychiat. 28, pp. 529 – 536.

Howells, F., Ives-Deliperi, V., Horn, N. and Stein, D. (2012). Mindfulness based cognitive therapy improves frontal control in bipolar disorder: a pilot EEG study, BMC Psychiatry, 12, (8 pages).

Hu, H. and Speizer, F.E. (1998). *Harrison's Principles of Internal Medicine* 14th Ed., eds. Fauci, A., Martin, J., Braunwald, E., Kasper, D., Isselbacher, K., Hauser, D., Wilson, J., Longo, D. and Jameson J., Chapter 5, "Influence of environmental and occupational hazards on disease," (McGraw Hill, New York) pp. 18 – 20.

Hyman, M. (2005). *A Physician's Guide to Return to Work* eds. Talmage, J.B, Melhorn, J.M. and Hyman, M., Chapter 15 "Working with common cardiopulmonary problems," (American Medical Association Press, Chicago) pp. 233 – 266.

Inanaga, K. (1998). Frontal midline theta rhythm and mental activity. Psychiatry Clin. Neurosci., 52, pp. 555 – 566.

Innstrand, S.T., Langballe, E.M. and Falkum, E. (2012). A longitudinal study of the relationship between work engagement and symptoms of anxiety and depression, Stress & Health, 28, pp. 1–10.

Inoue, A., Kawakami, N., Haratani, T., Kobayashi, M., Ishizaki, M., Hayashi, T., Fujita, O., Aizawa, Y., Miyazaki, S., Kiro, H., Masumoto, T., Hashimoto, S. and Araki, S. (2010). Job stressors and long-term sick leave due to depressive disorders among Japanese male employees: findings form the Japan Work Stress and Health Cohort study, J. Epidemiol. Community Health, 64, pp. 229–235.

Isaksson Rø, K., Gude, T., Tyssen, R. and Aasland, O.G. (2008). Counseling for burnout in Norwegian doctors: one year cohort study, BMJ., 337, a2004 (8 pages).

Ishizaki, M., Tsuritani, I., Noborisaka, Y., Yamada, Y., Tabata, M. and Nakagawa, H. (1996). Relationship between job stress and plasma fibrinolytic activity in male Japanese workers. Int. Arch. Occup. Environ. Health, 68, pp. 315–320.

Iskra-Golec, I., Folkard, S., Marek, T. and Noworol, C. (1996). Health, well-being and burnout in ICU nurses on 12- and 8-h shifts, Work & Stress, 10, pp. 251–256.

Israel, B., Goldenhar, L., Baker, E. and Heaney, C. (1996). Occupational stress, safety and health: conceptual framework and principles for effective prevention interventions, J. Occup. Health Psychol., 1, pp. 261 – 286.

Israel, J.B., Wickens, C.D. and Donchin, E. (1980) *Motivation, Motor and Sensory Processes in the Brain—Electrical Potentials, Behavior and Clinical Use*, eds. Kornhumber, H.H., and Deeke, L., Chapter, "The dynamics of P300 during dual-task performance," (North Holland, Amsterdam), pp. 416 – 421.

Ivanitsky, A.M., (1980). Evoked potentials and mental processes. Electroencephalogr. Clin. Neurophysiol. 48, pp. 727 – 32.

Jahoda, M. (1982). *Employment and Unemployment: A Social Psychological Analysis*, (Cambridge University Press, Cambridge).

Jahoda, M., Lazarsfeld, P.F. and Zeisel, H. (1933). *Die arbeitslosen von Marienthal: Ein soziographischer versuch*, (Hirzel, Leipzig).

Jahshan, C., Wynn, J., Mathis, K., Altshuler, L., Glahn, D. and Green, M. (2012). Cross-diagnostic comparison of duration mismatch negativity and P3a in bipolar disorder and schizophrenia, Bipolar Dis., 14, pp. 239 – 248.

Jakobsson, B., Ekholm, J., Bergroth, A. and Schüldt Ekholm, K. (2010). Improved employment rates after multiprofessional cross-sector cooperation in vocational rehabilitation: a 6-year follow-up with comparison groups. Int. J. Rehab. Res., 33, pp. 72 – 80.

Jakobsson, R., Gustavsson, P. and Lundberg, I. (1997). Increased risk of lung cancer among male professional drivers in urban but not rural areas of Sweden, Occup. Environ. Med., 54, pp. 189–193.

Jamison, K.R. (2006). The many stigmas of mental illness, Lancet, 367, pp. 533–534.

Janlert, U., Asplund, K., and Weinehall, L. (1991). Unemployment and cardiovascular risk indicators, Scand. J. Soc. Med., 20, pp. 14 – 18.

Järvholm, B. (2012). How should methods for return to work be evaluated? Scand. J. Work Environ. Health, 38, pp. 89 – 91.

Johansson, G. and Aronsson, G. (1984). Stress reactions in computerized administrative work, J. Occup. Behav., 5, pp. 159 – 181.

Johansson, G., Johnson, J. and Hall, E. (1991). Smoking and sedentary behavior as related to work organization, Soc. Sci. Med., 32, pp. 837–846.

John, E.R. and Prichep, L.S. (2006). The relevance of QEEG to the evaluation of behavioral disorders and pharmacological interventions. Clin. EEG Neurosci., 37, pp. 135 – 143.

Johnson, J.V. and Hall, E.M. (1988) Job strain, workplace social support and cardiovascular disease: A cross-sectional study of a random sample of the Swedish working population, Am. J. Public Health, 78, pp. 1336–1342.

Johnson, J.V., Hall, E.M. and Theorell, T. (1989). Combined effects of job strain and social isolation on the cardiovascular disease morbidity and mortality in a random sample of the Swedish male working population. Scand. J. Work. Environ. Health, 15, pp. 271–279.

Johnson, J.V., Hall, E.M., Ford, D.E., Mead, L.A., Levine, D.M., Yang, N-Y. and Klag, M.J. (1995). The psychosocial work environment of physicians. The impact of demands and resources on job dissatisfaction and psychiatric distress in a longitudinal study of Johns Hopkins Medical School graduates, J. Occup. Environ. Med., 37, pp. 1151–1159.

Johnson, J.V. and Stewart W. (1993). Measuring work organization exposure over the life course with a job-exposure matrix, Scand. J. Work Environ. Health, 19, pp. 21–28.

Johnson, S.B., Langlieb, A.M., Teret, S.P., Gross, R., Schwab, M., Massa, J., Ashwell, L. and Geyh, A.S. (2005). Rethinking first response: effects of the clean up and recovery effort on workers at the world trade center disaster site, J. Occup. Environ. Med., 47, pp. 386–391.

Johnsson, A. (2003). Rehabilitation from breast cancer—women who have undergone surgery and were afflicted by lymphedema—development of multidisciplinary care. Report to Cancerfonden, Stockholm.

Johnston, R.V. (2007). *Fitness for Work: The Medical Aspects* 4th Ed., eds. Palmer, K.T., Cox, R.A.F., and Brown, I., Appendix 1 "Civil aviation," (Oxford University Press, Oxford) pp. 625 – 628.

Johnston, V.S., Burleson, M.H., and Miller, D.R. (1987). Emotional value and late positive components of ERPs, Current Trends in Event-Related Potential Research, Suppl. 40, pp.198 – 203.

Jokela, M., Ferrie, J., Gimeno, D., Chandola, T., Shipley, M., Head, J., Vahtera, J., Westerlund, H., Marmot, M. and Kivimäki M. (2010). From midlife to early old age: Health trajectories associated with retirement, Epidemiology, 21, pp. 284–290.

Josephson, M., Lagerstrom, M., Hagberg, M. and Wigaeus Hjelm, E. (1997). Musculoskeletal symptoms and job strain among nursing personnel: a study over a three year period, Occup. Environ. Med., 54, pp. 681–685.

Josiassen, R.C., Roemer, R.A., Shagass, C. and Straumanis, J.J. (1986) *Brain Electrical Potentials and Psychopathology*, eds. Shagass, C., Josiassen, R.C. and Roemer, R., Chapter "Attention-related effects on somatosensory evoked potentials in nonpsychotic dysphoric psychiatric patients," (Elsevier, New York), pp. 259 – 277.

Journal of the National Cancer Institute (1998) Surveys show employers and employees have misgivings about workers with cancer, J. Natl. Cancer Inst., 90, pp.191–192.

Joy, M. (1992). Introduction and summary of principal conclusions to the first European workshop in aviation cardiology, Eur. Heart J., 13 Suppl H, pp. 1– 9.

Kagan, A.R. and Levi, L. (1974). Health and environment--psychosocial stimuli: a review, Soc. Sci. Med., 8, pp. 225–241.

Kageyama, T., Kobayashi, T., Nishikido, N., Oga, J. and Kawashima, M. (2005). Associations of sleep problems and recent life events with smoking behaviors among female staff nurses in Japanese hospitals, Ind. Health, 43, pp. 133–141.

Kales, S., Soteriades, E., Christoudias, S. and Christiani, D. (2003). Firefighters and on-duty deaths from coronary heart diease: a case control study, Environ. Health, 2: 14 pages.

Kales, S., Soteriades, E., Christophi, C. and Chriatiani, D. (2007). Emergency duties and deaths from heart disease among firefighters in the Unites States, New Engl. J. Med., 356, pp. 1207–1215.

Kales, S., Tsismenakis, A., Zhang, C. and Soteriades, E. (2009). Blood pressure in firefighters, police officers and other emergency responders, Am. J. Hypertension, 22, pp. 11–20.

Kalkanis, S.N., Quinones-Hinojosa, A., Buzney, E., Ribaudo, H.J. and Black, P.M. (2000). Quality of life following surgery for intracranial meningiomas at Brigham and Women's Hospital: a study of 164 patients using a modification of the functional assessment of cancer therapy-brain questionnaire, J Neuro-Oncology, 48, pp. 233 – 241.

Kalsbeek, J. (1967). Measurement of mental work load and acceptable load, possible applications in industry, Int. J. Production Research, 7, pp. 33 – 45.

Kalsbeek, J. (1971). Standards of acceptable load in ATC tasks, Ergonomics, 14, pp. 641 – 650.

Kalsbeek, J. and Ettema, T. (1963). Continuous recording of heart rate and the measurement of perceptual load, Ergonomics, 6, pp. 306 – 307.

Karaaslan, F., Gonul, A., Oguz, A., Erdinc, E. and Esel, E. (2003). P300 changes in major depressive disorders with and without psychotic features, J. Affect. Disord., 73, pp. 283 – 287.

Karasek, R.A. (1979). Job demands, job decision latitude and mental strain: implications for job redesign, Adm. Sci. Q., 24, pp. 285–308.

Karasek, R.A., Baker, D., Marxer, F., Ahlbom, A. and Theorell, T. (1981). Job decision latitude, job demands and cardiovascular disease: A prospective study of Swedish men. Am. J. Public Health, 71, pp. 694–70.

Karasek, R.A., Brisson. C., Kawakami, N., Houtman, I., Bongers, P. and Amick, B. (1998). The Job Content Questionnaire (JCQ): An instrument for internationally comparative assessments of psychosocial job characteristics, J. Occup. Health Psychology, 3, pp. 322–355.

Karasek, R.A., Russell, R.S. and Theorell, T. (1982) Physiology of stress and regeneration in job-related cardiovascular illness, J. Hum. Stress, 8, pp. 29–42.

Karasek, R.A. and Theorell, T. (1990) *Healthy Work: Stress, Productivity and the Reconstruction of Working Life*. (Basic Books, Inc., New York).

Karasek, R.A. and Theorell, T. (2000). The Demand-Control-Support Model and CVD, Occup. Med. State of the Art Reviews, 15, pp. 78–83.

Karl, A., Malta, L.S. and Maercker, A. (2006). Meta-analytic review of event-related potential studies in post-traumatic stress disorder, Biol. Psychol., 71, pp. 123–147.

Karlson, B., Jönsson, P., Pålsson, B., Åbjörnsson, G., Malmberg, B., Larsson, B. and Österberg, K. (2010). Return to work after a workplace-oriented intervention for patients on sick-leave for burnout-a prospective controlled study, BMC Public Health, 10, p. 301 (10 pages).

Karlsson, B., Knutsson, A., Lindahl, B. and Alfredsson, L. (2003). Metabolic disturbances in male workers with rotating three-shift work. Results of the WOLF study, Int. Arch. Occup. Environ. Health, 76, pp. 424–430.

Kaur, M., Battisti, R., Lagopoulos, J., Ward, P., Hickie, I. and Hermens, D. (2012). Neurophysiological biomarkers support bipolar-spectrum disorders within psychosis cluster, J. Psychiatry Neurosci, 37, pp. 313 – 321.

Kawada, T. (2011). Overtime working hours and depression: Questionnaire survey using the Patient Health Questionnaire, Chronobiol. Int., 28, pp. 474–454.

Kawakami, N., Araki, S., Kawashim, M., Masumoto, T. and Hayashi, T. (1997). Effects of work-related stress reduction on depressive symptoms among Japanese blue-collar workers, Scand. J. Work Environ. Health, 23, pp. 54–59.

Kawakami, N., Haratani, T. and Araki, S. (1998). Job strain and arterial blood pressure, serum cholesterol, and smoking as risk factors for coronary heart disease in Japan. Int. Arch. Occup. Environ. Health, 71, pp. 429–432.

Kawakami, N., Araki, S., Takatsuka, N., Shimizu, H. and Ishibashi, H. (1999). Overtime, psychosocial working conditions, and occurrence of non-insulin dependent diabetes mellitus in Japanese men, J. Epidemiol. Community Health, 53, pp. 359 – 363.

Kenny, D.T., Davis, P. and Oates, J. (2004). Music performance anxiety and occupational stress amongst opera chorus artists and their relationship with state and trait anxiety and perfectionism. J. Anxiet. Disord. 18, pp. 757–777.

Keough, M.E., Porter, E., Kredlow, M.A., Worthington, J.J., Hoge, E.A., Pollack, M.H., Shear, M.K. and Simon, N.M. (2012). Anchoring the Panic Disorder Severity Scale Assessment,. 19, pp. 257–259.

Kessler, R., Akiskal, H., Ames, M., Birnbaum, H., Greenberg, P., Hirschfeld, R., Jin, R., Merikangas, K., Simon, G. and Wang, P. (2006). Prevalence and effects of mood disorders on work performance in a nationally representative sample of U.S. workers, Am. J. Psychiatry, 163, pp. 1561 –1568.

Kidd, S., Boyd, G., Bielingm P., Pike, S. and Kazarian-Keith, D. (2008). Effect of a vocationally-focused brief cognitive behavioural intervention on employment-related outcomes for individuals with mood and anxiety disorders, Cognit. Behav. Therapy, 37, pp. 247 – 251.

Kim, S-S., Subramanian, S., Sorensen, G., Perry, M. and Christiani, D. (2012). Assocation between change in employment status and new-onset depressive symptoms in South Korea—a gender analysis, Scand. J. Work Environ. Health, e-publication ahead of print, doi: 10.5271/sjweh.3286.

Kissane, D.W., Maj, M., Sartorius, N., Clarke, D.M. (2010) *Depression and Cancer* eds. Kissane D. W., Maj M. and Sartorius N., Chapter 2 "Psychological adaptation, demoralization and depression in people with cancer" (John Wiley & Sons, Ltd, Chichester) doi: 10.1002/9780470972533.ch2 (published on line)

Kivimäki, M., Leino-Arjas, P., Luukkonen, R., Riihimäki, H., Vahtera, J. and Kirjonen, J. (2002). Work stress and risk of cardiovascular mortality: prospective cohort study of industrial employees. BMJ, 325, 1386-1390.

Kivimäki, M., Virtanen, M., Elovainio, M., Kouvonen, A., Väänänen, A. and Vahtera, J. (2006). Work stress in the etiology of coronary heart disease—a meta-analysis, Scand. J. Work Environ. Health, 32, pp. 431–442.

Kleppa, E., Sanne, B. and Tell, G.S. (2008). Working overtime is associated with anxiety and depression: the Hordaland Health Study, J. Occup. Environ. Med., 50, pp. 658–666.

Klimek, E.H. (2011). *A Physician's Guide to Return to Work,* eds Talmage, J.B, Melhorn, J.M. and Hyman, M., Chapter 16 "Working with common neurologic problems," (American Medical Association Press, Chicago) pp. 317 – 337.

Klimesch, V. (1999). EEG alpha and theta oscillations reflect cognitive and memory performance: a review and analysis, Brain Res. Rev., 29, pp. 169 – 195.

Klorman, R., and Ryan, R.M. (1980). Heart rate, contingent negative variation and evoked potentials during anticipation of affective stimulation, Psychophysiology, 17, pp. 513 – 523.

Knežević, A. (2011). Getting retired—Relief or misfortune? Med Pregl., 64, pp. 437–438.

Knott, V.J. and Lapierre, Y.D. (1987). Electrophysiological and behavioral correlates of psychomotor responsivity in depression, Biol. Psychiatry, 22, pp. 313 – 324.

Knutsson, A. (2003). Health disorders in shift workers. Occup. Med. (London), 53, pp. 103 – 108.

Knutsson, A., Alfredsson, L., Karlsson, B., Åkerstedt. T., Fransson. E., Westerholm. P. and Westerlund, H. (2012). Breast cancer among shift workers: results of the WOLF longitudinal cohort study. Scand. J. Work Environ. Health, 2012 e-publication ahead of print doi: 10.5271/SJWEH.

Knutsson, A., Hallquist, J., Reuterwall, C., Theorell, T., and Åkerstedt ,T. (1999). Shiftwork and myocardial infarction: a case-control study, Occup. Environ. Med., 56, pp. 46 – 50.

Kok, A. and Kramer, A. (1997). Event-related-potential (ERP) reflections of mental resources: a review and synthesis, Biol. Psychol., 45, pp. 19 – 56.

Kolassa, I-T., Musial, F., Kolassa, S. and Miltner, W. (2006). Event-related potentials when identifying or color-naming threatening schematic stimuli in spider phobic and non-phobic individuals. BMC Psychiatry, 6, pp. 38.

Kompier, M., Aust, B., van den Berg, A.M. and Siegrist, J. (2000). Stress prevention in bus drivers: evaluation of 13 natural experiments, J. Occup. Health Psychol., 5, pp. 11 – 31.

Kompier, M. and Di Martino, V. (1995). Review of bus drivers' occupational stress and stress prevention, Stress Med., 11, pp. 253 – 262.

Korunka, C., Wenzel, T. and Bauer, H. (1993). The 'oddball CNV' as an indicator of different information processing in patients with panic disorders, Int. J. Psychophys., 15, pp. 207– 215.

Kouvonen, A., Kivimäki, M., Virtanen, M., Pentti, J. and Vahtera, J. (2005).Work stress, smoking status and smoking intensity: an observational study of 46 190 employees. J. Epidemiol. Community. Health, 59, pp. 63–69.

Kozlowski, M. (1998). *Modeling the Stress-Strain Relationship in Work Settings*, (Routledge, London).

Kramer, A.F., Sirevaag, E. and Braune, R. (1987). A psychophysiological assessment of operator workload during simulated flight missions, Human Factors, 29, pp. 145 – 160.

Krause, N., Ragland, D.R., Greiner, B.A., Syme, S.L. and Fisher, J.M. (1997a). Psychosocial job factors associated with back and neck pain in public transit operators, Scand. J. Work Environ. Health, 23, pp. 179–186.

Krause, N., Ragland, D.R., Fisher, J.M., Holman, B.L. and Selvin, S. (1997b). Physical workload and ergonomic factors associated with prevalence of back and neck pain in urban transit operators, Spine 22, pp. 2117 – 2127.

Krause, N., Ragland, D.R., Fisher, J.M. and Syme, S.L. (1998). Psychosocial job factors, physical workload, and incidence of work-related spinal injuries, Spine, 23, pp. 2507 – 2516.

Kristal-Boneh, E., Raifel, M., Froom, P. and Ribak, J. (1995). Heart rate variability in health and disease, Scand. J. Work Environ. Health, 21, pp. 85 – 95.

Kristensen, T.S. (1996). Job stress and cardiovascular disease: A theoretic critical review, J. Occup. Health Psychol., 1, pp. 246 – 260.

Kristensen, T.S. (2000). Workplace intervention studies, Occup. Med. State of the Art Reviews, 15, pp. 293 – 305.

Kropp, P. and Gerber, W-D. (2005). Slow cortical potentials in migraine. Predictive value and possible novel therapeutic strategies to prevent an attack, Functional Neurology, 20, pp. 193 – 197.

Kruggel, F., Wiggins, C.H., Hermmann, C.S. and von Cramon, D.Y. (2000). Recording of the event-related potentials during functional MRI at 3.0 Tesla Field strength, Magn. Reson. Med., 44, pp. 277 – 282.

Kubo, T., Ozasa, K., Mikami, K., Wakai, K., Fujino, Y., Watanabe, Y., Miki, T., Nakao, M., Hayashi, K., Suzuki, K., Mori, M., Washio, M., Sakauchi, F., Ito, Y., Yoshimura, T. and Tamakoshi, A. (2006). Prospective cohort study of the risk of prostate cancer among rotating-shift workers: findings from the Japan collaborative cohort study, Am. J. Epidemiol., 164, pp. 358–366.

Kubzansky, D.L. and Kawachi, I. (2000). Going to the heart of the matter: do negative emotions cause coronary heart disease? J. Psychosom. Res. 48, pp. 323 – 337.

Kügler, C.F.A., Taghavy, A. and Platt, D. (1993). The event-related P300 potential analysis of cognitive human brain aging: A review, *Gerontology*, 39, pp.280 – 303.

Kulbertus, H. and Frank, G. (1988) *Neurocardiology*. (Futura Publishing Co., Mt. Kisco).

Kumar, S., Hatcher, S. and Huggard, P. (2005). Burnout in psychiatrists: an etiological model. Int. J. Psychiatry Med., 35, pp. 405–416.

Kuper, H., Marmot, M. and Hemingway, H. (2002). Systematic review of prospective cohort studies of psychosocial factors in the etiology and prognosis of coronary heart disease, Sem. Vasc. Med. 2, pp. 266 – 314.

Kupfer, D., Reynolds, C., Ulrich, R. and Grochocinski, V. (1986). Comparison of automated REM and slow-wave sleep analysis in young and middle-aged depressed subjects, Biol. Psychiatry, 21, pp. 189 – 200.

Kurimori, S. and Kakizaki, T. (1995). Evaluation of work stress using psychological and physiological measures of mental activity in a paced calculating task, Ind. Health, 33, pp. 7 – 22.

Kushnir, T., Levhar, C. and Cohen, A.H. (2004). Are burnout levels increasing? Experience of Israeli primary care physicians. Israel Med. Assoc. J. 6, pp. 451–455.

Laflamme, N., Brisson, C., Moisan, J., Milot, A., Mâsse, B. and Vézina, M. (1998). Job strain and ambulatory blood pressure among female white-collar workers, Scand. J. Work Environ. Health, 25, pp. 334–343.

Landsbergis, P. (1998). *Encyclopaedia of Occupational Health and Safety* ed. Stellman J. 4th Ed. Chapter 102 "Case studies of air traffic controllers in the United States and Italy," (International Labour Organization, Geneva), pp. 102– 109.

Landsbergis, P. (2003). The changing organization of work and the safety and health of working people: A commentary, J. Occup. Environ. Med., 45, pp. 61 – 72.

Landsbergis, P., Cahill, J., and Schnall, P.L. (1999). The impact of lean production and related new systems of work organization on worker health, J. Occup. Health Psychol., 4, pp. 1 – 23.

Landsbergis, P., Dobson, M, Koutsouras, G. and Schnall, P. (2013). Job strain and ambulatory blood pressure: A meta-analysis and systematic review, Am. J. Public Health, 103, pp. e61 – e71.

Landsbergis, P., Schnall, P., Warren, K., Pickering, T.G, Schwartz, J. (1994). Association between ambulatory blood pressure and alternative formulations of job strain, Scand. J. Work Environ. Health, 20, pp. 349–363.

Landsbergis, P., Schnall, P., Dietz, D., Warren, K., Pickering, T.G. and Schwartz, J. (1998). Job strain and health behaviors: results of a prospective study, Am. J. Health Promot., 12, pp. 237–245.

Landsbergis, P., Schnall, P., Belkić, K., Schwartz, J., Baker, D. and Pickering, T.G. (2008). Working conditions and masked (hidden) hypertension: Insights into the global epidemic of hypertension, Scand. J. Work Environ. Health, (Suppl 6), pp. 41–51.

Landsbergis, P., Theorell, T., Schwartz, J., Greiner, B.A. and Krause N. (2000) Measurement of psychosocial workplace exposure variables, Occup. Med. State of the Art Reviews, 15, pp. 163–188.

Lang, M., Lang, W., Diekmann, V. and Kornhuber, H.H. (1987). The frontal theta rhythm indicating motor and cognitive learning, Electroencephalogr. Clin. Neurophysiol., Suppl. 40, pp. 322 – 327.

Lásló, K.D., Ahnve, S., Hallqvist, J., Ahlbom, A. and Janszky, I. (2010). Job strain predicts recurrent events after a first acute myocardial infarction: the Stockholm Heart Epidemiology Program, J. Intern. Med. 267, pp. 599 – 611.

Lazarus, R.S. (1967) *Emotional Stress Physiological and Psychological Reactions Medical, Industrial and Military Implications*. ed. Levi, L. (editor), Chapter "Stress theory and psychophysiological research," (Forsvarsmedicin 3, Stockholm), pp. 152 – 177.

Lazarus, R.S., and Folkman, S. (1984). *Stress, Appraisal and Coping*, (Springer, New York).

Leigh, J.P. (2006). Expanding research on the economics of occupational health, Scand. J. Work Environ. Health, 32, pp. 1 – 4.

Leigh, J.P. and Robbins, J.A. (2004). Occupational disease and workers' compensation: coverage, costs, and consequences, Milbank Quart. 2004; 82, pp. 689 – 721.

Leigh, J.P. and Schnall, P. (2000). Costs of occupational circulatory disease, Occup. Med. State of the Art Reviews, 15, pp. 257 – 267.

Lesić, A.R., Stefanović, N.P., Peruničić, I., Milenković, P., Toševski, D.L. and Bumbaširević, M.Z. (2009). Burnout in Belgrade orthopaedic surgeons and general practitioners: A preliminary report, Acta Chir. Iugoslavica, 56, pp. 53–59.

Leslie, D. and Butz, D. (1998). GM suicide: flexibility, space, and the injured body. Economic Geography, 74, pp. 360–378.

Levav, I. (2009). *Psychiatric and Behavioral Disorders in Israel*. (Geffen Publishing House, Jerusalem).

Levi, L. (1972). Stress, distress and psychosocial stimulation, *Acta Med. Scand.*, Suppl 528, pp. 1 – 166.

Levi, L. (1981). *Preventing Work Stress*, (Addison-Wesley Publishing Co., Reading).

Levi, L. (2006). *Stress and Quality of Working Life: Current Perspectives in Occupational Health*, eds. Rossi, A.M., Perrewé, P.L. and Sauter, S.L.,"The European Commission's guidance on work-related stress and related initiatives: From words to action," Chapter 12 (Information Age Publishing, Charlotte) pp. 167-182.

Levy, B. (2013). Autonomic nervous system arousal and cognitive funcitoning in bipolar disorder, Bipolar Dis., 15, pp. 70 – 79

Leymann, H. (1996). The content and development of mobbing at work, Eur. J. Work. Org. Psychology, 5, pp. 165–184.

Li, J., Yan, W., Cheng, Y., Siegrist, J. and Cho, S-I. (2005). Effort-reward imbalance at work and job dissatisfaction in Chinese healthcare workers: a validation study, Int. Arch. Occup. Environ. Health, 78, pp. 198–204.

Lindfors, P.M., Meretoja, O.A., Luukkonen, R.A., Elovainio, M.J. and Leino, T.J. (2009). Suicidality among Finnish anaesthesiologists, Acta Anaesthesiol. Scand., 53, pp. 1027–1035.

Lindsten, H., Stenlund, H., Edlund, C. and Forsgren, L. (2002). Socioeconomic prognosis after a newly diagnosed unprovoked epileptic seizure in adults: A population-based case-control study, Epilepsia, 43, pp. 1230 – 1250.

Liu, T., and Waterbor, J.W. (1994). Comparison of suicide rates among industrial groups, Am. J. Indust. Med., 25, pp. 197–203.

Loisel, P., Buchbinder, R., Hazard, R., Keller, R., Scheel, I., van Tulder, M. and Webster, B. (2005). Prevention of work disability due to musculoskeletal disorders: The challenge of implementing evidence, J. Occup. Rehabil., 15, pp. 507 – 524.

Lourel, M., Abdellaoui, S., Chevaleyre, S., Paltrier, M. and Gana, K. (2008). Relationships between psychological job demands, job control and burnout among firefighters. N. Am. J. Psychology, 10, pp. 489–496.

Lown, B. (1990). Role of higher nervous activity in sudden cardiac death, Japanese Circul. J., 54, pp. 581 – 602.

Lutgendorf, S., Johnsen, E., Cooper, B., Anderson, B., Sorosky, J., Buller, R. and Sood, A. (2002). Vascular endothelial growth factor and social support in patients with ovarian carcinoma, Cancer, 95, pp. 808–815.

Luczak, H. (1971). The use of simulators for testing individual mental working capacity, Ergonomics, 14, pp. 651 – 660.

Luczak, H. and Lauring, W. (1973). An analysis of heart rate variability, Ergonomics 16, pp. 85 – 97.

Lydell, M., Grahn, B., Månsson, J., Baigi, A. and Marklund, B. (2009). Predictive factors of sustained return to work for persons with musculoskeletal disorders who participated in rehabilitation, Work, 33, pp. 317 – 328.

Mahan, P.L., Mahan, M.P., Park, N.J., Shelton, C., Brown, K.C. and Weaver, M.T. (2010). Work environment stressors, social support, anxiety and depression among secondary school teachers, AAOHN Journal, 58, pp. 197–205.

Main, D.S., Nowels, C.T., Cavender, T.A., Etschmaier, M. and Steiner, J.F. (2005). A qualitative study of work and work return in cancer survivors, Psycho-oncology, 14, pp. 992 – 1004.

Maisano, G. (1988). Summary and conclusions towards guidelines for retun to work after myocardial infarction and myocardial revascularization, Eur. Heart J., 9 Suppl. L, pp. 120 – 122.

Mäki, N. and Martikainen, P. (2009). The role of socioeconomic indicators on non-alcohol and alcohol-associated suicide mortality among women in Finland. A register-based follow-up study of 12 million person-years, Soc. Sci. Med., 68, pp. 2161–2169.

Mann, J., Ellis, S.P, Waternaux, C., Liu, X., Oquendo, M., Malone KM, Brodsky, B., Haas, G. and Currier, D. (2008). Classification trees distinguish suicide attempters in major psychiatric disorders: a model of clinical decision making, J. Clin. Psychiatry, 69, pp. 23–31.

Manning, C. and White, P. (1995). Attitudes of employers to the mental ill, Psychiatr. Bull., 19, pp. 541 – 543.

Markowitz, S.B. (1998). *Environmental and Occupational Medicine*. ed. Rom, W.N., Chapter 3 "The role of surveillance in occupational health," (Lippincott-Raven Publishers, Philadelphia), pp. 19 – 29.

Maron, D, Ridker P. and Pearson, T. (1998). *Hurst's The Heart, Arteries and Veins*, 9th Ed., eds. Alexander, R. and Hurst, W., Chapter "Risk factors and the prevention of coronary heart disease," (McGraw Hill, New York), pp. 1175 – 1195.

Martin, F., Siddle, D.A.T., Gourley, M., Taylor, J. and Dick, R. (1992). P300 and traffic scenes: The effect of temazepam, Biol. Psychol., 33, pp. 225 – 240.

Martin, M., Williams, R.M. and Clark, D.M. (1991). Does anxiety lead to selective processing of threat-related information? Behav. Res., 29, pp. 147 – 160.

Marzano, C., Ferrara, M., Sforza, E. and De Gennaro, L. (2008). Quantitative electroencephalogram (EEG) in Insomnia: A new window on pathophysiological mechanisms, Curr. Pharmaceut. Des., 14, pp. 3446 – 3455.

Maslach, C., Schaufeli, W.B. and Leiter, M.P. (2001). Job burnout, Annu. Rev. Psychol., 52, pp. 397–422.

Maslach, C., Jackson, S.E. and Leiter, M.P. (1996). *Maslach Burnout Inventory Manual*. 3rd Ed. (Consulting Psychology Press, Palo Alto).

Maslach, C. and Leiter, M.P. (2008). Early predictors of job burnout and engagement, J. Appl. Psychol., 93, pp. 498–512.

Mason, L., O'Sullivan, N., Blackburn, M., Bentall, R. and El-Deredy, W. (2012). I want it now! Neuronal correlates of hypersensitivity to immediate reward in Hypomania, Biol. Psychiatry, 71 pp. 530 – 537.

Mathalon, D. and Ford, J. (2002). The long and short of it: influence of interstimulus interval on auditory P300 abnormalities in schizophrenia, Clin Electroencephalogr., 33, pp. 125 – 135.

McCallum, W.C. and Abraham, P. (1973). The contingent negative variation in psychosis. Electroenceph. Clin. Neurophysiol Suppl 33, pp. 329 – 335.

McCallum, W., Cooper, R. and Pocock, P. (1988). Brain slow potential and ERP changes associated with operator load in a visual tracking. EEG. Clin. Neurophysiol., 69, pp. 453 – 468.

McCarthy, G. and Donchin, E. (1981). A metric for thought: A comparison of P300 latency and reaction time, Science, 211, pp. 77 – 80.

McEwen, B.S. (1998). Protective and damaging effects of stress mediators, New Engl. J. Med., 338, pp. 171 – 179.

McFarlane, A.C., Weber, D.L. and Clark, C.R. (1993). Abnormal stimulus processing in posttraumatic stress disorder, Biol. Psychiatry, 34, pp. 311 – 320.

McMichael, A.J. (1976) Standardized mortality ratios and the "healthy worker effect". Scratching the surface, J. Occup. Med., 18, pp. 165–168.

Medin, J., Barajas, J. and Ekberg, K. (2006). Stroke patients' experiences of return to work, Disab Rehab., 28, pp. 1051 – 1060.

Meijman, T.F. and Mulder, G. (1998) *Handbook of Work and Organizational Psychology*, eds. Drenth, P.J., Thierry, H., and de Wolff, C.J., Chapter "Psychological aspects of workload," (Psychology Press Ltd., Hove) pp. 5 – 33.

Melamed, S., Kristal-Boneh, E., Harari, G., Froom, P. and Ribak, J. (1998). Variation in the ambulatory blood pressure response to daily work load--the moderating role of job control, Scand. J. Work Environ. Health, 24, pp. 190–196.

Melamed, S., Shirom, A.,Toker, S., Berliner, S. and Shapira, I. (2006). Burnout and risk of cardiovascular disease: Evidence, possible causal paths, and promising research directions, Psych. Bull., 132, pp. 327 – 353.

Merkel, J. (1885). Die zeitlichen Verhaltrisse der Willenstatigkeit, Philosophie Studion, 2, pp. 73 – 127.

Messing, K. (2000) *Women's Health*, eds., Goldman, M.B., and Hatch, M.C., Chapter 36 "Multiple roles and complex exposures: hard-to-pin-down risks for working women," (Academic Press, San Diego) pp. 455 - 462.

Messing, K., Seifert, A.M. and Escalona, E. (1997). The 120-S minute: using analysis of work activity to prevent psychological distress among elementary school teachers, J. Occup. Health. Psychol., 2, pp. 45–62.

Messing, T. (2008). *Händelser vid Ratten* (Tine Messing, Visby).

Metzger, L., Carson, M., Paulus, L., Lasko, N., Paige, S., Pitman, R. and Orr, S.P. (2002). Event-related potentials to auditory stimuli in female Vietnam nurse veterans with post-traumatic stress disorder, Psychophysiology, 39, pp. 46 – 63.

Mezuk, B., Bohnert, A., Ratliff, S. and Zivin, K. (2011). Job strain, depressive symptoms and drinking behavior among older adults: Results from the Health and Retirement Study, J. Gerontology, 66, pp. 426–434.

Michaels, D. and Zoloth, S.R. (1991). Mortality among urban bus drivers, Int. J. Epidemiol., 20, pp. 399–404.

Michie, S., and Cockcroft, A. (1996). Overwork can kill: especially if combined with high demand, low control, and poor social support, BMJ., 312, pp. 921 – 922.

Miller, G.A., Simons, R.F. and Lang, P.J. (1984). Electrocortical measures of information processing deficit in anhedonia, Ann. N.Y. Acad. Sci., 425, pp. 598 – 602.

Miller, S.C., Pandi, P., Esquifino, A., Cardinali, D. and Maestroni, G. (2006). The role of melatonin in immuno-enhancement: potential application in cancer, Int. J. Exp. Path., 87, pp. 81 – 87.

Milutinović, D., Golubović, B., Brkić, N. and Prokeš, B. (2012). Professional stress and health among critical care nurses in Serbia. Arh. Hig. Rada Toksikol., 63, pp. 171–180.

Mizock, L. (2012). The double stigma of obesity and serious mental illnesses: promoting health and recovery, Psychiatr. Rehabil. J., 35, pp. 466 – 469.

Mokran, V., Ciganek, L. and Kabatnik Z. (1971). Electroencephalographic theta discharges in the midline. Eur. Neurol. 5, pp. 288 – 293.

Molloy, R. and Parasuraman, R. (1996). Monitoring an automated system for a single failure: vigilance and task complexity effects, Human Factors, 38, pp. 311 – 322.

Morikawa, Y., Nakagawa, H., Ishizaki, M., Tabata, M., Nishijo, M., Miura, K., Kawano, S., Kido, T., and Nogawa, K. (1997). Ten-year follow-up study on the relation between the development of non-insulin-dependent diabetes mellitus and occupation, Am. J. Ind. Med., 31, pp. 80 – 84.

Morikawa, Y., Nakagawa, H., Miura, K., Ishizaki, M., Tabata, M., Nishijo, M., Higashiguchi, K., Yoshita, K., Sagara, T., Kido, T., Naruse, Y. and Nogawa, K.

(1999) Relationship between shift work and onset of hypertension in a cohort of manual workers, Scand. J. Work Environ. Health, 25, pp. 100 – 104.

Morris, J., Kagan, A., Pattison, D., Gardner, M. and Raffle, P. (1966). Incidence and prediction of ischaemic heart disease in London busmen, Lancet, 2, pp. 553–559.

Morselli, P.L., Elgie, R. and Cesana, B.M. (2004). GAMIAN-Europe/BEAM survey II: cross-national analysis of unemployment, family history, treatment satisfaction and impact of the bipolar disorder on life style, Bipolar Disord., 6, pp. 487 – 497.

Moruzzi, G. and Magoun, H.W. (1979). Brainstem reticular formation and activation of the EEG. EEG Clin. Neurophysiol. 1, pp. 455 – 473.

Mulder, G. and van der Meulen, M. (1973). Mental load and the measurement of heart rate variability. Ergonomics, 16, pp. 69 – 83.

Mulder, G. and Wijers, A.A. (1991). Selective attention and mental chronometry, Electroencephalogr. Clin. Neurophysiol., Suppl. 42, pp. 228 – 243.

Mullan, R.J. and Murthy, L.K. (1991).Occupational sentinel health events: an updated list for physician recognition and public health surveillance, Am. J. Ind. Med., 19, pp. 775 –799.

Murata, K., Araki, S., Yokoyama, K., Uchida, E. and Fujimura, Y. (1993). Assessment of central, peripheral and autonomic nervous system functions in lead workers: neuroelectrophysiologic studies, Environ. Res. 61, pp. 323 – 336.

Mustard, C., Bielecky, A., Etches, J., Wilkins, R., Tjepkema, M., Amick, B.C., Smith, P.M., Gnam W.H. and Aronson, K.J. (2010). Suicide mortality by occupation in Canada, 1991-2001, Can. J. Psychiatry, 55, pp. 369–376.

Muzi, G. Locati, E. H., Murgia, N. Ambrosio, G. and Abbritti, G. (2004). Evaluation of the effects of occupational noxae on the cardiovascular system, Med. Lav., 95, pp. 145 – 57.

Myers, A.H., Baker, S.P., Li, G., Smith, G.S., Wiker S, Liang, K-Y. and Johnson, J.V. (1999). Back injury in municipal workers: A case-control study, Am. J. Public Health, 89, pp. 1036–1041.

Näätänen, R. and Alho, K. (1995). Mismatch negativity-a unique measure of sensory processing in audition, Int. J. Neurosci., 80, pp. 317 – 337.

Nagel-Leiby, S., Dandrea, G., Grunfeld, S. and Brown, E. (1990). Event-related slow potential and associated catecholamine function in migraine, Cephalgia, 10, pp. 317 – 329.

Nakata, A. (2011). Work hours, sleep sufficiency, and prevalence of depression among full-time employees: a community-based cross-sectional study, J. Clin. Psychiatry, 72, pp. 605–614.

Natelson, B.H. (1985). Neurocardiology: An interdisciplinary area for the 80s, Arch. Neurol., 42, pp. 178 – 184.

Natelson, B. and Chang, Q. (1993). Sudden death: A neurocardiologic phenomenon. Neurol. Clin., 11, pp. 293 – 308.

Nedić, O. (2006a). Occupational Stressors and Physician Health with a Focus upon Cardiovascular Disease, PhD Thesis, Medical Faculty of the University of Novi Sad, Novi Sad, 228p.

Nedić, O. (2006 b). Restoring dignity and respect to health care workers, Med. Pregl., 59, 515–521.

Nedić, O., Belkić, K., Filipović, D. and Jocić, N. (2008a). Gender as an important effect modifier between exposure to work stressors among physicians of various specialties and the occurence of cardiovascular disease, Med. Pregl. 61, pp. 343–349.

Nedić, O., Belkić, K., Filipović, D. and Jocić, N. (2008b). Work stressors among physicians with the acquired cardiovascular disorders. Assessment using the occupational stress index, Med, Pregl., 61, pp. 226 – 234.

Nedić, O., Belkić, K., Filipović, D., and Jocić, N. (2010). Job Stressors among female physicians: Relation to having a clinical diagnosis of hypertension, Int. J. Occup. Environ. Health, 16, pp. 330–340.

Nedić, O., Filipović, D. and Solak, Z. (2001). Job stress and cardiovascular diseases among health workers, Med. Pregl., 54, pp. 423–431.

Neerincx, M.A. and Griffioen, E. (1996). Cognitive task analysis: harmonizing tasks to human capacities, Ergonomics, 39, pp. 543 – 561.

Nelson, D.L., Burke, R.J. and Michie, S. (2002). *Gender, Work Stress and Health.* eds. Nelson, D.L. and Burke, R.J., Chapter 14 "New directions for studying gender, work stress, and health," (American Psychological Association, Washington D.C.) pp. 229 - 242.

Nerrière, E., Vercambre, M.N., Gilbert, F. and Kovess-Masfety, V. (2009). Voice disorders and mental health in teachers: a cross-sectional nationwide study, BMC Public Health, 9, 370 doi: 10.1186/1471-2458-9-370.

Netterstrøm, B. and Juel, K. (1988). Impact of work-related and psychosocial factors on the development of ischemic heart disease among urban bus drivers in Denmark, Scand. J. Work. Environ. Health, 14, pp. 231 – 238.

Netterstrøm, B., and Juel, K.(1990). Peptic ulcer among urban bus drivers in Denmark, Scand. J. Soc. Med., 18, pp. 97 – 102.

Netterstrøm, B., Kristensen, T., Damsgaard, M., Olsen, O. and Sjol, A. (1991). Job strain and cardiovascular risk factors: A cross sectional study of employed Danish men and women. Br. J. Indust. Med., 48, pp. 684–689.

Niedhammer, I., Goldberg, M., Leclerc, A., Bugel, I. and Landre, M.F. (1998). Psychosocial work environment and cardiovascular risk factors in an occupational cohort in France, J. Epidemiol. Commun. Health, 52, pp. 93–100.

Nielsen, M., Bültmann, Madsen, I., Martin, M., Christensen, U., Diderichsen, F. and Rugulies, R. (2012). Health, work and personal-related predictors of time to return to work among employees with mental health problems, Disab. Rehab., 34, pp. 1311 – 1316.

Noordik, E., van der Klink, J.J., Geskus, R.B., de Boer, M.R., van Dijk, F.J.H. and Nieuwenhuijsen, K. (2012). Effectiveness of an exposure-based return-to-work program for workers on sick leave due to common mental disorders: a cluster-randomized controlled trial, Scand. J. Work Environ. Health, doi: 10.5271/sjweh.3320.

Nordmark, B., Blomqvist, P., Andersson, B., Hägerström, M., Nordh-Grate, K., Rönnqvist, R., Svensson, H. and Klareskog, L. (2006). A two-year follow-up of work capacity in early rheumatoid arthritis: a study of multidisciplinary team care with emphasis on vocational support, Scand. J. Rheumatol., 35, pp. 7 – 14.

Norman, C. (2006). The Fountain House movement, an alternative rehabilitation model for people with mental health problems, Scand. J. Caring Sci. 20, pp. 184 – 192.

Norrefalk, J., Linder, J., Ekholm, J. and Borg, K. (2007). A 6-year follow-up study of 122 patients attending a multiprofessional rehabilitation programme for persistent musculoskeletal-related pain, Int. J. Rehab. Res., 30, pp. 9 – 18.

Nyssen, A.S., Hansez, I., Baele, P., Lamy, M. and De Keyser, V. (2003). Occupational stress and burnout in anaesthesia, Br. J. Anaesthesia, 90, pp. 333–337.

Nyström, L., Kolmodin-Hedman, B., Jonsson, E. and Thomasson, L. (1990). Mortality from circulatory diseases, especially ischaemic heart disease in sea pilots and boatmen in Sweden 1951-1984: a retrospective cohort study, Br. J. Indust. Med., 47, pp. 122–126.

Öhman, A. (1986). Face the beast and fear the face: animal and social fears as prototypes for evolutional analyses of emotion, Psychophysiology, 23, pp. 123 – 145.

Oksanen, T., Vahtera, J., Westerlund, H., Pentti, J., Sjösten, N., Virtanen, M., Kawachi, I. and Kivimäki, M. (2011). Is retirement beneficial for mental health? Antidepressant use before and after retirement. Epidemiology, 22, pp. 553–559.

Olkinuora, M., Asp, S., Juntunen,J., Kauttu, K., Strid, L. and Äärimaa, M. (1992). Stress symptoms, burnout and suicidal thoughts of Finnish physicians, Scand. J. Work Environ. Health, 18 Suppl 2, pp. 110–112.

Orris, P., Hartman, D.E., Strauss, P., Anderson, R.J., Collins, J., Knopp, C., Xu, Y. and Melius, J. (1997). Stress among package truck drivers, Am. J. Indust. Med., 31, pp. 202 – 210.

Orrison, W.W., Lewine, J.D, Sanders, J.A. and Jartshoren, M.F. (1995). *Functional Brain Imaging*, (Mosby, St. Louis).

Ostojić,P., Zivojinović, S., Reza, T. and Damjanov, N. (2010). Symptoms of depression and anxiety in Serbian patients with systemic sclerosis. Impact of disease severity and socioeconomic factors, Mod. Rheumatol., 20, pp. 353 – 357.

Oyama, I., Kubo, T., Fujino, Y., Kadowaki, K., Kunimoto, M., Shirane, K., Tabata, H., Sabanai, K., Nakamura, T. and Matsuda, S. (2012). Retrospective cohort study of the risk of impaired glucose tolerance among shift workers, Scand. J. Work Environ. Health, 38, pp. 291–297.

Palmer, K.T., and Greenough, C.G. (2007). *Fitness for Work: The Medical Aspects* 4th Ed., eds. Palmer, K.T., Cox, R.A.F., and Brown, I., Chapter 11 "Spinal disorders," (Oxford University Press, Oxford) pp. 233 – 260.

Palmer, K.T. and Pearson, S.B. (2007). *Fitness for Work: The Medical Aspects* 4th Ed., eds. Palmer, K.T., Cox, R.A.F., and Brown, I., Chapter 18 "Respiratory disorders," (Oxford University Press, Oxford) pp. 401 – 427.

Papart, P., Ansseau, M., Devoitille, J.M., Manatanus, M. and Timsit-Berthier, M.(1990). *Psychiatry: a world perspective*. eds. Stephanis CN, Rabavilas AD, Soldatos CR, Chapter "Contingent negative variation and severity of depression," (Elsevier Science, Amsterdam) pp. 402 – 408.

Pas, E.T., Bradshaw, C.P. and Hershfeldt, P.A. (2012). Teacher- and school-level predictors of teacher efficacy and burnout: identifying potential areas of support, J. School Psychology, 50, pp. 129 –145.

Pavlov, I.P. (1951). *Complete collected works*. (Moscow-Leningrad) 1951.

Pelfrene, E., Vlerick, P., Moreau, M., Mak, R., Kornitzer, M. and De Backer, G. (2004). Use of benzodiazepine drugs and perceived job stress in a cohort of working men and women in Belgium. Results form the BELSTRESS-study, Soc. Sci. Med., 59, pp. 433–442.

Pellouchoud, E., Smith, M., McEvoy, L. and Gevins, A. (1999). Mental effort-related EEG modulation during video-game play: comparison between juvenile subjects with epilepsy and normal control subjects, Epilepsia, 40(Suppl. 4) , pp. 38 – 43.

Perakis, C.R. (2010). Soul sickness: a frequently missed diagnosis, J. Am. Osteopath. Assoc. 110, pp. 347–349.

Peter, R., Alfredsson, L., Hammar, N., Siegrist, J., Theorell, T. and Westerholm, P. (1998). High effort, low reward and cardiovascular risk factors in employed Swedish men and women: Baseline results from the WOLF study, J. Epidemiol. Community Health, 52, pp. 540–547.

Peter, R., Siegrist, J., Stork, J., Mann, H. and Labrot, B. (1991). Cigarette smokers and psychosocial work stress in middle managers, Soz. Präventiv. Med., 36, pp. 315–321.

Peter, R. and Siegrist, J. (1997). Chronic work stress, sickness absence, and hypertension in middle managers: General and specific sociological explanations? Soc. Sci. Med., 45, pp. 1111–1120.

Peter, R., Siegrist, J., Hallqvist, J., Reuterwall, C., Theorell, T. and the SHEEP Study Group. (2002). Psychosocial work environment and myocardial infarction: improving risk estimation by combining two complementary job stress models in the SHEEP study, J. Epidemiol. Community Health, 56:294–300.

Petersen, M.R. and Burnett, C.A. (2008). The suicide mortality of working physicians and dentists. Occup. Med. (London), 58, pp. 25–29.

Pfurtscheller, G., Neuper, C. and Mohl, W. (1994). Event-related desynchronization (ERD) during visual processing, Int. J. Psychophysiol., 16, pp. 147 – 153.

Pickering, T., Shimbo, D. and Haas, D. (2006). Ambulatory blood pressure monitoring, New Engl. J. Med. 354, pp. 2368 – 2374.

Pikhart, H., Bobak, M., Pajak, A., Malyutina, S., Kubinova, R., and Marmot, M., (2002). An association between depression, effort-reward imbalance and job demand-control model in three post-Communist Countries. *3rd Int. Conf. Work Environment & Cardiovascular Diseases—ICOH.*

Piko, B.F. (2006). Burnout, role conflict, job satisfaction and psychosocial health among Hungarian health care staff: a questionnaire survey, Int. J. Nurs. Studies, 43, pp. 311 – 318.

Pokorny, M.L.I., Blom, D.H.J. and van Leeuwen, P. (1987). Shifts, duration of work and accident risk of bus drivers, Ergonomics, 30, pp. 61 – 88.

Polich, J. and Kok, A. (1995). Cognitive and biological determinants of P300: an integrative review, Biol. Psychol., 41, pp. 103 – 146.

Potter, B.A. (1987). *Preventing job burnout. Transforming work pressure into productivity.* (Crisp Publications, Inc., Menlo Park).

Pramuka, M., Hendrickson, R., Zinski, A. and Van Cott A.C. (2007). A psychosocial self-management program for epilepsy: A randomized pilot study in adults, Epilepsy Behav., 11, pp. 533 – 545.

Pransky, G., Berndt, E., Finkelstein, S., Verma, S. and Agrawal, A. (2005). Performance decrements results from illness in the workplace: The effect of headaches, J. Occup. Environ. Med., 47, pp. 34 – 40.

Price, A.E. and Petch, M.C., *Fitness for Work: The Medical Aspects* 4th Ed., eds. Palmer, K.T., Cox, R.A.F., and Brown, I., Chapter 17 "Cardiovascular disorders," (Oxford University Press, Oxford) pp. 381 – 399.

Prichep, L.S. (2005). Use of normative data bases and statistical methods in demonstrating clinical utility of QEEG: Importance and cautions, Clinical EEG Neurosci., 36, pp. 82 – 98.

Pro, J.D. (2005). *A Physician's Guide to Return to Work* eds. Talmage, J.B, Melhorn, J.M. and Hyman, M., Chapter 18 "Working with common psychiatric problems," (American Medical Association Press, Chicago) pp. 305 – 320.

Proctor, S.P., White, R.F., Robins, T.G., Echeverria, D. and Rocskay, A.Z. (1996). Effect of overtime work on cognitive function in automotive workers, Scand. J. Work. Environ. Health, 22, pp. 124 – 132.

Proulx, G.B. and Picton, T.W. (1984). The effects of anxiety and expectancy on the CNV, Ann. NY Acad. Sci., 425, pp. 617 – 622.

Punnett, L. and Bergqvist, U. (1997). Visual display unit work and upper extremity musculoskeletal disorders. A review of epidemiological findings. National Institute for Working Life—Ergonomic Expert Committee Document No. 1, 10, Stockholm.

Quesnel-Vallée, A., DeHaney, S. and Ciampi, A. (2010). Temporary work and depressive symptoms: A propensity score analysis, Soc. Sci. Med., 70, pp. 1982–1987.

Quinlan, M., Mayhew, C. and Bohle, P. (2001). The global expansion of precarious employment, work disorganization and consequences for occupational health: A review of recent research, Int. J. Health Services, 31, pp. 335 – 414.

Rafnsson, V. and Gunnarsdóttir, H. (1991). Mortality among professional drivers, Scand. J. Work Environ. Health, 17, pp. 312 – 317.

Ragland, D., Greiner, B., Holman, B. and Fisher, J. (1997). Hypertension and years of driving in transit vehicle operators, Scand. J. Soc. Med., 25, pp. 271–279.

Ragland, D., Greiner, B., Krause, N., Holman, B. and Fisher, J. (1995). Occupational and non-occupational correlated of alcohol consumption in urban transit operators, Prev. Med., 24, pp. 634–645.

Ragland, D., Winkleby, M., Schwalbe, J., Holman, B., Morse, L., Syme, S.L. and Fisher, J.M. (1987). Prevalence of hypertension in bus drivers, Int. J. Epidemiol., 16, pp. 208–214.

Rajalin, S. and Summala, H. (1997). What surviving drivers learn from a fatal road accident. Accid. Anal. Prev. 29, pp. 277 – 283.

Rantanen, J. (2000). Sven Hernberg—profile in high-quality research and publishing, Scand. J. Work Environ. Health, 26, pp. 1–3.

Ravitch, D. (2010). *The Death and Life of the Great American School System*, (Basic Books, USA).

Razmjou, S. (1996). Mental workload in heat: Toward a framework for analyses of stress states, Aviat. Space Environ. Med., 67, pp. 530 – 538.

Reed, D., LaCroix, A., Karasek, R., Miller, D. and MacLean C. (1989). Occupational strain and the incidence of coronary heart disease. Am J Epidemiol., 129, pp. 495–502.

Riecansky, J., Milichercik, J., Kasper, J., Zelenay, J. and Havlinova, K. (1988). Myocardial infarction at young age, Czech Med., 11, pp. 123–130.

Ritter, W., Vaughan, H.G. and Costa, L.D. (1968). Orienting and habituation to auditory stimuli: A study of short term changes in averaged evoked responses, Electroencephalogr. Clin. Neurophysiol., 25, pp. 550 – 556.

Roberts, R. and Lee, E. (1993). Occupation and the prevalence of major depression, alcohol and drug abuse in the United States, Environ. Res., 61, pp. 266–278.

Robroek, S., Schuring, M., Croezen, S., Stattin, M. and Burdorf A. (2012). Poor health, unhealthy behaviors and unfavorable work characteristics influence pathways of exit from paid employement among older workers in Europe: a four year follow-up study, Scand. J. Work Environ. Health, e-publication ahead of print, doi: 10.5271/sjweh.3319.

Roffwarg, H.P. (1979). Diagnostic classification of sleep and arousal disorders, Sleep, 2, pp. 1 – 137.

Rohmert, W. (1971). An international symposium on objective assessment of workload in air traffic control tasks: Introduction, Ergonomics, 14, pp. 545-547.

Rosenberg, R. and Godhramji, P.P. (2001). Is shift work making your patient sick? Emerging theories and therapies for treating shift work disorder, Postgrad. Med., 123, pp.106–115.

Rosengren, A., Anderson, K. and Wilhelmsen, L. (1991). Risk of coronary heart disease in middle-aged male bus and tram drivers compared to men in other occupations: A prospective study, Int. J. Epidemiol., 20, pp. 82–87.

Roth, T. (2012). Shift work disorder: Overview and diagnosis, J. Clin. Psychiatry, 73, e09.

Rothman, K.J. and Greenland, S. (1998) *Modern Epidemiology* eds. Rothman, K.J. and Greenland, S. 2nd Edition, Chapter 2 "Causation and causal inference" (Lippincott-Raven, Philadelphia) pp. 7–28.

Rotshtein, P., Pichardson, M.P., Winston, J.S., Kiebel, S.J., Vuilleumier, P., Eimer, M., Driver, J. and Dolan, R.J. (2010). Amygdala demage affects event-related potentials for fearful faces at specific time windows, Hum. Brain Mapp. 31, pp. 1089 – 1105.

Rozanski, A., Blumenthal, J.A. and Kaplan, J. (1999). Impact of psychological factors on the pathogenesis of cardiovascular diseases and implications for therapy, Circulation, 99, pp. 2192 – 2217.

Russek, H.I., and Zohman, B.I. (1958). Relative significance of heredity, diet, and occupational stress in coronary heart disease of young adults, Am. J. Med. Sci., 235, pp. 266 – 275.

Ryder, S.J. and Bird, H.A. (2007). *Fitness for Work: The Medical Aspects* 4th Ed., eds. Palmer, K.T., Cox, R.A.F., and Brown, I., Chapter 13 "Rheumatological disorders," (Oxford University Press, Oxford) pp. 294 – 310.

Rydstedt, L.W., Johansson, G., Evans, G.W. (1998). The human side of the road: Improving the working conditions of urban bus drivers, J. Occup. Health Psychology, 3, pp. 161 – 171

Saarni, H., Niemi, L., Koskela, R., Pentti, J., Hartiala, J. and Kuusela, A. (1996). Cardiac status and cardiovascular risk factors among Finnish sea pilots, Int. J. Occup. Med. Environ. Health, 9, pp. 53–58.

Sackett, D.L. (1979). Bias in analytic research, *J. Chron. Dis.*, 32, pp. 51 – 63.

Saijo, Y., Ueno, T. and Hashimoto, Y. (2007). Job stress and depressive symptoms among Japanese fire fighters. Am. J. Indust. Med., 50, pp. 470–480.

Saijo, Y., Ueno, T. and Hashimoto, Y. (2008). Twenty-four hour shift work, depressive symptoms and job dissatisfaction among Japanese firefighters. Am. J. Indust. Med., 51, pp. 380–391.

Saijo, Y., Ueno, T. and Hashimoto, Y. (2012). Post-traumatic stress disorder and job stress among firefighters of urban Japan. Prehospital Disaster Med., 27, pp. 59–63.

Salm, M. (2009). Does job loss cause ill health? Health Econ., 18, pp. 1075–1089.

Salo, P., Sivertsen, B., Hall, M., Pentti, J., Virtanen, M., Vahtera, J. and Kivimäki, M. (2010). Sleep disturbances as a predictor of cause-specific work disability and delayed return to work, Sleep, 33, pp. 1323 – 1331.

Sancho, F.N. and Ruiz, C.N. (2010). Risk of suicide amongst dentists: myth or reality? Int. Dental J., 60, pp. 411–418.

Sanderson, K., Nicholson, J., Graves, N., Tilse, E. and Oldenburg, B. (2008). Mental health in the workplace: Using the ICF to model the prospective associations between symptoms, activities, participation and environmental factors, Disab.Rehab., 30, pp. 1289 – 1297.

Sandmark, H. (2011). Health, sleep and professional career in female white-collar workers back to work after long-term sick-listing due to minor mental disorders, Scand. J. Public Health, 39, pp. 823 – 829.

Sansone, R.A. and Sansone, L.A. (2010), Demoralization in patients with medical illness, Psychiatry (Edgmont)., 7, pp. 42–45.

Saunders, D. (2006). The older anaesthetist, Best Practice Res. Clin. Anaesthesiol., 20, pp. 645-651.

Savić, Č. (2002). The physician and stress. *Proc. 17th Medical Meeting in Sombor Medical Society of Vojvodina*, pp. 52–54.

Savić, Č. (1993). Application of Cognitive-Evoked Potentials in an Occupational Group at High Risk for Developing Acquired Cardiovascular Disease. PhD Thesis, University of Priština, 114 p.

Savić, Č. and Belkić, K. (1995). *Central Stress Mechanisms and Cardiovascular Response: Clinical Neurophysiologic Investigations using Laboratory Simulation of Occupational Stressors,* (Savremena Administracija, Belgrade).

Savić, Č. and Belkić, K. (1998). *Event-related Potentials: Clinical Applications in Psychiatry and Neurology*, (Službeni List, Belgrade).

Savić, Č. and Rajšić, N. (1996). Eye closure epileptiform discharges among epileptic patients on treatment in the Institute for Mental Health in Belgrade, *2nd Eur. Cong. Epileptology*, p. 54.

Schernhammer, E.S. and Colditz, G.A. (2004). Suicide rates among physicians: a quantitative and gender assessment (meta-analysis), Am. J. Psychiatry, 161, pp. 2295–2302.

Schernhammer, E.S., Laden, F., Speizer, F.E., Willett, W., Hunter, D., Kawachi, I. and Colditz, G. (2001). Rotating night shifts and risk of breast cancer in the women participating in the nurses' health study, J. Natl. Cancer Inst., 93, pp. 1563–1568.

Schernhammer, E.S., Laden, F., Speizer, F.E., Willett, W.C., Hunter, D.J., Kawachi, I., Fuchs, C. and Colditz, G. (2003). Night-shift work and risk of colorectal cancer in the Nurses' Health Study, J. Natl. Cancer Inst., 95, pp. 825 – 828.

Schnall, P. and Belkić, K. (2000). Obtaining a CVD history: obstacles and challenges, Occup. Med. State of the Art Reviews, 15, pp. 189 – 190.

Schnall, P.L., Landsbergis, P.A. and Baker, D. (1994). Job strain and cardiovascular disease, Annu. Rev. Public Health, 15, pp. 381 – 411.

Schnall, P., Schwartz, J., Landsbergis, P., Warren, K. and Pickering, T.G. (1992). Relation between job strain, alcohol and ambulatory blood pressure, Hypertension, 19, pp. 488–494.

Schnall, P., Schwartz, J., Landsbergis, P., Warren, K. and Pickering, T.G. (1998). A longitudinal study of job strain and ambulatory blood pressure: results of a three year follow-up, Psychosom. Med., 60, pp. 697–706.

Schneiderman, N. (1978). *Coronary-Prone Behavior.* ed. Dembroski, T.M. Chapter "Animal models relating behavioral stress and cardiovascular pathology," (Springer-Verlag, New York) pp. 155-181.

Schonfeld, I.S. (1992). A longitudinal study of occupational stressors and depressive symptoms in first-year female teachers, Teaching, Teacher Educ., 31, pp. 151 – 158.

Schurman, S.J. and Israel, B.A. (1995). *Job Stress Interventions* eds. In: Murphy, L.R., Hurrell, J.J., Sauter, S.L. Puryear Keita, G. Chapter 16 "Redesigning work systems to reduce stress. A participatory action research approach to creating change," (American Psychological Association, Washington, D.C., 1995) pp. 235 – 263.

Schwartz, J.E. (2000). Imputation of job characteristics scores, Occup. Med. State of the Art Reviews, 15, pp. 172–175.

Schwartz, J., Belkić, K., Schnall, P. and Pickering, T. (2000) Mechanisms by which work stress may lead to hypertension and cardiovascular morbidity, Occup. Med. State of the Art Reviews, 15, pp. 121–132.

Schwartz, J., Pickering, T. and Landsbergis, P. (1996).Work-related stress and blood pressure: Current theoretical models and considerations from a behavioral medicine perspective, J. Occup. Health Psychol., 1, pp. 287–310.

Schweitzer, B. (1994). Stress and burnout in junior doctors, So. African Med. J., 84, pp. 352–354.

Seeman, T.E., McEwen, B.S., Rowe, J.W., and Singer, B.H. (2001). Allostatic load as a marker of cumulative biological risk: MacArthur studies of successful aging, Proc. National Acad. Sci., 98, pp. 4770 – 4775.

Sega, R., Cesana, G., Costa, G., Ferrario, M., Bombelli, M. and Mancia, G. (1998). Ambulatory blood pressure in air traffic controllers, Am. J. Hyperten., 11, pp. 208–212.

Selye, H. (1976) *Stress in Health and Disease*, (Butterworths, Boston).

Shafer, A. (2005). Meta-analysis of the brief psychiatric rating scale factor structure, Psychol. Assess., 17, pp. 324 - 335.

Shanafelt, T.D., Balch, C.M., Bechamps, G., Russell, T., Dyrbye, L., Satele, D., Collicott, P., Novotny, P., Sloan, J. and Freischlag, J. (2009). Burnout and career satisfaction among American surgeons, Ann. Surg., 250, pp. 463–471.

Shanafelt, T.D., Balch, C.M., Dyrbye, L., Bechamps, G., Russell, T., Satele, D., Rummans, T., Swartz, K., Novotny, P.J., Sloan, J. and Oreskovich, M.R. (2011). Suicidal ideation among American surgeons, Arch. Surg., 146, pp. 54–62.

Shanafelt, T.D., Boone, S., Tan, L., Dyrbye, L., Sotile, W., Satele, D., West, C.P., Sloan, J. and Oreskovich, M.R. (2012). Burnout and satisfaction with work-life balance among US physicians relative to the general US population, Arch. Intern. Med., 172, pp. 1377–1385.

Sherman, A.C., Edwards, D., Simonton, S. and Mehta, P. (2006). Caregiver stress and burnout in an oncology unit, Palliat. Support. Care, 4, pp. 65–80.

Shields, M. (1999). Long working hours and health. Health Rep., 11, pp. 33–48.

Shimomitsu, T. and Levi, L. (1992). Recent working life change in Japan, Eur. J. Public Health, 1992; 2, pp. 76 – 86.

Shimomitsu, T., and Odagiri, Y. (2000). Working life in Japan, Occup. Med. State of the Art Reviews, 15, pp. 280–281.

Shirom, A. (2011). *Handbook of Occupational Health Psychology*, eds. Campbell Quick, J. and Tetrick, L., Chapter 12, "Job-related burnout: A review of major research foci and challenges" (American Psychological Association, Washington D.C.) pp. 223 – 242.

Siegrist, J. (1996). Adverse health effects of high-effort/low-reward conditions, J. Occup. Health Psychol. 1, pp. 27–41.

Siegrist, J. and Peter, R. (1999). *Measuring Effort-Reward Imbalance:Guidelines*. (University of Düsseldorf, Düsseldorf).

Siegrist, J., Peter, R., Georg, W., Cremer, P. and Seidel, D. (1991). Psychosocial and biobehavioral characteristics of hypertensive men with elevated atherogenic lipids, Atherosclerosis, 86, pp. 211–218.

Simons, R.F. (1982). Physical anhedonia and future psychopathology: An electrocortical continuity? Psychophysiology, 19, pp. 433 – 441.

Singh, M., Clements, P., Furst, D., Maranian, P. and Khanna, D. (2012). Work productivity in scleroderma: analysis from the University of California, Los Angeles Scleroderma Quality of Life Study, Arthritis Care Res., 64, pp. 176 – 183.

Siniatchkin, M., Gerber-von Müller, G., Darabaneanu, S., Petermann, F., Stephani, U. and Gerber, W-D. (2010). Behavioural treatment programme contributes to normalization of contingent negative variation in children with migraine, Cephalalgia 31, pp. 562 – 572.

Singleton, W.T. (1974). *Introduction to Ergonomics*, (World Health Organization, Geneva).

Sirevaag, E.J., Kramer, A.F., Coles, M.G.H. and Donchin, E. (1984). P300 amplitude and resource allocation, Psychophysiology, 21, pp. 589 – 599.

Skov, T., Borg, V. and Orhede, E. (1996). Psychosocial and physical risk factors for musculoskeletal disorders of the neck, shoulders, and lower back in salespeople. Occup. Environ. Med. 53, pp. 351–356.

Slobounov, S.M., Fukada, K., Simon, R., Rearick, M. and Ray, W. (2000). Neurophysiologic and behavioral indices of time pressure effects on visuomotor task performance, Cogn. Brain Res., 9, pp. 287 – 298.

Sluiter, J.K., van der Beek, A.J., and Frings-Dresen, M.H.W. (1999). The influence of work characteristics on the need for recovery and experienced health. A study on coach drivers, Ergonomics, 42, pp. 573 – 583.

Smallwood Sherrer, Y. (2005). *A Physician's Guide to Return to Work* eds. Talmage, J.B, Melhorn, J.M. and Hyman, M., Chapter 17 "Working with common rheumatologic disorders," (American Medical Association Press, Chicago) pp. 289 – 304.

Smith, D., Devine, S., Leggat, P. and Ishitake, T. (2005). Alcohol and tobacco consumption among police officers. Kurume Med. J., 52, pp. 63–65.

Smith, G.F. and Toonen T.R. (2007). Primary care of the patient with cancer, Am. Fam. Physician, 75, pp. 207 –1214.

Sokejima, S. and Kagamimori, S. (1998).Working hours as a risk factor for acute myocardial infarction in Japan: case-control study, BMJ, 317, pp. 775 –780.

Sonnenschein, M., Sorbi, M., Verbraak, M., Schaufeli, W., Maas, C. and van Doornen, L. (2008). Influence of sleep on symptom improvement and return to work in clinical burnout, Scand. J. Work Environ. Health, 34, pp. 23 – 32.

Soteriades, E., Smith, D., Tsismenakis, A., Baur, D. and Kales, S. (2011). Cardiovascular disease in US firefighters, Cardiol. Rev., pp. 19: 202–215.

Speizer, F.E. (1998). *Harrison's Principles of Internal Medicine* 14th Ed., eds. Fauci, A., Martin, J., Braunwald, E., Kasper, D., Isselbache, K., Hauser, D., Wilson, J., Longo, D. and Jameson J., Chapter 254, "Environmental lung disease," (McGraw Hill, New York) pp. 1429 – 1436.

Spielberger, C.D., Gorusch, R.L., Lushene, P.R., Vagg, P.R. and Jacobs, A.G. (1983) *Manual for the State-Trait Anxiety Inventory STAI (Form Y)* (Consulting Psychologists Press, Inc. Palo Alto).

Spurgeon, A., Harrington, J.M. and Cooper, C.L. (1997). Health and safety problems associated with long working hours: a review of the current position, Occup. Environ. Med., 54, pp. 367–375.

Stack, S. (2004). Suicide risk among physicians: A multivariate analysis, Arch. Suicide Res., 8, pp. 284–292.

Stanford, M.S., Vasterling, J.J., Mathias, C.W., Constans, J.I. and Houston, R.J. (2001). Impact of threat relevance on P3 event-related potentials in combat-related post-traumatic stress disorder, Psychiatry Res.,102, pp. 125 – 137.

Stansfeld, S. and Candy, B. (2006). Psychosocial work environment and mental health—a meta-analytic review, Scand. J. Work Environ. Health, 32, pp. 443–62.

Steiger, A. and Kimura, M. (2010). Wake and sleep EEG provide biomarkers in depression. J. Psychiat. Res. 44, pp. 242 – 252.

Steinberg, J. (2011). *A Physician's Guide to Return to Work* 2nd Ed. eds. Talmage, J.B, Melhorn, J.M. and Hyman, M., Chapter 22 "Working with common psychiatric problems," (American Medical Association Press, Chicago) pp. 411 – 426.

Stewart, W.F., Lipton, R.B. and Simon, D. (1995). Work-related disability: results of the American migraine study, Cephalgia, 16, pp. 231 – 238.

Stokols, K., Allen, J. and Bellingham, R.L. (1996). The social ecology of health promotion: Implications for research and practice, Am. J. Health. Promot., 10, pp. 247 – 251.

Stokols, D., Pelletier, K. and Fielding, J. (1995). Integration of medical care and worksite health promotion, JAMA, 273 , pp. 1136 – 1142.

Strine, T.W., Kobau, R., Chapman., D.P., Thurman, D.J., Price, P. and Balluz, L.S. (2005). Psychological distress, comorbidities and health behaviors among US adults with seizures: results form the 2002 health survey interview. Epilepsia, 46, pp. 1133 – 1139.

Sudak, H., Maxim, K. and Carpenter, M. (2008). Suicide and stigma: A review of the literature and personal reflections, Acad. Psychiatry, 32, pp. 136–142.

Suetsugi, M., Mizuki, Y., Ushijima, I., Yamada, M. and Imaizumi, J. (1998). Anxiolytic effects of low-dose clomipramine in highly anxious healthy volunteers assessed by frontal midline theta activity. Prog. Neuro. Psychopharmacol. Biol. Psychiatry, 22, pp. 97 – 112.

Suetsugi, M., Mizuki, Y., Ushijima, I., Kobayashi, T., Tsuchiya, K., Aoki, T. and Watanabe, Y. (2000). Appearance of frontal midline theta activity in patients with generalized anxiety disorder, Neuropsychobiology, 41, pp. 108 – 112.

Sutton, S., Braren, M., Zubin, J. and John, E.R. (1965). Evoked potential correlates of stimulus uncertainty, Science, 150, pp. 1187 – 1188.

Sutton, S. and Ruchkin, D.S. (1984). The late positive complex: Advances and new problems, Ann. N. Y. Acad. Sci., 42, pp. 1 – 23.

Takeda, F. (1994). Depressive state and related factors in nursery teachers and guidance workers in homes for mentally retarded children, Japanese J. Indust. Health, 36, pp. 183–193.

Talmage, J. (2005). *A Physician's Guide to Return to Work* eds. Talmage, J.B, Melhorn, J.M. and Hyman, M., Chapter 19 "Working with common functional syndromes: Fibromyalgia and chronic fatigue syndrome," (American Medical Association Press, Chicago) pp. 321– 325.

Tamminga, S., de Boer, A., Verbeek, J. and Frings-Dres, M.H. (2012). Breast cancer survivors' views of factors that influence the return-to-work process-a qualitative study. Scand. J. Work Environ. Health, 38, pp. 144 – 154.

Task Force of the European Society of Cardiology and the North American Society of Pacing and Electrophysiology. (1996). Heart rate variability standards of measurement, physiological interpretation, and clinical use, Eur. Heart J. 17, pp. 354 – 381.

Tasto, D.L., Colligan, M.J., Skjei, E.W. and Polly, S.J. (1978). Health consequences of shift work. (National Institute of Occupational Safety & Health, US Department of Health Education and Welfare, Cincinnati).

Taylor, P.J. and Pocock, S.J. (1972). Mortality of shift and day workers 1956-1958, Br. J. Ind. Med., 29, pp. 201 – 207.

Teasdale, E.L. and Deahl, M.P., *Fitness for Work: The Medical Aspects* 4th Ed., eds. Palmer, K.T., Cox, R.A.F., and Brown, I., Chapter 7 "Mental health and psychiatric disorders," (Oxford University Press, Oxford) pp. 147 – 168.

Tecce, J.J., and Cattanach, L., (1987). *Electroencephalography Basic principles, clinical applications and related fields.* 2nd Ed. eds. Niedermeyer, E., and Lopes da Silva, F., Chapter "Contingent negative variation (CNV)," (Urban & Schwarzenberg, Baltimore-Munich) pp. 657 – 679.

Thelin, A. (1991). Morbidity in Swedish farmers, 1978-1983, according to national hospital records, Soc. Sci. Med., 32, pp. 305 – 309.

Theorell, T., Leymann, H. and Jodko, M. (1992). Person under train incidents: Medical consequences for subway drivers, Psychosom. Med., 54, pp. 480 – 488.

Theorell, T., Leymann, H., Jodko, M., Konarski, K., Norbeck, H.E. and Eneroth, P.E. (1994). Person under train incidents: from the subway driver's point of view-a prospective one-year follow-up study: The design, and medical and psychiatric data, Soc. Sci. Med., 38, pp. 471 - 475.

Theorell, T., Perski, A., Åkerstedt, T., Sigala, F., Ahlberg-Hulten, G., Svensson, J. and Eneroth, P. (1988). Changes in job strain in relation to changes in physiological states A longitudinal study, Scand. J. Work Environ. Health, 14, pp. 189–196.

Theorell, T., Perski, A., Orth-Gomér, K., Hamsten, A. and deFaire, U. (1991). The effects of the strain of returning to work on the risk of death after a first myocardial infarction before age of 45, Int. J. Cardiol., 30, pp. 61–67.

Tiedtke, C., Donceel, P., Knops, L., De´siron, H., Dierckx de Casterle, B. and de Rijk, A. (2012). Supporting return-to-Work in the face of legislation: Stakeholders' experiences with return-to-work after breast cancer in Belgium, J. Occup. Rehabil., 22, pp. 241 – 251.

The Tokyo Declaration (1998). The Tokyo Declaration on work-related stress and health in three postindustrial settings–the European Union, Japan and the United States of America, J. Tokyo Med. Univ., 56, pp. 760–767

Toomingas, A., Theorell, T., Michelsen, H. and Nordemar R. (1997). Associations between self-rated psychosocial work conditions and musculoskeletal symptoms and signs, Scand. J. Work Environ. Health, 23, pp. 130 – 139.

Torre, D.M., Wang, N.Y., Meoni, L.A., Young, J.H., Klag, M.J. and Ford, D.E. (2005). Suicide compared to other causes of mortality in physicians, Suicide Life Threat. Behav. 35, pp.146–153.

Tse, S. (2002). Practice guidelines: Therapeutic interventions aimed at assisting people with bipolar affective disorder achieve their vocational goals, Work, 19, pp. 167 – 179.

Tse S. and Yeats M. (2002). What helps people with bipolar affective disorder succeed in employment: Grounded theory approach, Work, 19, pp. 47 – 62.

Tüchsen, F. (1997). Stroke morbidity in professional drivers in Denmark 1981-1990, Int. J. Epidemiology, 26, pp. 989 – 994.

Tüchsen, F., (2000). High-risk occupations for cardiovascular disease, Occup. Med. State of the Art Reviews, 15, pp. 57 – 60.

Tüchsen, F., Hannerz, H., Roepstorff, C., and Krause, N. (2006). Stroke among male professional drivers in Denmark 1994-2003, Occup. Environ. Med. 63, pp. 456 – 460.

Tunc, T. and Kutanis, R.O. (2009). Role conflict, role ambiguity, and burnout in nurses and physicians at a university hospital in Turkey, Nurs. Health Sci., 11, pp.410–416.

Tyssen, R. (2007). Health problems and use of health services among physicians, Ind. Health. 45, pp. 599–610.

Uchiyama, S., Kurasawa, T., Sekizawa, T. and Nakatsuka, H. (2005). Job strain and risk of cardiovascular events in treated hypertensive Japanese workers: hypertension follow-up group study, J. Occup. Health, 47, pp. 102–111.

Uglješić, M., Belkić, K., Bošković, S., Avramović, D. and Micković, Lj. (1992). Rise in arterial blood pressure during work and risk factor profile of workers in stressful occupations, Kardiologija, 13, pp. 150–154.

Uglješić, M., Belkić, K., Simeunovic-Micković, Lj. and Vukajlović, M. (1992). Implementation of a plan for cardiac prevention among professional drivers as a high-risk group, Srp. Arh. Lek. 120 (Suppl. 1), pp. 49 – 51.

Ullsperger, P., Metz, A.M. and Gille, H.G. (1988). The P300 component of the event-related potential and mental effort, Ergonomics, 31, pp.1127 – 1137.

U.S. Department of Labor. (1948). The performance of physically impaired workers in manufacturing industries. U.S. Department of Labor Bulletin No. 293, (US Government Printing Office, Washington, D.C.).

Vahtera, J. and Pentti J. (1996). The effect of objective job demands on registered sickness absence spells: do personal, social and job-related resources act as moderators? Work & Stress, 10, pp. 286–308.

van Amelsvoort, L.G.P.M. (1995). Coronary heart disease among truck drivers. Report of the International Workshop on the Epidemiology of Coronary Heart Disease among European Truck Drivers (European Commission, Bilthoven).

van der Berghe, R. and Huberman, A.M. (1999). *Understanding and preventing teacher burnout. A Sourcebook of International Research and Practice,* (Cambridge University Press, Cambridge).

van der Hulst, M. (2003). Long workhours and health, Scand. J. Work Environ. Health, 29, pp. 171–188

Van Dijk, F.J.H. (1995). Work-related musculoskeletal and mental disorders. Central Europ. J. Occup. Environ. Med., 1, pp. 292 – 305.

van Dujin, M., Lötters, F., and Burdorf, A. (2005). Influence of modified work on return to work for employees on sick leave due to musculoskeletal complaints, J. Rehabil. Med., 37, pp. 172 – 179.

van Loon, A., Tihjuis, M., Surtees, P. and Ormel, J. (2000). Lifestyle risk factors for cancer: the relationship with psychosocial work environment, Int. J. Epidemiol., 29, pp. 785–792.

van Luijtelaar, G., Verbraak, M., van den Bunt, M., Keijsers, G. and Arns M. (2010). EEG findings in burnout patients, J Neuropsychiatry Clin. Neurosci., 22, pp. 208–217.

Van Winsum, W., Sergeant, J. and Geuze, R. (1984). The functional significance of event-related desynchronization of alpha rhythm in attentional and activating tasks, EEG Clin. Neurophysiol., 58, pp. 519 – 524.

Vedantham, K., Brunet, A., Boyer, R., Weiss, D.S., Metzler, T.J., and Marmar, C.R. (2001). Posttraumatic stress disorder, trauma exposure, and the current health of Canadian bus drivers, Can. J. Psychiatry, 46, pp. 149–155.

Ventura, J., Lukoff, D., Nuechterlein, K., Liberman, R., Green, M. and Shaner, A. (1993). Manual for the Expanded Brief Psychiatric Rating Scale, Int. J. Methods Psychiatr. Res., 3, pp. 227 – 244.

Vercambre, M-N., Brosselin, P., Gilbert, F. and Nerrière, E. (2009). Individual and contextual covariates of burnout: a cross-sectional nationwide study of French teachers, BMC Public Health, 9, 333 (12 pages).

Verrotti, A., Striano, P., Belcastro, V., Matricardi, S., Villa, M.P. and Parisi, P. (2011). Migralepsy and related conditions: Advances in pathophysiology and classification, Seizure, 20 pp. 271 – 275.

Villarem, D., Thieuleux, F., LaBlanche, J., Tilmant, P. and Bertrand, M. (1982). Myocardial infarction in subjects less than 30 years of age, Ann. Cardiol. Angeiol., 31, pp. 263–268.

Vlahov, D., Galea, S., Ahern, J., Resnick, H., Boscarino, J., Gold, J., Bucuvalas, M. and Kilpatrick, D. (2004). Consumption of cigarettes, alcohol and marijuana among

New York City residents 6 months after the September 11 terrorist attacks. Am. J. Drug Alcohol Abuse, 30, pp. 385–407.

Vlasveld, M., van der Feltz-Cornelis, C., Adèr, H., Anema, J., Hoedeman, R., van Mechelen, W. and Beekman, A. (2012). Collaborative care for sick-listed workers with major depressive disorder: a randomized controlled trial from the Netherlands Depression Initiative aimed at return to work and depressive symptoms, Occup. Environ. Med., doi: 10.1136/oemed-2012-100793.

Volpert, W. (1982). *Cognitive and Motivational Aspects of Action*. eds. Hacker, W., Volpert, W. and von Cranach, M. Chapter "The model of hierarchical-sequential organization of action," (North-Holland, Amsterdam), pp. 35 – 51.

Von Thiele, U., Lindfors, P. and Lundberg, U. (2006). Self-rated recovery from work stress and allostatic load in women, J. Psychosom. Res., 61, pp.237 – 242.

Voss. M., Floderus, B. and Diderichsen F. (2004). How do job characteristics, family situation, domestic work and lifestyle factors relate to sickness absence? A study based on Sweden Post, J. Occup. Environ. Med., 46, pp. 1134–1143.

Waclawski, E.R. (1989). Employment and diabetes: a survey of the prevalence of diabetic workers known by occupational physicians, and the restrictions placed on diabetic workers in employment, Diabetic Med., 6, pp. 16 – 19.

Waclawski, E.R. and Gill, G.V. (2007). *Fitness for Work: The Medical Aspects* 4th Ed., eds. Palmer, K.T., Cox, R.A.F., and Brown, I., Chapter 15 "Diabetes and other endocrine disorders," (Oxford University Press, Oxford) pp. 345 – 360.

Wada, K., Kawata, Y., Murakami, T., Kamata, A., Zhu, G., Mizuno, K., Okada, M. and Kaneko, S. (2001). Sociomedical aspects of epileptic patients: Their employment and marital status. Psychiatry Clin. Neurosci., 55, pp. 141–146.

Wagner, D., Heinrichs, M. and Ehlert, U. (1998). Prevalence of symptoms of posttraumatic stress disorder in German professional firefighters, Am. J. Psychiatry, 155, pp. 1727–1732.

Waldenström, K. and Härenstam, A. (2008). Does the job demand-control model correspond to externally assessed demands and control for both women and men? Scand. J. Public Health, 36, pp. 242–249.

Waldron, H.A. (1996). Sickness in the medical profession, Ann. Occup. Hyg., 40, pp. 391–396.

Walitzer, K.S. and Sher, K.J. (1996). A prospective study of self-esteem and alcohol use disorders in early adulthood: evidence for gender differences, Alcohol. Clin. Exp. Res., 20, pp.1118 – 1124.

Walton, P., Callaway, E., Halliday, R. and Naylor, H. (1987). Stimulus intensity, contrast, and complexity have additive effects on P300 latency, Electroencephalogr. Clin. Neurophysiol. Supplement No.40, pp. 284 – 292.

Wang, J.L. (2006). Perceived work stress, imbalance between work and family/personal lives and mental disorders, Soc. Psychiatry Psychiatr. Epidemiol., 4155, pp. 541–548.

Wang, J.L., Patten, S.B., Currie, S., Sareen, J. and Schmitz N. (2012). A population-based longitudinal study on work environmental factors and the risk of major depressive disorder, Am. J. Epidemiol., 176, pp. 52–59.

Wang, J.L., Smailes, E., Sareen, J., Schmitz, N., Fick, G. and Patten, S. (2012). Three job-related stress models and depression: a population-based study, Soc. Psychiatry Psychiatr. Epidemiol., 47, pp.185–193.

Watson, M., Haviland, J.S., Greer, S., Davidson, J. and Bliss, J.M. (1999). Influence of psychological response on survival in breast cancer: a population-based cohort study, Lancet, 354, pp. 1331 – 1336.

Wehr, T. (2000) *Kaplan & Sadock's Comprehensive Textbook of Psychiatry.* 7th Ed. eds. Sadock, B.J. and Sadock, V.A. Chapter 1.13 "Chronobiology," (Lippincott Williams & Wilkins, Philadelphia) pp.133–142.

Weinstein, A.M. (1995). Visual ERPs evidence for enhanced processing of threatening information in anxious university students, Biol. Psychiatry, 37, pp. 847 – 858.

Welford, A.T. (1960). The measurement of sensory-motor performance: Survey and reappraisal of twelve years' progress, Ergonomics, 3, pp. 189 – 230.

Wenckebach, K.R. and Winterberg, H. (1927). *Die Unregelmassige Hertzatigkend.* (Engelman, Leipzig).

Wennberg, A., Iregren, A., Struwe, G., Cizinsky, G., Hagman, M. and Johansson, L. (1991). Manganese exposure in steel smelters: A health hazard to the nervous system, Scand. J. Work Environ. Health, 17, pp. 255 – 262.

Westman, M. and Eden, D. (1997). Effects of a respite from work on burnout: vacation relief and fade-out, J. Appl. Psychol., 82, pp. 516 – 527.

Westman, M., Eden, D. and Shirom, A. (1985). Job stress, cigarette smoking and cessation: the conditioning effects of peer support, Soc. Sci. Med., 20, pp. 637 – 644.

Westmoreland, B. and Klass, D. (1986). Midline theta rhythm, Arch. Neurol. 43, pp. 139 – 141.

Wieclaw, J., Agerbo, E., Mortensen, P.B., Burr, H., Tüchsen, F. and Bonde, J.P. (2008). Psychosocial working conditions and the risk of depression and anxiety disorders in the Danish workforce. BMC Public Health, 8, 280 doi:10.1186/1471-2458-8-280.

Willcox, R., and Hardy, R.J., (2007). *Fitness for Work: The Medical Aspects* 4th Ed., eds. Palmer, K.T., Cox, R.A.F., and Brown, I., Chapter 6 "Neurological disorders," (Oxford University Press, Oxford) pp. 105 – 146.

Winkleby, M., Ragland, D., Fisher, J. and Syme, S. (1988). Excess risk of sickness and disease in bus drivers: a review and synthesis of epidemiological studies, Int. J. Epidemiol., 17, pp. 255–262.

Wirtz, A., Lombardi, D.A., Willetts, J.L., Folkard, S. and Christiani, D.C. (2012). Gender differences in the effect of weekly working hours on occupational injury risk in the United States working population, Scand. J. Work. Environ. Health, doi:10.5271/sjweh.3295.

Woestenburg, J., Kramer, C., Orlebeke, J., and Passchier, J. (1993) Brain potential differences related to spatial attention in migraineurs with and without aura symptoms support supposed differences in activation, Headache, 33, pp. 413 – 416.

Wolf, M.M., Varigos, G.A., Hunt, D. and Sloman, J.G. (1978). Sinus arrhythmia in acute myocardial infarction, Med. J. Australia, 2, pp. 52 – 53.

Wolf, S. (1995). Discrete, patterned and purposeful adaptive physiological adjustments integrated by forebrain influences, Integ. Physiol. Behav. Sci., 30, pp. 190-20.

Wolf, S. and Belkić, K. (2000). The central nervous system: bridge between the external milieu and the cardiovascular system, Occup. Med. State of the Art Reviews, 15, pp. 107 – 116.

Wolfersdorf, M. (2007). Suicide and suicide prevention for female and male physicians, MMW Fortschr. Med. 149, pp. 34 – 36.

Woodside, H., Schell, L. and Allison-Hedges, J. (2006). Listening for recovery: the vocational success of people living with mental illness, Can. J. Occup. Ther., 73, pp. 36 – 43.

World Health Organization. (1993). *The ICD-10 Classification of Mental and Behavioural Disorders: Diagnostic Criteria for Research* (World Health Organization, Geneva).

Wu, S., Schuler, T., Edwards, M., Yang, H-C. and Brothers B. (2012). Factor analytic and item response theory evaluation of the Penn State Worry Questionnaire in women with cancer, Qual. Life Res., DOI 10.1007/s11136-012-0253-0.

Wynn, J., Jahshan, C., Altshuler, L., Glahn, C. and Green, M. (2012). Event-related potential examination of facial affect processing in bipolar disorder and schizophrenia. Psychological Med., (9 pages) doi: 10.1017/

Yamamoto, S. and Matsuoka, S. (1990). Topographic EEG study of visual display terminal (VDT) performance with special reference to frontal midline theta waves, Brain Topogr., 4, pp. 257 – 267.

Yang, H., Schnall, P., Jauregui, M., Su, T. and Baker, D. (2006). Work hours and self-reported hypertension among working people in California, Hypertension, 48, pp. 744–750.

Yee, C.M. and Miller, G.A. (1987) Affective valence and information processing, Current Trends in Event-Related Potential Research, EEG Suppl. 40, pp. 300 – 307.

Young, R., Biggs, J, Ziegler, V. and Meyer, D. (1978). A rating scale for mania: reliability, validity and sensitivity, Br. J. Psychiatry, 133, pp. 429 – 435.

Zapoli, R., Papini, M. and Cabras, P. (1969). Influence of spontaneous gernalized and focal temporal epileptic EEG discharges on the contingent negative variation, Electroencephalography Clin. Neurophysiol., 27, pp. 662 – 663.

Zapoli, R., Papini, M. Pasquinelli, A., Martinetti, M., Guerri, S. and Thyrion, E. (1977). Event-related slow potentials (ERSPs) of the brain in cases of temporal psychomotor and petit mal status, Riv. Patol. Nerv. Ment., 98, pp. 119 – 132.

Zee, P. (2012). Struggling with shift work disorder, www.medscape.org.

Zeier, H. (1979). Concurrent physiological activity of driver and passenger when driving with and without automatic transmission in heavy city traffic, Ergonomics, 22, pp. 799 – 810.

Zenger, M., Brähler, E., Berth, H. and Stöbel-Richter, Y. (2011). Unemployment during working life and mental health of retirees: Results of a representative survey, Aging & Mental Health, 15, pp. 178–185.

Zhan, Y., Wang, M., Liu, S. and Shultz, K.S. (2009). Bridge employment and retirees' health: a longitudinal investigation, J. Occup. Health Psychol., 14, pp. 374–389.

Zorn, E., Harrington, J. and Goethe, H. (1977). Ischaemic heart disease and stress in West German sea pilots, J. Occup. Med. 19, pp. 752–755.

Zubin, J., Sutton, S. and Steinhauer, S.R. (1986) *Brain Electrical Potentials and Psychopathology*, eds. Shagass, C., Josiassen, R.C., and Roemer, R., Chapter 7 "Event-related potential and behavioral methodology in psychiatric research," (Elsevier, New York) pp. 1 - 26.

Zyzanski, S. and Jenkins, C. (1970). Basic dimensions within the coronary-prone behavior pattern, J. Chron. Dis., 22, pp. 781 – 795.

Index